Concise Clinical Immunology for Healthcare Professionals

Clinical immunology is relevant to all medical disciplines and all healthcare professionals need a basic understanding of the subject. This textbook offers the healthcare professional in training or practice a clear and simple introduction to immunology. It covers:

- Essential basic immunology
- Clinical immunology
- Laboratory investigations of immunological disorders
- Treatments used in immunological disorders

Concise Clinical Immunology for Healthcare Professionals focuses on clinical problems seen in practice. It includes self-assessment questions and case histories to aid learning and understanding. It is suitable for doctors, undergraduate medical students, undergraduate and postgraduate biomedical scientists as well as nurses, nutritionists, pharmacists and physiotherapists working in specialist areas.

Mary T. Keogan is Consultant Clinical Immunologist at Beaumont Hospital, Dublin and Senior Lecturer in Pathology, Royal College of Surgeons in Ireland.

Eleanor M. Wallace is Senior Scientist in the Department of Immunology, St James's Hospital, Dublin and Visiting Lecturer at the Dublin Institute of Technology, Dublin, Ireland.

Paula O'Leary is Senior Lecturer and Consultant Physician, Department of Medicine, University College Cork and Cork University Hospital, Cork, Ireland.

Concise Clinical Immunology for Healthcare Professionals

Mary T. Keogan, Eleanor M. Wallace and Paula O'Leary

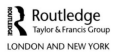
Routledge
Taylor & Francis Group

LONDON AND NEW YORK

First published 2006
by Routledge
2 Park Square, Milton Park, Abingdon, Oxon OX14 4RN

Simultaneously published in the USA and Canada
by Routledge
270 Madison Ave, New York, NY 10016

Routledge is an imprint of the Taylor & Francis Group, an informa business

© 2006 Mary T. Keogan, Eleanor M. Wallace and Paula O'Leary

Typeset in Sabon by
Newgen Imaging Systems (P) Ltd, Chennai, India
Printed and bound in Great Britain by
The Cromwell Press, Trowbridge, Wiltshire

British Library Cataloguing in Publication Data
A catalogue record for this book is available from the British Library

Library of Congress Cataloging in Publication Data
A catalog record for this book has been requested

ISBN10: 0–415–29829–6 (hbk)
ISBN10: 0–415–29830–X (pbk)

ISBN13: 978–0–415–29829–2 (hbk)
ISBN13: 978–0–415–29830–8 (pbk)

For our nearest and dearest

Andrew, James, Eva
MK

Fiona
EW

Denis, Daniel, Julia and Robbie,
and for my late mother, Helen, who helped me in
ways she never could have imagined
PO'L

Contents

PART 1   BASIC IMMUNOLOGY   1

PART 2   CLINICAL IMMUNOLOGY   127

PART 3   IMMUNOTECHNIQUES AND DIAGNOSTIC TESTS USED IN
CLINICAL IMMUNOLOGY   253

PART 4 TREATMENT OF IMMUNOLOGICAL DISORDERS 361

CLINICAL IMMUNOLOGY – FUTURE PROSPECTS 404

List of Figures

List of Tables

List of Case Studies

Acknowledgements

The authors wish to extend sincere thanks to all who facilitated them in the completion of this textbook. Our colleagues at the Immunology Departments at Beaumont Hospital, St James's Hospital and at the Department of Medicine University College Cork were tremendously supportive in many ways. Practical assistance in the form of reading, printing, image generation and photography, and circulating interim and final drafts of the book material was given by staff at each of the sites. Our colleagues, publishers and reviewers offered enthusiastic critical appraisal which we believe has elevated the final version to a very high standard and for that we are grateful. MK and PO'L acknowledge the important input of EW in relation to the translation of their hand-drawn diagrams into the final computer-generated illustrations used throughout the book. Finally, we thank our long-suffering family and friends, without whose patience this book may never have seen the light of day.

Abbreviations

6-MP	6-Mercaptopurine
AA	Aplastic anaemia
ABO	ABO blood group system
ABPA	Allergic bronchopulmonary aspergillosis
ACA	Anti-cardiolipin antibody
ACE	Angiotensin converting enzyme
AChR	Acetylcholine receptor
AD	Atopic Dermatitis/Eczema
ADCC	Antibody-dependent cellular cytotoxicity
AGA	Anti-gliadin antibody
AIDS	Acquired immunodeficiency syndrome
AIHA	Autoimmune haemolytic anaemia
AIRE	Autoimmune regulator
ALL	Acute lymphoblastic leukaemia
AMA	Anti-mitochondrial antibody
AML	Acute myeloid leukaemia
ANA	Anti-nuclear antibody
ANCA	Anti-neutrophil cytoplasmic antibody
ANF	Anti-nuclear factor
ANNA	Anti-neuronal nuclear antibody
APC	Antigen presenting cell
APGS	Autoimmune polyglandular syndrome
APR	Acute phase response
APS	Antiphospholipid syndrome
APTT	Activated partial thromboplastin time
ARA	American Rheumatological Association
ATG	Anti-thymocyte globulin
BALT	Bronchial associated lymphoid tissue
BBB	Blood brain barrier
BCG	Bacillus Calmette-Guérin
B-CLL	B cell chronic lymphocytic leukaemia
BCR	B cell receptor
β_2-GP1	β_2-glycoprotein 1
BJP	Bence–Jones protein
β_2-M	β_2-microglobulin
BMT	Bone Marrow Transplantation
BMZ	Basement membrane zone
BP	Bullous pemphigoid

BPI	Bactericidal permeability increasing protein
C	Constant
C1	Complement component 1
C1,C2, . . . , C9	Complement component 1, etc.
C1-Inh	C1-Inhibitor
CAH	Chronic autoimmune hepatitis
C-ANCA	Cytoplasmic ANCA
CCIE	Counter-current immunoelectrophoresis
CCR	Chemokine receptor
CD	Cluster of differentiation
CD40L	CD40 ligand
CDC	complement-dependent cytotoxicity
CDR	Complementarity determining region
CGD	Chronic granulomatous disease
CH50	Haemolytic complement assay
CID	Combined immunodeficiency
CIDP	Chronic inflammatory demyelinating polyneuropathy
CLL	Chronic lymphocytic leukaemia
CML	Chronic myeloid leukaemia
CMV	Cytomegalovirus
CNS	Central nervous system
COX	Cyclooxygenase
CP	Cyclophosphamide
CR1	Complement receptor 1
CREST	Calcinosis, Raynaud's phenomenon, oesophageal dysmotility, sclerodactyly, telangiectasiae
CRM	Certified Reference Material
CRP	C-reactive protein
CRS	Cytokine release syndrome
CSF	Cerebrospinal fluid
CTD	Connective tissue disease
CTL	Cytotoxic T lymphocyte
CVID	Common variable immunodeficiency
D	Diversity
DBPCAC	Double-blind placebo-controlled allergen challenge
DBPCFC	Double-blinded placebo-controlled food challenge
DC	Dendritic cell
DEJ	Dermoepidermal junction
DH	Dermatitis herpetiformis
DIF	Direct immunofluorescence
DLE	Discoid lupus erythematosus
DM	Diabetes mellitus
DNA	Deoxyribonucleic acid
DRVVT	Dilute Russell viper venom test
dsDNA Abs	Double-stranded DNA antibodies
EAA	Extrinsic allergic alveolitis
EBV	Epstein Barr Virus
EDTA	Ethylenediaminetetra acetic acid
ELISA	Enzyme-linked immunosorbent assay
EMA	Endomysial antibodies
ENA	Extractable nuclear antigens
ER	Endoplasmic reticulum

ESR	Erythrocyte sedimentation rate
Fab	Antigen binding fragment of Ig
FAB classification	French American British classification
FasL	Fas Ligand
FBC	Full blood count
Fc	Constant fragment (of immunoglobulin)
FcR	Fc Receptor
FITC	Fluorescein isothiocyanate
FKBP-12	FK binding protein – 12
GAD	Glutamic acid decarboxylase
GALT	Gut associated lymphoid tissues
GBM	Glomerular basement membrane
GBS	Guillain–Barré syndrome
G-CSF	Granulocyte colony stimulating factor
GIT	Gastrointestinal tract
GM-CSF	Granulocyte monocyte-colony stimulating fragment
GN	Glomerulonephritis
GPC	Gastric parietal cell
GvHD	Graft versus Host disease
HAART	Highly active anti-retroviral therapy
HACA	Human anti-chimeric antibodies
HAE	Hereditary angioedema
HD	Hodgkin's disease
hdIVIg	High dose IVIg
HDN	Haemolytic disease of the newborn
HEp-2	Human epithelial cell line-2
HHV-8	Human herpesvirus-8
HiB	Haemophilus influenzae Type B
HIV	Human immunodeficiency virus
HLA	Human leucocyte antigen
HSC	Haemopoietic Stem Cell
HTLV-1	Human T cell lymphotropic virus-1
HUS	Haemolytic uraemic syndrome
HV	Hypervariable
IBD	Inflammatory bowel disease
ICs	Immune complexes
ICS	Intercellular substance
IDDM	Insulin dependent DM
IEF	Isoelectric focussing
IF	Intrinsic factor
IFN	Interferon
Ig	Immunoglobulin
IgA	Immunoglobulin A
IgD	Immunoglobulin D
IgE	Immunoglobulin E
IgG	Immunoglobulin G
IgH	Immunoglobulin heavy chain
IgM	Immunoglobulin M
Ii	Invariant chain
IIF	Indirect immunofluorescence
IL	Interleukin
IL-1ra	IL-1 receptor antagonist

IMIg	Intramuscular immunoglobulin
ITP	Immune thrombocytopaenic purpura
IU	International unit
IVIg	Intravenous immunoglobulin
J	Joining
KCT	Kaolin clotting time
KIR	Killer inhibitory receptor
LAD	Leucocyte adhesion deficiency
LFTs	Liver function tests
LKM	Liver kidney microsomal antibody
LKS	Liver kidney stomach
LPS	Lipopolysaccharide
MAb	Monoclonal antibody
MAC	Membrane attack complex
MALT	Mucosa associated lymphoid tissue
MBL	Mannose binding lectin
MCTD	Mixed Connective Tissue Disease
MenC	Meningococcus Type C (used in relation to vaccine)
MG	Myasthenia gravis
MGUS	Monoclonal gammopathy of uncertain significance
MHC	Major histocompatibility complex
MM	Multiple myeloma
MMF	Mycophenolate mofetil
MMR	Measles mumps rubella vaccine
MPGN	Membranoproliferative glomerulonephritis
MPO	Myeloperoxidase
MS	Multiple sclerosis
MTX	Methotrexate
NBT	Nitroblue tetrazolium
NHL	Non-Hodgkins lymphoma
NIDDM	Non-insulin dependent DM
NK	Natural killer
NPV	Negative predictive value
NSAIDs	Non-steroidal anti-inflammatory drugs
OPSI	Overwhelming post-splenectomy infection
PA	Pernicious anaemia
PALS	Periarteriolar lymphoid sheath
PAN	Polyarteritis nodosa
P-ANCA	Perinuclear ANCA
PBC	Primary biliary cirrhosis
PBMC	Peripheral blood mononuclear cell
PBSC	Peripheral blood stem cell
PCC	Purkinje cell cytoplasm antibody
PCP	Pneumocystis carinii pneumonia
PCR	Polymerase chain reaction
PE	Phycoerythrin
PHA	Phytohaemagglutinin
PMA	Phorbol myristate acetate
PMN	Polymorphonuclear (leucocytes)
Pm-Scl	Polymositis/scleroderma
POEMS	Polyneuropathy, organomegaly, endocrine abnormalities, monoclonal gammopathy and skin rashes

PP	Plasmapheresis
PPV	Positive predictive value
PR-3	Proteinase 3
PRA	Panel reactive antibody
PRM	Pattern recognition molecules
PTLD	Post-transplant lymphoproliferative disorder
RA	Rheumatoid arthritis
RAG	Recombinase activating genes
RBC	Red blood cell
REAL classification	Revised European American Lymphoma classification
RF	Rheumatoid factor
Rh	Rhesus
Rho	Anti-D immunoglobulin
RIA	Radioimmunoassay
RID	Radial immunodiffusion
RNA	Ribonucleic acid
RNP	Ribonucleoprotein
RPGN	Rapidly Progressive Glomerulonephritis
RSV	Respiratory syncitial virus
SBE	Subacute bacterial endocarditis
SC	Secretory component
SCID	Severe combined immunodeficiency
Scl-70	Scleroderma 70/topoisomerase
SCLE	Subacute cutaneous lupus erythematosus
SD	Standard deviation
SI	Stimulation index
sIg	Surface immunoglobulin
SLA	Soluble liver antibodies
SLE	Systemic lupus erythematosus
SLVL	Splenic lymphoma with villus lymphocytes
SMA	Smooth muscle antibody
SPT	Skin prick test
SRP	Signal recognition proteins
ssDNA	Single-stranded DNA
SSO	Sequence-specific oligonucleotide
SSP	Sequence-specific polymorphism
STD	Sexually transmitted disease
T3	Triiodothyronine
T4	Thyroxine
TAA	Tumour associated antigen
TAP	Transporters associated with antigen processing
T_C	Cytotoxic T cells
TCR	T cell receptor
TD	T dependent
TG	Thyroglobulin
TGF	Transforming growth factor
T_H	T helper cell
T_H1	T helper cell, type 1
T_H2	T helper cell, type 2
TI	T independent
TLR	Toll-like receptor
TM	Thyroid microsomal

TNF	Tumour necrosis factor
TOR	Target of Rapamycin
TPN	Total parenteral nutrition
TPO	Thyroid peroxidase
T$_R$	T regulatory cell
TSA	Tumour specific antigen
TSH	Thyroid Stimulating Hormone
TSST	Toxic shock syndrome toxin
tTg	Tissue transglutaminase
UC	Ulcerative colitis
UV	Ultraviolet
V	Variable
VDRL	Venereal disease reference laboratory
VZV	Varicella zoster virus
WHO	World Health Organization

Introduction

The impetus to write this book came from the many healthcare professionals who asked for a book that explained the immune system – 'but only the bits I really need to know'. Immunology impinges on all areas of medicine and therefore all healthcare professionals need a working knowledge of clinical immunology. Unfortunately, however, the medical curriculum is so overloaded that most students have very limited time to devote to each discipline. This book aims to provide a simple summary of clinical immunology, and to give students a framework, to which further knowledge can be added as appropriate.

The book is divided into four parts, each of which is further divided into many small subsections. Part 1 outlines the workings of the immune system in health and disease. The emphasis is on knowledge that is essential to understand immunological disease, investigation and management. We aim to include the essentials; for the more interested student, we hope that this section will provide a good start. There are many excellent textbooks, which provide much more detail on the workings of the immune system, and we would urge you to expand your knowledge.

Part 2 describes the most commonly encountered immunological disorders, including allergy, immunodeficiency, autoimmunity, transplantation and lymphoproliferative disorders. The emphasis is on immunological aspects of disease and we aim to use outlines of clinical disease to illustrate several aspects of basic immunology. We hope that this section will help to remind students about the workings of the immune system, usually taught at an earlier point in the course. For laboratory scientists and other healthcare professionals this section should provide a straightforward account of the diseases encountered.

Part 3 describes commonly requested immunological investigations and tests. Understanding the indications, methods, interpretation and pitfalls of assays should improve the value gained from the Clinical Immunology Laboratory. Laboratory scientists will need to consult additional methodological texts, however, we hope that this section will provide a useful overview.

Part 4 describes commonly used immunological therapies. The emphasis is on understanding the effects of these agents on the immune system, as well as practical aspects of using these therapies.

The book is laid out in small sections, and is extensively cross-referenced. This should allow readers to dip into the book to clarify a particular aspect of basic immunology, clinical immunology, laboratory immunology or treatment of immunological disorders, as they arise in daily practice. We have also arranged the sections in logical sequence so that readers new to immunology can work through the sections.

Clinical Immunology is a fascinating clinical science, which impacts on the care of many patients. With the advances in our understanding of immunology in the last decade we can now explain much more about the workings of the human immune system. While animal experiments have generated many ideas and hypotheses, detailed molecular investigation of patients with immunological disease has provided an understanding of human immunology. We now know enough about human immunology to illustrate principles in a clinically relevant way.

Our aim was to write a straightforward, concise clinical immunology text. This of course led to the frustration of omitting many fascinating aspects and details of clinical immunology. However, we hope that you will gain a useful working knowledge of immunology that will encourage you to delve more deeply into the areas of immunology relevant to your area of clinical practice.

MK, EW, PO'L

BASIC IMMUNOLOGY

INTRODUCTION

This part outlines basic aspects of how the immune system functions to protect us against pathogens. Some basic mechanisms underlying allergy and hypersensitivity are also included. The aim of this part is to provide a concise summary of essential aspects of immunity required to understand immunological diseases, investigations and treatment. There are many excellent textbooks available, which provide additional detail and more detailed explanation. We have, however, aimed to include sections describing clinically relevant aspects of basic immunology that are frequently scattered, such as ontogeny of the immune response, as well as sections aimed at integrating information.

REFERENCES

Davies, D. H., Halablab, M. A., Clarke, J., Fox, F. E. G. and Young, T. W. K. (1999) *Infection and Immunity*, London: Taylor & Francis.
Janeway, C. A., Travers, P., Hunt, S. and Walport, M. (2000) *Immunobiology: The Immune System in Health and Disease*, New York: Garland Publishing.
Nairn, R. and Helbert, M. (2002) *Immunology for Medical Students*, London: Mosby.
Parham, P. (2000) *The Immune System*, London: Elsevier Science.

KEY DEFINITIONS

Every effort has been made to explain new terms as this part progresses. However occasionally, particularly in the early chapters, fully explaining each term was too cumbersome. This list is not a complete glossary, merely a list of key definitions with which you should be familiar before reading this section.

Acute phase response (APR)   Changes in metabolism occurring in response to inflammation, including inflammation caused by infection. The APR results in fever and changes in protein production. Production of transport proteins (such as albumin) is reduced, while production of protective proteins (immune system molecules, clotting factors and protease inhibitors) is increased. Proteins which increase during inflammation are known as **acute phase reactants** or **acute phase proteins**.

Antibody   Immunoglobulin, secreted by plasma cells. Antibodies are key effectors in the humoral limb of the adaptive immune response. See Immunoglobulins.

Antigen   Originally used to describe any molecule, which could lead to production of an antibody (**antibody gen**erators). The term antigen now includes any molecule which generates an adaptive immune response. Antigens which elicit hypersensitivity or allergic responses may be referred to as **allergens**.

Antigen presenting cell (APC)   A cell capable of presenting antigen to a helper T cell. Competent antigen presentation requires expression of *M*ajor *H*istocompatability *C*omplex (MHC) Class II as well as co-stimulatory molecules. **Professional APCs** are required to present antigen to naïve T cells, and antigen presentation is the cells primary function (e.g. dendritic cells). **Non-professional APCs** can present antigen to antigen experienced T cells, but have other functions in addition to antigen presentation (e.g. macrophages, B cells).

Chemokine   A chemical messenger, the primary function of which is to control the movement of cells of the immune and haemopoietic systems.

Cytokine   A chemical messenger which coordinates a function/functions of the immune system. Cytokines usually have highly localised effects. Cytokines may be divided into **monokines** (produced by monocytes/macrophages) or **lymphokines** (produced by lymphocytes).

Epitope   The precise portion of an antigen which evokes an immune response. Antigens can contain many copies of the same epitope (common in carbohydrate antigens) or contain several different epitopes (common in protein antigens). B cells epitopes are **conformational** (i.e. affected by the three-dimensional structure of the antigen), while T cell epitopes are short peptides, not affected by antigen conformation.

Human leucocyte antigen (HLA) complex   HLA is the human MHC. The term HLA may be used with reference to the chromosome region, the genes or protein molecules.

Immunoglobulins   These are antigen-binding molecules produced by B cells. Immunoglobulins may be bound to the surface of the B cell, acting as an antigen receptor for the cell, or may be secreted, acting as the effector portion of the humoral response. Immunoglobulins (Ig) are divided into five functionally distinct major classes; IgG, IgA, IgM, IgD and IgE.

Interleukin (IL)   A general term for cytokines produced by leucocytes.

Leukotriene   Family of inflammatory mediators, produced by metabolism of arachidonic acid.

Lymphocytes   Cells of the immune system, which are essential for all adaptive immune responses. Lymphocytes are subclassified as **B lymphocytes** (produce antibody response), **T lymphocytes** (produce cellular adaptive response) and **Natural Killer or NK cells** which usually form part of the innate immune response.

MHC   Complex of genes which encode surface bound molecules which are involved in antigen presentation. The MHC molecules can be divided into Class I molecules, which are expressed on all nucleated cells and platelets, and MHC Class II molecules normally only expressed on specialised immune cells which present antigen to helper T cells. The human MHC is termed the HLA complex.

Monokines   See under **cytokines**.

Opsonin   A molecule which binds to pathogens or particles to make it more susceptible to phagocytosis. The process of coating particles to enhance phagocytosis is **opsonisation**. Opsonins include natural opsonins such as mannan binding lectin (MBL) and C-reactive protein, complement, as well as antibodies produced as part of the adaptive immune response.

Phagocyte   A cell capable of ingesting a particle by **phagocytosis**, an active process involving formation of pseudopodia which engulf the particle. The vesicle so formed in the cell is called the **phagosome**. The principal phagocytes are neutrophils, monocytes and macrophages.

Introduction

WHY DO WE NEED AN IMMUNE SYSTEM?

We encounter many thousands of microbes every day – many harmless, many beneficial but some that cause disease. The immune system defends us against infections caused by the huge variety of microorganisms we encounter, including viruses, bacteria, fungi and parasites. Microbes divide rapidly, each division allowing genetic variation and change. Thus microbes can change within days or even hours. It takes years for humans to reproduce and generate genomic variation. The immune system has developed elegant mechanisms that facilitate somatic change without genomic variation in response to infection and other stimuli.

THE MAJOR DEFENCE MECHANISMS AGAINST INFECTIONS

Microorganisms come in all shapes and sizes, with some penetrating into cells and others entering the body but remaining outside the cells. Thus the immune system has had to develop several different mechanisms to recognise and kill microbes depending on their characteristics. From the immune systems point of view, microbes can be divided according to type of infection caused.

Extracellular infection

- Bacteria enter tissues but usually remain outside the cells. However, as they are smaller than cells of the immune system, specialised immune cells can ingest, kill and digest the bacteria.
- Multi-cellular parasites also remain outside cells, however, as they are larger than immune cells, they cannot be ingested and so additional immune mechanisms are required to fight infection.

Intracellular infection

- Viruses enter the cytoplasm, hijack the host cells protein synthesis machinery and assemble new virus particles, which bud from the cell surface and infect new cells. Immune mechanisms which act in the extracellular space are ineffective once virus enters the cells.
- Intra-vesicular organisms (e.g. *Mycobacteria*) are taken up into cells but remain within vesicles, never entering the cytoplasm. Immune mechanisms that kill virus-infected cells are ineffective as the organisms are in a different cell compartment – therefore requiring an additional immune strategy.

Infecting organisms must first breach the body's natural defences (skin, mucous membranes etc.). The pathogen then faces the two major types of immune response, the innate immune response, and the adaptive or specific immune response. When thinking about how these systems work it is helpful to consider (1) the recognition phase where the micro-organism/pathogen is recognised as foreign, and (2) the effector phase, which kills the organism.

The innate immune response is immediately available to fight pathogens without the requirement for prior exposure to the pathogen. This is the first line of defence against pathogens, recognising microbes by the presence of molecular patterns not present on mammalian cells. Innate immunity is moderately effective at controlling infection and does not improve with repeated exposure to a particular organism.

The adaptive immune response is refined and expanded after infection, taking several days to provide protection on first exposure to a particular pathogen. The cells and molecules produced are highly specific for the pathogen. The adaptive immune system remembers when a microbe has previously invaded the body resulting in a rapid and efficient removal of the pathogen on the second and third time that it invades the body (immunological memory).

Innate and adaptive immunity depend on white blood cells or leucocytes. Innate immunity involves granulocytes and macrophages. Adaptive immune responses depend on lymphocytes, which provide the lifelong immunity that can follow exposure to disease or vaccination. However, the two systems do not operate independently – there are many examples of co-operation. Killing of microorganisms by the adaptive immune response frequently depends upon linking antigen-specific recognition to activation of effector mechanisms that are also used in the innate response.

Together, the innate and adaptive immune systems provide an amazing defence system. Despite the fact that we are surrounded by a multitude of potentially pathogenic micro-organisms, we rarely succumb to infection. Many infections are eliminated by the innate immune system and cause no disease. Infections that cannot be resolved by innate immunity trigger adaptive immunity, which usually eliminates the infection (often before we are aware of it) and generates immunological memory.

WHAT HAPPENS WHEN THE IMMUNE SYSTEM GOES WRONG?

The immune system is only apparent when it goes wrong, and virtually any clinical presentation may be the sign of an underlying immunological disorder. The immune system must find a balance between producing a life-saving response to infection and tissue-damaging reactions. It is also essential that the immune system only mounts a vigorous response to pathogens that pose a threat, and ignores our own tissues, as well as environmental substances including foods and medicines.

Immunodeficiency diseases

Immunodeficiency means a failure of the immune system to protect us from infection. It may be primary (due to an intrinsic defect in the immune system) or secondary, (due to drugs, infection, malnutrition etc.).

Overactivity of part of the immune system

The immune response can cause incidental tissue damage as well as the intended removal and/or destruction of microorganisms. Additionally the immune system may fail to distinguish between pathogens and innocuous stimuli such as pollen or self-tissue. In this case a vigorous immune response causes disease.

Allergy

An over-response to environmental stimuli, which pose no threat, is called allergy. Several different immune mechanisms may be involved. The most common mechanism causes rapid responses varying in severity from hayfever to potentially fatal anaphylactic shock.

Autoimmunity

Autoimmune diseases can affect any tissue in the body, and occur when the immune system fails to distinguish between self (which should be ignored) and non-self (which should be attacked). Many autoimmune diseases can be diagnosed by testing for immune products (antibodies) against self-tissues in patients' blood.

Transplantation

Transplantation involves transfer of cells, tissues or solid organs from one person to another. As the transplanted tissue is seen as non-self, the immune system attempts to eliminate it. Powerful immunosuppression has been required to make clinical transplantation a reality. Transplantation of bone marrow, kidney, pancreas, liver, heart and lung are now routine treatments for irreversible organ failure.

VACCINATION

Vaccination is one of the great success stories of immunology. By generating an adaptive immune response that leads to immunological memory, people can be protected from severe disease. Vaccination has led to the eradication of smallpox, and the World Health Organization aims to eradicate poliomyelitis in the near future. The incidence of many severe infectious diseases has been hugely reduced by vaccination campaigns.

Clinical immunology is the specialty that focuses on diagnosis and treatment of immune mediated disease. An understanding of the immune system and how it works is essential for treating patients with these disorders. However, immunological disorders impinge on all medical specialties to a greater or lesser degree. Thus all healthcare professionals require some understanding of basic and clinical immunology.

Overview of Defence Mechanisms

THE DEFENCE SYSTEMS OF THE BODY FALL INTO THREE CATEGORIES

- Non-immunological external defences
- Innate immunity
- Adaptive immunity.

The principle difference between innate and adaptive immune responses is in pathogen recognition. Many effector mechanisms used to kill pathogens are shared by both systems.

NON-IMMUNOLOGICAL EXTERNAL DEFENCES

Skin and mucus membranes form physical barriers to infectious organisms. When breached (e.g. burn victims) infection is common despite normal immune function. Pathogens must attach to epithelial cells and migrate through the epithelium to establish infection. Surface epithelia provide mechanical, chemical and microbiological barriers as a first line of defence against infection (Figure 1.2.1).

Mechanical barriers prevent microbial attachment and include

- Flow of secretions across epithelium – when flow is obstructed infection is common.
- Mucociliary elevator. Inhaled organisms are trapped by mucus, which is moved by the coordinated action of cilia on the surface of ciliated epithelium. In the respiratory tract, mucus and organisms are moved to the oropharynx and swallowed or expectorated.

Chemical barriers

Chemical barriers include the acid environment in the stomach, together with digestive enzymes and the antimicrobial effect of lysozyme found in tears and sweat, as well as defensins (bactericidal peptides found in the respiratory and gastrointestinal tracts).

Figure 1.2.1 External defences of the body.

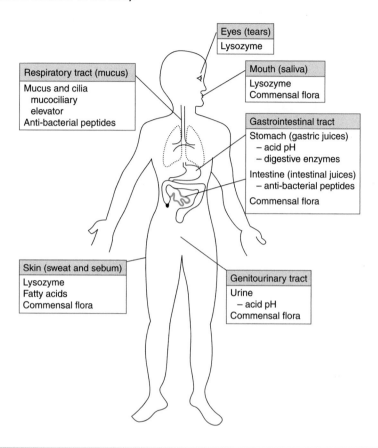

Microbial barrier

Commensal flora, found on skin and mucosal membranes, form a microbial barrier by competing for nutrients and attachment sites on cells. Some also produce anti-bacterial substances.

INNATE IMMUNE RESPONSES

When microorganisms penetrate epithelial surfaces they are usually killed by the innate immune response (Figure 1.2.2). Innate immunity acts immediately, recognises broad microbial patterns rather than unique specificities and does not produce immunological memory.

Macrophages and neutrophils have surface receptors that recognise and bind common constituents of many bacteria. Binding induces engulfment, killing and degradation of bacteria – termed phagocytosis.

Following phagocytosis, activated macrophages secrete chemical messengers (cytokines), which initiate inflammation. Inflammation increases blood vessel permeability, rapidly

Figure 1.2.2 The innate immune response: overview.

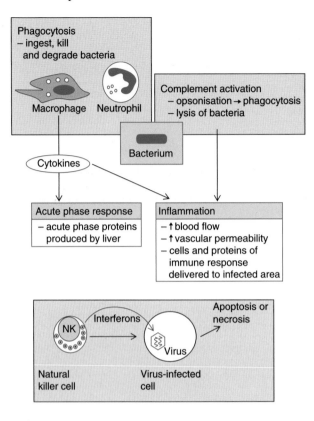

increasing delivery of cells and proteins of the immune system to the infected area. Activation of complement, a system of plasma proteins, generates fragments that coat or opsonise bacteria increasing the efficiency of phagocytes. Complement also lyses some bacteria, and releases small pro-inflammatory peptides.

Macrophage activation results in cytokine release, causing a rise in body temperature and an acute phase response. Acute phase proteins are produced in the liver and contribute to inflammation and host defence.

NK cells recognise and kill virus-infected cells. NK cells are activated by cytokines (TNF-α and IL-12) produced by macrophages. Virus infected cells produce interferon-α and β (IFN-α and β), which inhibit viral replication within cells, make surrounding cells more resistant to viral entry, and also activate NK cells.

The innate immune response makes a crucial contribution to activation of adaptive immunity

◆ Macrophages enhance the adaptive immune response by acting as antigen presenting cells (APCs).
◆ Cytokines produced by cells (macrophages and NK cells) of innate immunity enhance responses by the adaptive immune response.
◆ The inflammatory response increases the flow of lymph containing antigen and APCs to the lymphoid tissue.

ADAPTIVE IMMUNE RESPONSES

Adaptive immunity provides protection when innate immunity fails to eliminate infection. Adaptive immunity develops slowly, has unique specificity for antigen and produces immunological memory (Figure 1.2.3).

Adaptive immunity results in selection of lymphocyte clones bearing highly antigen-specific receptors (recognition molecules). Each lymphocyte expresses cell-surface receptors of a single specificity. B cell receptors (immunoglobulins) bind extracellular molecules and pathogens, while T cell receptors (TCR) bind peptide fragments bound to MHC molecules on cell surfaces.

Following initiation of an immune response, the antigen-specific lymphocyte(s) proliferate and its progeny differentiate into effector cells that can eliminate the pathogen. A subset of these proliferating lymphocytes differentiates into memory cells capable of responding rapidly if the same pathogen is encountered again.

Adaptive immunity can be divided into humoral (antibody-mediated) immunity, and cell-mediated immunity. Both types of immune response require activation of helper T cells (TH), a pivotal lymphocyte subset that are essential for the development of effective adaptive immune responses.

Figure 1.2.3 The adaptive immune response: overview.

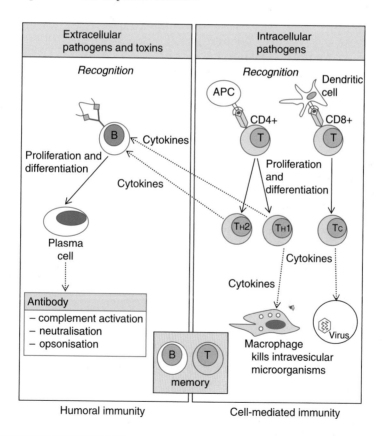

Table 1.2.1 Features of innate and adaptive immunity

CHARACTERISTICS	CELLS	MOLECULES
Innate immunity		
Rapid response within hours	Macrophages	Cytokines
No unique specificity	Neutrophils	Complement
No memory	NK cells	Acute phase proteins
		Natural opsonins
Adaptive immunity		
Slower reponse ~5–6days	T and B lymphocytes	Antibodies
Highly specific	Plasma cells	Cytokines
Memory		

B cells differentiate into plasma cells that make antibody, or secreted immunoglobulin. Antibodies bind extracellular pathogens or toxins, bringing about their destruction. This is termed humoral immunity.

Cell-mediated immunity provides protection against intracellular pathogens. Antigen-specific cytotoxic T cells kill virally infected cells in an attempt to eliminate the virus. Another T cell subset (helper T cells) activates macrophages to kill microorganisms that reside within intracellular vesicles. Both mechanisms are included in the term cell-mediated immunity.

The features of innate and adaptive immunity are summarised in Table 1.2.1.

INNATE AND ADAPTIVE IMMUNITY SHARE SOME EFFECTOR MECHANISMS

The effector functions of antibody depend on recruiting cells and molecules of the innate immune system. Antibodies target pathogens and their toxic products for disposal by phagocytes.

♦   Antibodies bind and neutralise bacterial toxins.
♦   Antibodies opsonise bacteria, facilitating their ingestion and destruction by macrophages or neutrophils.
♦   Antibodies activate complement, which can lyse bacteria or opsonise microbes.

Macrophages become more effective at killing organisms after interaction with helper T cells.

CROSS REFERENCES

Section 1.4   Innate Immune Responses I
Section 1.5   Innate Immune Responses II – The Complement System
Section 1.7   Inflammation
Section 1.11   How Does the Immune System See Antigen?
Section 1.15   Immunoglobulin Function
Section 1.17   Helper T Cell Activation
Section 1.18   Cytotoxic T Cells

Cells and Organs of the Immune System

Cells of the immune system originate in the bone marrow. Once mature these cells patrol tissues, circulating in blood and lymphatic vessels. Haematopoietic stem cells (HSCs) found mainly in the bone marrow give rise to all blood cells and cells of the immune system. HSCs differentiate into both myeloid and lymphoid progenitors (Figure 1.3.1).

MYELOID CELLS

Myeloid cells are involved in innate and adaptive immunity. They include granulocytes (neutrophils, eosinophils, basophils), monocytes and macrophages, dendritic cells and mast cells.

Granulocytes

Granulocytes have densely staining cytoplasmic granules and have multilobed nuclei (hence also known as polymorphonuclear leucocytes or PMNs).

Neutrophils are short-lived, mobile phagocytes, which circulate in the bloodstream until recruited to sites of inflammation. They are the most numerous cells of the innate immune response, but also interact with antibodies playing an effector role in adaptive responses. Eosinophils play a role in defence against parasitic infections and are also recruited to sites of allergic inflammation. The function of basophils is uncertain.

Monocytes and macrophages

Monocytes circulate in the blood, migrate into tissues and differentiate into macrophages. Macrophages are part of the mononuclear phagocyte system (previously known as the reticuloendothelial system) and are distributed widely in body tissues. Macrophages play an important role in innate immunity and also present antigen to T cells.

Figure 1.3.1 Origin of blood cells.

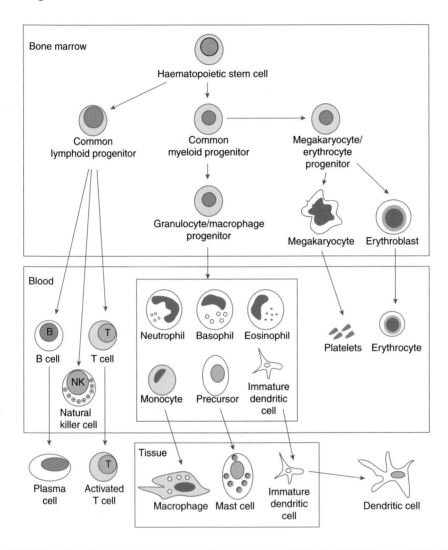

Dendritic cells

Dendritic cells are professional APCs, which migrate from blood into tissues. On encountering a pathogen, dendritic cells ingest antigen by phagocytosis, mature and migrate to lymph nodes where they present antigen to T cells and activate T cells.

Mast cells

Mast cells are found in connective tissue and close to mucosal surfaces. They trigger local inflammatory responses to antigen by rapidly releasing inflammatory mediators including histamine. Mast cells play a pivotal role in allergic responses.

LYMPHOID CELLS

The common lymphoid precursor matures into lymphocytes, including B and T cells which generate adaptive immune responses.

B cells and T cells

B cells develop in the bone marrow. T cell precursors leave the bone marrow and mature in the thymus. B and T lymphocytes cannot be distinguished morphologically – both are small cells with condensed chromatin and few cytoplasmic organelles. B and T lymphocytes can be distinguished by assessing expression of lineage-specific molecules (see Section 3.3). Mature B and T cells circulate between the blood and peripheral lymphoid tissues. Encounter with antigen triggers proliferation and differentiation into cells with specialised effector functions. Both B and T cells have a large repertoire of receptors that can recognise a wide diversity of antigens.

Plasma cells

B cells mature into plasma cells, terminally differentiated cells which secrete antibody.

NK cells

NK cells are large granular lymphocytes found throughout the tissues of the body but predominantly in the circulation. They lack antigen-specific receptors and are part of the innate immune system. NK cells kill tumour cells and virus-infected cells.

LYMPHOID ORGANS

Lymphoid organs are specialised tissues where lymphocytes develop, mature and differentiate. They are divided into primary lymphoid organs, where lymphocytes develop, and secondary lymphoid organs, where adaptive immune responses are initiated (Figure 1.3.2).

Primary lymphoid organs – bone marrow and thymus

B and T cells originate in the bone marrow but only B cells mature here (bone marrow derived). T cells migrate to the thymus for maturation (thymus derived). Once maturation is complete, both types of cells enter the bloodstream and migrate to the peripheral lymphoid organs.

Secondary lymphoid organs

Secondary lymphoid organs are organised to trap antigen from sites of infection, facilitate antigen presentation to lymphocytes and provide the optimal microenvironment for lymphocyte maturation. They include lymph nodes, spleen and mucosa-associated lymphoid tissue (MALT) and all share the same basic structure. Immune responses are initiated in secondary lymphoid tissues.

Lymph nodes

Lymph nodes trap antigens from sites of infection in tissue (Figure 1.3.3). Afferent lymphatic vessels transport extracellular tissue fluid (lymph) carrying antigen and APCs to

Figure 1.3.2 Primary and secondary lymphoid organs.

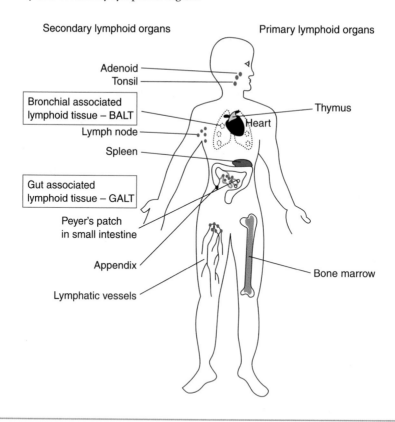

Secondary lymphoid organs   Primary lymphoid organs

Adenoid

Tonsil

Bronchial associated
lymphoid tissue – BALT

Thymus

Heart

Lymph node

Spleen

Gut associated
lymphoid tissue – GALT

Peyer's patch
in small intestine

Appendix

Bone marrow

Lymphatic vessels

the lymph nodes. In lymph nodes, B cells are concentrated in follicles and T cells are distributed in the surrounding paracortical area (T cell zone). When B cells encounter their specific antigen and antigen-specific helper T cells, they proliferate in germinal centres of the follicles. The organisation of lymph nodes and other secondary lymphoid tissues promotes B cell interaction with helper T cells, which is essential for antibody responses.

Spleen

The spleen collects antigens from the blood. The main bulk of the spleen is red pulp, the site of red blood cell (RBC) disposal. Lymphocytes surround arterioles entering the spleen forming areas of white pulp, which are divided into the peri-arteriolar lymphoid sheath (PALS), containing mostly T cells, and the B cell corona. Lymphocytes and antigen-loaded dendritic cells come together in the PALS.

Mucosal-associated lymphoid tissue

MALT includes the gut-associated lymphoid tissue (GALT), bronchial-associated lymphoid tissue (BALT) and aggregates of lymphocytes in other mucosae. GALT collects antigen from the epithelial surfaces of the gastrointestinal tract (GIT) and includes the tonsils, adenoids, appendix and specialised structures called Peyers patches in the small intestine.

Figure 1.3.3 A lymph node.

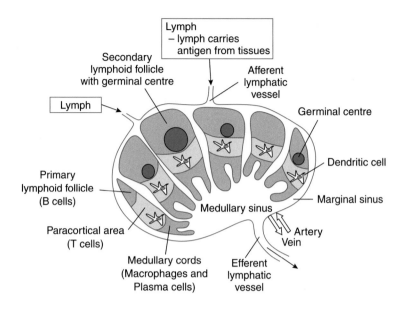

LYMPHOCYTE TRAFFICKING

Lymphocytes express adhesion molecules, with which they attach to endothelial cells prior to migrating into tissues or lymphoid organs. Some lymphocytes have specific adhesion molecules (addressins), which bind to ligands on endothelial cells in particular vascular beds, for example, mucosal lymphocytes express addressins which favour migration into MALT.

Naïve T and B cells are mature lymphocytes that have not yet encountered antigen. These cells continually migrate into the secondary lymphoid tissues via the bloodstream. They return to the blood via the (efferent) lymphatic vessels and the thoracic duct. Naïve lymphocytes recirculate until they meet their cognate antigen. If this does not occur they die.

When pathogens enter the body, APCs (e.g. dendritic cells) take up and process antigen. APCs and free antigen are carried in afferent lymphatics to regional lymph nodes. Here APCs display processed antigen to recirculating T lymphocytes, activating antigen-specific cells. Activated T cells proliferate and differentiate into antigen-specific effector cells and leave the lymph node via efferent lymphatics, re-enter the blood stream and migrate to the site of infection.

Recirculating B cells that encounter antigen are activated, proliferate and differentiate into antibody-secreting plasma cells. Plasma cells may remain in the lymph node or return to the bone marrow (via efferent lymphatics and bloodstream).

All secondary lymphoid tissues trap APCs and antigen, present it to migratory lymphocytes thus stimulating an adaptive immune response. B cell follicles of the lymph nodes expand and proliferate to form germinal centres and the entire lymph node enlarges – giving rise to swollen glands.

Innate Immune Responses I

The innate immune response detects organisms using pattern recognition molecules (PRMs), which recognise molecules present on microorganisms, but absent from mammalian cells. There is a limited repertoire of PRMs, and they do not vary during the course of the immune response. The innate immune response is capable of mounting a rapid response to an invading microbe and frequently augments the adaptive immune response.

Components of the innate immune response include:

- Cells

  — Phagocytes (neutrophils and macrophages)
  — Degranulating cells (mast cells and eosinophils)
  — NK cells

- Proteins

  — Complement
  — Natural opsonins (Mannan binding lectin, MBL; C reactive protein, CRP)
  — Acute phase reactants

- Chemical messengers

  — Cytokines
  — Interferons (IFNs)

This section will focus on phagocytosis and natural opsonins, which play a role in the innate immune response to bacteria, and NK cells and IFNs, which are the principle innate defences against viral pathogens. The next two sections describe other aspects of the innate response.

PHAGOCYTES AND PHAGOCYTOSIS

Neutrophils, monocytes and macrophages are all phagocytic cells. Macrophages may develop special phenotypes depending on their location. At sites of inflammation they

Figure 1.4.1 **Phagocytosis.**

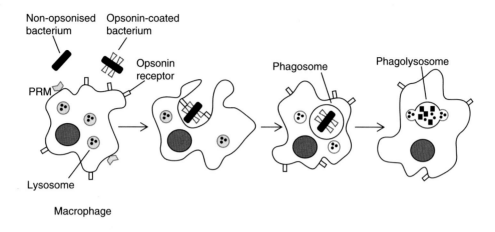

may become giant cells and epitheloid cells. Fixed macrophages are found in the sinusoids of the liver and spleen and remove particulate and antibody coated matter from the blood. Specialised macrophages are found in bone (osteoclasts), brain (glial cells) and lungs (alveolar macrophages).

Phagocytosis is the process whereby these cells ingest particulate matter, including pathogens and cellular debris (Figure 1.4.1). Phagocytic cells recognise debris using PRMs or receptors that bind complement, immunoglobulin or other opsonins. Engagement of receptors on the phagocyte's surface induces formation of pseudopodia, which surround and engulf particles. The ingested particle is contained in a vesicle called a phagosome. Fusion with lysosomes forms phagolysosomes resulting in acidification of the phagosome and release of proteases, and ultimately microbial killing and digestion. Phagocyte activation results in increased oxygen consumption termed the respiratory burst, associated with production of toxic reactive oxygen intermediates (superoxide, hydrogen peroxide).

Phagocytosis can result from engagement of PRMs on phagocytes in the absence of opsonins. However, the process is more efficient in the presence of opsonins including immunoglobulin, which binds to Fc receptors or complement, which engages complement receptors on phagocytes. Natural opsonins do not require activation to acquire activity, behaving as soluble PRMs binding to microbe-specific molecular signatures. These include MBL, which binds mannan residues, a type of carbohydrate not expressed by mammalian cells. CRP is a protein produced in large amounts during episodes of inflammation, and widely measured clinically as a marker of inflammation. It binds to C protein, found on Streptococci, opsonising this group of organisms.

INNATE IMMUNITY TO VIRAL INFECTIONS – INTERFERONS

Interferons (IFNs) are divided into Type I IFNs (IFN-α and β) and Type II IFN (IFN-γ). Type I IFNs are produced by many cells following viral infection. In contrast, IFN-γ is only produced by selected immune cells including some helper T (TH1) cells and NK cells.

Type I IFN production is induced by the double-stranded RNA generated by viruses, but not normally present in mammalian cells. Interferon is produced within hours of infection.

Protective effects of IFN include:

- Inhibition of viral replication within the infected cell
- Rendering neighbouring cells more resistant to viral entry
- NK cell activation
- Upregulation of viral peptide processing, which bind to MHC Class I molecules. This alerts the adaptive immune response that the cell is infected by a virus.

IFN-γ has little direct antiviral activity but has potent immunostimulatory actions. Actions of IFN-γ will be described in more detail when T cell function is considered. However NK cells can also produce IFN-γ.

INNATE IMMUNITY TO VIRAL INFECTIONS – NK CELLS

NK cells are large granular lymphocytes that constitute about 10% of lymphocytes. They do not rearrange antigen receptor molecules, in contrast to B and T lymphocytes. NK cells can kill without activation by cytokines, but they proliferate in response to IL-2 and become more effective at killing infected cells in the presence of Type I IFNs, IL-12 and IFN-γ.

NK cells detect virus-infected cells or tumour cells through a complex system of receptors, some delivering negative and some positive signals. Positive signals stimulate NK cells to kill and they originate from binding abnormal PRMs on infected cells. However, if the cell expresses adequate amounts of MHC Class I, the NK cell receives a negative signal through killer inhibitory receptors (KIRs). This negative signal may override the positive signal to the NK cell – however, an MHC Class I bearing infected cell will later be killed by cytotoxic T cells. Some virally infected cells and tumour cells downregulate MHC

Figure 1.4.2 NK cells kill target cells by two mechanisms.

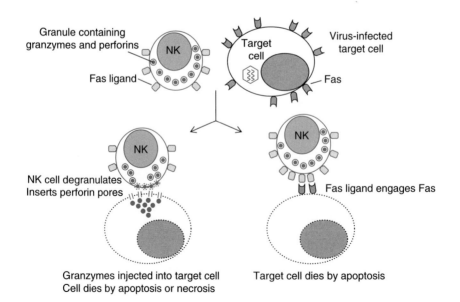

Class I, as a mechanism to evade cytotoxic T cells. However, this strategy may result in killing by NK cells.

NK cells also have Fc receptors and bind to antibody-coated target cells. This activates the NK cell, resulting in target cell killing. This is called antibody-dependent cellular cytotoxicity (ADCC).

NK cells kill target cells in two ways that are similar to the mechanisms used by cytotoxic T cells (Figure 1.4.2). NK cells express Fas ligand (FasL) and thus can bind Fas on target cells inducing programmed cell death or apoptosis in the target cell. Alternatively, NK cells can insert pores into target cells, using perforin. Perforin forms pores by polymerising on the target cell surface. These pores allow granzymes (proteolytic enzymes) enter the target cell where they degrade host cell proteins. Pores also render the cell susceptible to osmotic lysis. The action of perforin and granzymes can result in apoptosis or necrosis of the target cell.

In addition to killing target cells, NK cells secrete cytokines including γ-IFN, biasing subsequent adaptive responses towards a cellular immune response, which is the effector mechanism required for recovery from viral infections.

CROSS REFERENCE

Section 1.24   Immune Responses to Infection

Innate Immune Responses II – The Complement System

The complement system is part of the innate immune system and includes over 20 functionally linked soluble plasma proteins. Complement components are acute phase proteins synthesised in the liver (hepatocytes) and by monocytes. Like other acute phase proteins, synthesis is increased after injury or during inflammation. Activation of complement generates molecules and complexes, important both in defence against bacterial infection and removal of circulating and deposited immune complexes (antibody–antigen). Complement circulates in inactive precursor forms and is activated in a cascade fashion. This is local, occurring on cell membranes or antigen–antibody complexes.

COMPLEMENT ACTIVATION

Complement activation can occur via three different pathways:

* Classical pathway
* Lectin pathway
* Alternative pathway.

The classical pathway (including complement components C1, C4, C2) is activated by antibodies bound to antigen (immune complexes). The lectin pathway (MBL, C4, C2) is activated by mannan-containing carbohydrates on bacteria or viruses. The alternative pathway (C3, factor B, factor D properdin) is constitutively minimally active, but is strongly activated when a transiently active complement component binds to polysaccharides on a pathogen. The alternative and mannan binding lectin pathways do not require antibody and therefore represent an early defence against microbial infection. Antibody activation of the classical pathway illustrates how the adaptive immune response harnesses elements of the innate immune response to augment effector responses.

C3 is the central component of the complement system. The first critical step in each pathway involves the generation of an enzyme ('C3 convertase') that splits the C3 molecule into C3a and C3b, the biologically active forms of C3. The next step involves the

Figure 1.5.1 Complement activation pathways.

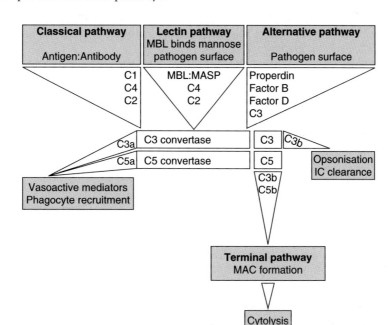

generation of another enzyme ('C5 convertase') that splits C5 into C5a and C5b, the biologically active forms of C5. This leads each pathway into same set of terminal steps generating the cytolytic membrane attack complex (MAC). An overview of these three pathways and their components is found in Figure 1.5.1.

THE BIOLOGICAL FUNCTIONS OF COMPLEMENT

Host defence against infection and foreign antigens

Opsonisation   C3b coats or opsonises bacteria. Phagocytosis is promoted and enhanced when C3b binds complement receptor 1 (CR1) expressed on neutrophils and macrophages.

Chemotaxis and activation of neutrophils   C5a attracts neutrophils and monocytes to the site of microbial infection or foreign antigen. C5a also augments cell adhesion, degranulation and activation of the respiratory burst in these cells.

Inflammation and vascular responses   The inflammatory peptides C3a and C5a (known as anaphylatoxins) activate mast cells resulting in histamine release. Histamine increases vascular permeability enhancing delivery of cells and proteins of the immune system.

Lysis of bacteria and cells   The MAC is formed by C5b–C9. This complex forms small pores that puncture cell membranes and cause cell death by lysis.

Solubilisation and phagocytic clearance of immune complexes

Immune complexes (ICs) form when the host mounts a vigorous antibody response to an abundant circulating antigen. Immune complexes are potentially harmful if deposited in vessel walls as they lead to inflammatory reactions that damage the surrounding tissue.

Complement affects immune complexes in two ways:

Solubilisation   Complement activation on immunoglobulin molecules inhibits immune complex growth by destabilising complex-forming reactions between adjacent immunoglobulin molecules.

Phagocytic clearance   Immune complexes bind and activate complement. C3b-coated immune complexes bind to CR1 that is expressed on red blood cells. Phagocytes in the liver and spleen strip and clear RBC-bound immune complexes.

REGULATION OF COMPLEMENT

The complement system is a potent mediator of inflammation and is tightly regulated to prevent injury to host cells. Complement cascades are tightly regulated at multiple steps: activated complement components are highly labile with short half-lives. This limits the range of destructive activity close to the activation site. Fluid phase inhibitors including C1-Inhibitor, Factor H, Factor I, C4-binding protein and membrane proteins including CR1, membrane cofactor protein, decay accelerating factor, and CD59, also play important regulatory roles. Most membrane regulatory proteins are expressed on host cells but not on microbes thus limiting the effects of complement activation to invading microorganisms.

CROSS REFERENCES

Section 2.6   Other Types of Hypersensitivity Reactions
Section 2.11   Complement Deficiency

REFERENCE

Walport, M. (2001) 'Advances in immunology: complement', *New Engl. J. Med.*, 344: 1058–66, 1140–4.

Innate Immune Responses III – Other Soluble Factors

THE ACUTE PHASE RESPONSE (APR)

Dramatic changes in vasculature, metabolism, temperature and plasma protein composition occur in response to tissue damage. Anti-microbial activity is enhanced. Pro-inflammatory cytokines (IL-1, IL-6 and TNF-α) released by phagocytes are the dominant mediators of these effects. Effects occur within hours and contribute to protection before and during the adaptive immune response. Adverse effects occur if the APR is inappropriately exaggerated or prolonged (Figure 1.6.1).

Key features include:

- Fever – inflammatory cytokines re-set hypothalamic temperature control. Microbial growth is impaired and specific immunity is more efficient at higher temperatures.
- Increased metabolism – release of energy from muscle and fat stores increases temperature. Weight loss is common.
- Vascular changes – TNF-α increases vascular permeability, facilitating movement of inflammatory cells and molecules into damaged tissue. Procoagulant effects localise inflammation at sites of injury.

During the APR the concentrations of many plasma proteins are altered – known as acute phase reactants. Some have anti-microbial properties.

Pro-inflammatory cytokines induce increased liver cell synthesis of the following proteins:

- CRP – natural opsonin
- MBL – natural opsonin
- Complement proteins (C3, C4)
- Ferritin – reduces levels of free iron which impedes some microbial growth
- Fibrinogen – procoagulant effects.

Immunoglobulin levels also increase slowly during chronic inflammation.

Figure 1.6.1 The acute phase response.

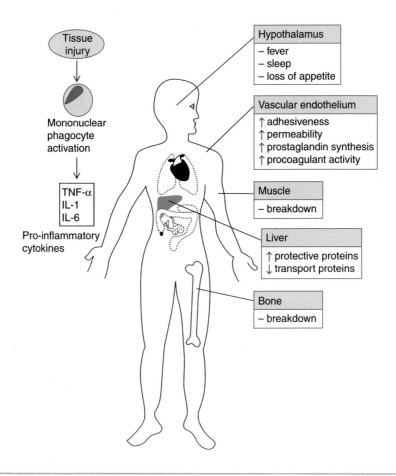

Reduced production of other proteins occurs in the APR:

- Albumin – hypoalbuminaemia can be pronounced in inflammatory states.
- Transferrin – like ferritin, reduces iron required for microbial growth.

The net effect is to shift hepatic protein synthesis towards production of protective proteins and away from storage and transport proteins. Elevation of plasma proteins, especially fibrinogen and immunoglobulins, increases the *Erythrocyte Sedimentation Rate* (ESR) in inflammatory states. Measurement of CRP is commonly used to monitor inflammation. Distinct patterns of plasma protein variations occur in different conditions. This is discussed further in Section 3.9.

CYTOKINES

Cytokines are small soluble proteins produced by cells (mainly of immune origin) that alter behaviour of that cell itself or of other cells.

Cytokines are categorised according to the cell of origin into:

- Interleukins (IL) – produced by blood cells and primarily influence leucocytes
- Lymphokines – produced by activated lymphocytes
- Monokines – produced by activated mononuclear phagocytes.

Common structural features allow cytokines to be classified into distinct families:

- Interferons – IFN-α and β, IFN-γ
- Chemokines – IL-8, RANTES etc.
- TNF family – TNF-α and β
- Haemopoietins – IL-2, IL-4, IL-6, granulocyte-colony stimulating factor (G-CSF), granulocyte monocyte-colony stimulating factor (GM-CSF), IL-3, IL-7.

Cytokines exert their effects through interaction with cytokine receptors on cell surfaces, and often use common signaling pathways within cells. Families of structurally related receptors interact with families of cytokines (above).

Cytokines can also be categorised according to the major effector functions they mediate.

- Innate immune response cytokines – initiate early immune responses. They also influence the type of subsequent specific immune response.
- Regulation of lymphocyte function – cytokines induce, direct and regulate lymphocytic responses.
- Inflammatory cell activation – mediate effector functions of macrophages and lymphocytes.
- Regulation of cell movement – chemokines are a distinct group of cytokines that share structural and functional characteristics. Chemokines are secreted by many cell types and influence the movement of immune cells.
- Haemopoietic growth factors – a number of cytokines influence haemopoietic differentiation.

Cytokines have a multitude of effects, but a number of features are common:

- Short duration of action – half-life is short and degradation is rapid.
- Locally active – most work on the cell of origin or on cells in the local microenvironment only. Others, like the haemopoietic factors and TNF-α act on distant cells.
- Multiple effects – most cytokines have many rather than one action (e.g. TNF-α – neutrophil activation, vascular effects, hepatic effects). Cytokine concentration also influences the pattern of the response.
- Overlapping effects – the same effect can be mediated by a number of cytokines (e.g. pro-inflammatory effects of IL-1 and TNF-α). This is an obstacle to the development of cytokine-directed therapies universally effective in inflammatory diseases.

All these factors make measurement of circulating cytokines both difficult and of dubious relevance in most situations.

Table 1.6.1 is not a complete list of all known cytokines but, rather highlights well-documented effects of some cytokines with critical roles in the induction, direction and regulation of inflammatory and immune responses.

Table 1.6.1 Cytokines and their functions

CYTOKINE	SOURCE	ACTIONS
Innate immunity and inflammatory responses		
IL-1	Macrophage	Vascular endothelial activation; neutrophil mobilisation, activation; APR activation; non-specific lymphocyte activation; increases IL-6 production
IL-6	Macrophages, T cells	APR induction; lymphocyte activation; enhanced antibody production
TNF-α	Macrophages, NK cells	Vascular endothelial activation; neutrophil activation; APR induction; energy release
IFN-α and β	White cells (α), Fibroblasts (β)	NK activation; enhanced antigen recognition; inhibition of viral replication
IFN-γ	T cells, NK cells	Macrophage, endothelial cell and NK activation
IL-5	TH2 T cells	Eosinophil growth and survival; B cell differentiation to IgE production
IL-8	Macrophages	Neutrophil chemoattractant
MIP-1 analogues	Macrophages, T cells	T cell and monocyte chemoattractant
MCP	Macrophages	Monocyte chemoattractant
RANTES	T cells	Memory T cell chemoattractant
Eotaxin	T cells	Eosinophil chemoattractant
Lymphocyte regulation		
IL-2	T cells	Lymphocyte proliferation and differentiation; IL-15 similar effects
IFN-γ	T cells, NK cells	Enhances CTL and TH1 pattern responses
IL-4	T cells, mast cells	TH2 cytokine; B cell activation and class switching to IgE; inhibit TH1 responses; IL-13 similar effects
IL-10	T regulatory cells	Inhibit TH1 responses; suppresses cytokine production by macrophages
TGF-β	T regulatory cells	Anti-inflammatory; pro-fibrotic
IL-12	Macrophages	NK cell activation; promote TH1 responses
Haemopoietic growth factors		
IL-3	Thymic epithelium, T cells	Early haemopoiesis
IL-7	Bone marrow stromal cells	Lymphocyte development
G-CSF	Fibroblasts	Neutrophil development
GM-CSF	Macrophages, T cells	Myeloid-monocytic development

CROSS REFERENCES

Section 1.2   Overview of Defence Mechanisms
Section 1.17   Helper T Cell Activation
Section 3.9   Measurement of the Acute Phase Response

Inflammation

Inflammation is the reaction of living tissue to injury or infection, and may be acute or chronic. Acute inflammation may be followed by resolution, or if the stimulus persists may become chronic (Figure 1.7.1). Clinically, acute inflammation is characterised by heat, redness, swelling and pain and often loss of function.

Inflammation has many beneficial functions including:

♦ Dilutes and removes toxins
♦ Limits spread of bacteria
♦ Facilitates influx of neutrophils, complement, opsonins and antibodies
♦ Provides a supply of inflammatory mediators
♦ Ensures an increased supply of nutrients for cells
♦ Promotes initiation of the immune response
♦ Initiates the healing process.

However acute inflammation also has harmful effects. Swelling may have a mechanical effect – for example, in acute epiglottitis where the airway may become obstructed by the swollen epiglottis. Swelling can impair function directly or by impairing blood flow, particularly when tissue expansion is limited (e.g. in intracranial inflammation). Inflammation also contributes to tissue damage. When acute inflammation fails to resolve, chronic inflammation can cause considerable tissue damage, which may result in scarring and loss of tissue function.

INITIATION OF INFLAMMATION

Inflammation results from a variety of insults, which lead to production of pro-inflammatory mediators. The nature of these mediators affects the nature of the inflammatory response. The type and severity of the injury and the genetic makeup of the individual affect inflammation.

Figure 1.7.1 Outcomes of inflammation.

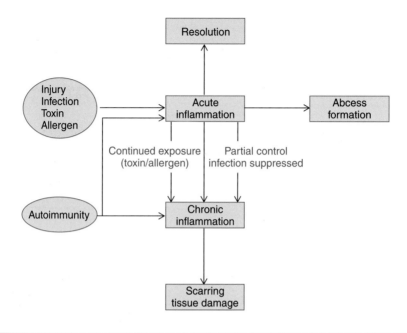

Inflammation may result from:

- Physical injury – trauma, burns
- Infection – organisms and toxins
- Allergy
- Autoimmune disease.

Components of the innate and adaptive immune response play pivotal roles in the inflammatory process.

THE INFLAMMATORY RESPONSE

Injury damages cells resulting in release of proinflammatory mediators such as prostaglandins and leukotrienes and leakage of cell contents. Bacterial components and toxins provide additional proinflammatory stimuli. Mast cell degranulation results from physical trauma and complement activation, releasing histamine. Tissue macrophages ingest particles and debris, become activated and release a number of proinflammatory cytokines such as IL-1, IL-6 and TNF-α. Macrophages also produce chemokines, which attract specific leucocytes to the site of injury.

Prostaglandins, histamine and complement components (particularly the anaphylatoxins C3a and C5a) cause vasodilation and increased vascular permeability. This increases extravasation of fluid, including macromolecules, which do not cross a normal vascular bed. Monokines also alter vascular endothelium locally, making it more 'sticky' by upregulating adhesion molecules, and increasing expression of procoagulant molecules. Enhanced clotting in local vessels helps to stop bleeding and also limits the ability of bacteria to spread.

Figure 1.7.2 Multi-stage leucocyte–endothelial interaction.

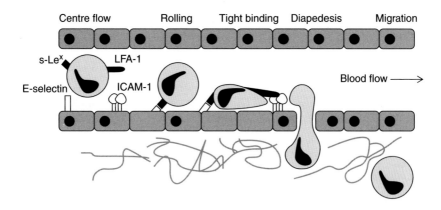

Leucocytes migrate to the area of inflammation, with neutrophils arriving rapidly, followed by monocytes and lymphocytes hours to days afterwards. Leucocytes normally travel in the centre of vessels, due to laminar flow. Leucocytes make contact with endothelium intermittently, rolling for some distance, and then detaching if no further adherent stimuli are encountered. If the *rolling* leucocyte encounters inflamed endothelium expressing activated integrin adhesion molecules, integrin-mediated firm adhesion ensues (*tight binding*). The leucocyte can then migrate through the endothelium, via the interaction of additional adhesion molecule pairs (*diapedesis*). Leucocytes reach the site of tissue injury by *chemotaxis* (directional cell migration) along gradients of chemotactic mediators. Chemotactic mediators which attract neutrophils include anaphylatoxins, leukotrienes, chemokines such as IL-8 (produced by macrophages) and bacterial products, particularly formyl peptides (Figure 1.7.2).

The precise composition of the inflammatory infiltrate is influenced by the initiating stimulus. Suppurative inflammation is commonly seen in response to infection with pyogenic bacteria. The inflammatory infiltrate is neutrophil dominated, and pus formation may result. Pus is a semi-liquid mixture containing bacteria, damaged cells and neutrophils. It is green because of the high content of neutrophil myeloperoxidase. A localised collection of pus is called an abscess. Allergic inflammation is discussed in detail in Section 1.30. However, mast cell degranulation plays a key role in initiating this type of inflammation, and the early phase is dominated by tissue oedema with a later influx of eosinophils. Pus formation does not occur.

Later in the course of inflammation monocytes and lymphocytes enter, attracted by chemokines released from macrophages and other cells in the inflammatory infiltrate.

If the stimulus is removed or eradicated acute inflammation may resolve, often leaving no tissue injury. Once the stimulus is removed, the rate of arrival of new cells decreases rapidly. Leucocytes present at the inflammatory site die by apoptosis and are removed by resident macrophages. Fibroblasts repair the connective tissue, and breaches in epithelium heal.

The physiological and cellular events underlying inflammation give rise to the clinical features outlined in Table 1.7.1.

Acute inflammation enhances antigen presentation to the immune system, eliciting an immune response to infecting organisms. APCs including dendritic cells and macrophages at the site of inflammation take up antigen and become activated. These

Table 1.7.1 Clinical and physiological features of acute inflammation

CLINICAL EFFECT	PHYSIOLOGICAL EFFECT	MEDIATORS
Heat	Increased blood flow Vasodilation	Histamine Prostaglandins (some)
Redness	Vasodilation	Anaphylotoxins (C3a, C5a)
Swelling	Vasodilation Extravasation of fluid	Histamine Bradykinin Anaphylatoxins Leukotrienes
Pain	Nerve stimulation Pressure on nerve endings	Prostaglandin E2 Bradykinin

Figure 1.7.3 Common types of inflammation.

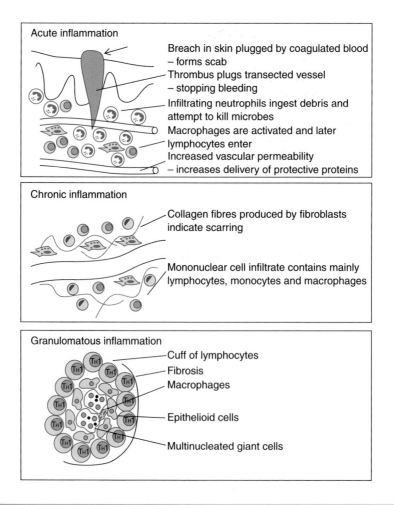

Acute inflammation

Breach in skin plugged by coagulated blood – forms scab
Thrombus plugs transected vessel – stopping bleeding
Infiltrating neutrophils ingest debris and attempt to kill microbes
Macrophages are activated and later lymphocytes enter
Increased vascular permeability – increases delivery of protective proteins

Chronic inflammation

Collagen fibres produced by fibroblasts indicate scarring

Mononuclear cell infiltrate contains mainly lymphocytes, monocytes and macrophages

Granulomatous inflammation

Cuff of lymphocytes
Fibrosis
Macrophages
Epithelioid cells
Multinucleated giant cells

APCs then migrate to regional lymph nodes where the chances of encountering antigen specific T and B cells are substantially increased. In the local nodes lymphocyte proliferation and differentiation occurs. Activated T cells then migrate back to the tissues, while B cells mature into plasma cells and produce antibody in the lymph nodes or bone marrow.

CHRONIC INFLAMMATION

Chronic inflammation usually follows unresolved acute inflammation, usually because of persistence of infection, allergen or other stimulus. Occasionally chronic inflammation can occur without preceding acute inflammation in some types of autoimmune disease. Chronic inflammation is characterised by ongoing tissue damage occurring at the same time as healing and repair (Figure 1.7.3).

Chronic inflammation is usually associated with impairment of function. Resolution is usually associated with fibrosis and scarring. When chronic inflammation cannot be fully controlled, progressive fibrosis may occur in association with progressive loss of organ function.

GRANULOMATOUS INFLAMMATION

Granulomatous inflammation is a special type of chronic inflammation associated with intense macrophage activation, driven by IFN-γ producing helper T cells.

Macrophages differentiate into epithelioid cells with enhanced secretory function, and diminished phagocytic capacity. Epithelioid cells fuse into multi-nucleated giant cells. This collection of epithelioid cells, giant cells and lymphocytes is called a granuloma (Figure 1.7.3). Granulomatous inflammation is associated with infections with organisms such as *Mycobacteria*, *Treponema pallidum* (which causes syphilis) and fungi. Granulomatous inflammation also occurs around foreign bodies, in some autoimmune disorders and idiopathic conditions such as sarcoidosis.

REFERENCE

Richard N. Mitchell and Ramzi S. Cotran (2003) 'Acute and chronic inflammation', in: *Robbins Basic Pathology*, 7th edn, V. Kumar, R. Cotran and S. L. Robbins, Saunders, Philadelphia, PA, pp. 33–59.

What the Immune System Recognises

ANTIGENS

The term antigen originally described any substance that could induce antibody formation. Antigens include proteins, carbohydrates, lipids and nucleic acids. Following characterisation of the cellular immune response, the use of the term antigen was expanded to include any substance that activated the immune response. Autoantigens are molecules found on host tissues that can induce an immune response.

Antigenic determinants and epitopes

Antibodies or lymphocytes produced in response to an antigen are directed against specific parts of the molecule called antigenic determinants or epitopes and not against the whole molecule. Epitopes are the smallest unit of antigens which can elicit an immune response. One molecule may have several identical or different epitopes, for example, a carbohydrate with repeating sugar units has several identical epitopes, while a large single chain protein has many different antigenic epitopes.

Conformational and linear epitopes

Antibodies usually bind conformational epitopes dependent on folding of the molecule (tertiary structure). Molecular folding brings different parts of a linear peptide chain close together, forming a single, discontinuous epitope. Many antibodies bind conformational epitopes in native proteins, but will not bind the denatured unfolded molecule. In contrast, T cell receptors recognise linear epitopes arising from the linear amino acid sequences of peptide antigens (primary structure) (Figure 1.8.1).

Haptens

Haptens are small molecules that can bind antibody but are incapable of inducing an adaptive immune response alone. Haptens must bind carrier molecules to elicit antibody

Figure 1.8.1 T and B cell epitopes.

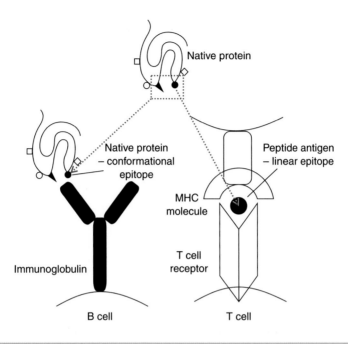

and T cell responses. Haptens such as drugs may elicit responses when bound to host proteins and anti-hapten antibodies may mediate allergic drug reactions.

IMMUNOGENICITY

Molecules that can stimulate an adaptive immune response are said to be immunogenic and can also be called immunogens. Factors other than antigen characteristics influence immunogenicity (Table 1.8.1). Substances that improve an immune response to antigens are called adjuvants. Purified proteins may be poorly immunogenic and carbohydrates, nucleic acids and other types of molecule usually require modification to induce an immune response. These issues are important for development and use of vaccines (Section 4.11).

WHAT DO THE INNATE AND ADAPTIVE IMMUNE RESPONSES RECOGNISE?

Targets of the innate immune response

Groups of organisms often have distinctive molecular patterns that are targets of the innate immune response. Table 1.8.2 summarises the most important of these targets and corresponding organisms, the pattern recognition receptor or molecule and their cellular location. PRMs are utilised by the innate immune response, to facilitate removal of pathogens.

Table 1.8.1 Factors that influence the immune response to an antigen

Nature of molecule	Protein content
	Size
	Solubility
	Large, complex, particulate, denatured proteins are most effective
Dose	Low dose – high antibody affinity + restricted specificity
	Moderate dose – varying affinity antibodies + broad specificity
	High dose – tolerance
	Moderate dose more immunogenic
Route of entry	Oral – Peyer's patches
	Inhalation – bronchial lymphoid tissue
	IV – spleen
	ID, IM, SC – regional lymph nodes
	Subcutaneous injection induces strongest responses
Substances with synergistic effects	Adjuvants
	Alum used in many human vaccines
	Bacterial products may provide stronger adjuvants in the future

Note: ID – intradermal; IM – intramuscular; SC – subcutaneous; IV – intravenous.

Table 1.8.2 Molecular targets of PRMs of the innate immune system

INNATE TARGETS	RECOGNITION MOLECULE: PATTERN RECOGNITION RECEPTOR	CELLULAR LOCATION
Mannosyl/fucosyl structures *Pseudomonas aeruginosa* *Mycobacterium tuberculosis* *Candida albicans* *Pneumocytsis carinii* *Klebsiella pneumoniae* *Leishmania donovani*	Mannose receptor	Macrophages Endothelial cells Dendritic cells

LPS
Gram-negative bacteria
  E. coli
  Neisseria
  Salmonella
	CD14
	LPS-binding protein (LBP),
	  an essential adaptor protein
		Macrophages

Carbohydrates or lipids Bacterial and yeast cell walls	Scavenger receptor	Macrophages
LPS Gram-negative bacteria	TLRs	APCs B cells Macrophages
Peptidoglycans, teichoic acids Gram-positive bacteria Arabinomannans, glucans		

Table 1.8.3 Thymus dependent and thymus independent antigens

TD-ANTIGEN	TI-1 ANTIGEN	TI-2 ANTIGEN
Diptheria toxin	Bacterial	Pneumococcal polysaccharide
Viral haemagglutinin	lipopolysaccharide	*Salmonella* polymerised flagellin
Purified proteins	*Brucella abortus*	Dextran
derivative (PPD) of		Hapten-conjugated Ficoll (polysucrose)
M. tuberculosis		*Haemophilus influenza* capsular polysaccharides

Antigen targets of the adaptive immune response: thymus-dependent and thymus-independent antigens

Thymus-dependent (TD) antigens (most proteins) require T cell help to induce antibody production. Thymus-independent (TI) antigens induce antibody production without T cell help; some bacterial polysaccharides, polymeric proteins and lipopolysaccharides can directly stimulate specific B cells. B cell responses to TI antigens are particularly important in organisms whose surface antigens elicit weak peptide-specific T cell responses. In children adequate responses to TI-antigens can take 4–6 years to develop (Table 1.8.3).

There are two types of TI-antigens that activate B cells by different mechanisms:

◆ TI-1 antigens possess intrinsic B cell stimulatory activity. At high concentrations TI-1 antigens activate the majority of B cells independently of their specific B cell receptor, acting as mitogens. At low concentrations, only B cells specific for the TI-1 antigen are activated. Bacterial lipopolysaccharides (LPS) are TI-1 antigens.
◆ TI-2 antigens are linear molecules with highly repetitive structures, for example, bacterial capsular polysaccharides. TI-2 antigens activate mature B cells by extensive cross-linking of their specific B cell receptors. The capsular polysaccharide of *Haemophilus influenzae* type B is a TI-2 antigen.

CROSS REFERENCE

Section 4.11   Vaccination and Passive Immunisation

37

Human Leucocyte
Antigen (HLA) Molecules

HLA molecules are the human MHC molecules. HLA molecules play a pivotal role in the normal immune response, and inability to express these molecules causes a lethal immunodeficiency. An individual's HLA type determines in part their ability to respond to infection and predisposition to autoimmune disease. Matching donor and recipient HLA types as closely as possible improves outcome in most types of transplantation.

HLA MOLECULES – STRUCTURE AND FUNCTION

HLA molecules are divided into two main classes, HLA Class I (including HLA-A, B and C) and HLA Class II molecules (including HLA-DR, DP and DQ). HLA Class I molecules have one variable α chain, and are stabilised by β_2-microglobulin. HLA Class II molecules are heterodimers, comprising 2 variable chains (α and β chains). Both Class I and Class II molecules have a peptide-binding groove (Figure 1.9.1). The physiological function of both classes of HLA molecules is to present short pathogen-derived peptides to T cells. This is the key interaction in initiating an antigen specific, adaptive immune response.

HLA molecules bind many different peptides stably as an integral part of the HLA molecule – HLA is unstable when peptides are not bound. The peptide binding domains of HLA Class I, and HLA Class II molecules are polymorphic; that is, particular amino acids in the peptide-binding grooves vary from allele to allele. These polymorphic residues make contact with the antigen-derived peptide. The peptide amino acids that bind HLA are called anchor residues. Peptides range in length from 8 to 10 residues for HLA Class I, to 12–20 residues for HLA Class II.

HLA Class I molecules are expressed on all nucleated cells and on platelets and present cytoplasmic peptides to CD8+ cytotoxic T cells. Widespread expression of HLA Class I molecules allows all cells to present peptides from intracellular pathogens to cytotoxic T cells of the immune system.

HLA Class II molecules are expressed on a restricted repertoire of immune cells including dendritic cells, monocytes and macrophages, B cells, activated T cells and thymic epithelial cells. HLA Class II molecules present antigen to CD4+ helper T cells to initiate adaptive immune responses, a role requiring restricted expression. At sites of inflammation, particularly in the

Figure 1.9.1 Structure of MHC (or HLA) Class I and Class II molecules.

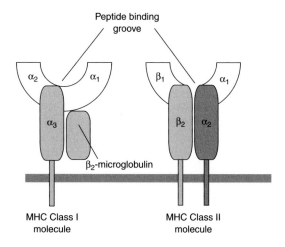

Figure 1.9.2 Chromosome 6: genes in the Major Histocompatibility region encode HLA molecules.

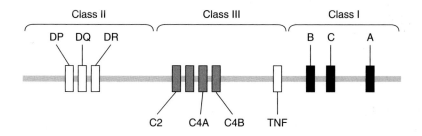

presence of IFN-γ, Class II molecules are induced on cells that do not normally express these molecules.

The genes encoding the HLA molecules are found in a small cluster on Chromosome 6 (Figure 1.9.2). This region contains in excess of 200 genes including both *HLA*, non-*HLA* genes involved in the immune response, and many genes with no apparent immunological role.

HLA MOLECULES – DIVERSITY

Within the population, there are hundreds of different *HLA* alleles. Most variability between different alleles of a HLA molecule resides around the peptide-binding groove. Expression of HLA molecules is polygenic (we each have several *HLA* genes) and polymorphic (at each *HLA* gene locus there are many possible alleles). Individuals of differing HLA type infected with the same organism will usually present different pathogen-derived peptides to initiate an immune response. The outcome of the immune response is often equivalent, however, possession of particular HLA types has been associated with disease resistance in some situations. For example, expression of *HLA*-B53 is associated with reduced mortality from severe malaria.

We inherit one set of *HLA* genes from each parent, and both maternal and paternal alleles are expressed on all cells. Within particular populations gene 'packages' known as haplotypes are frequently identified. Thus some *HLA* genes may be found almost exclusively associated with typical haplotypes within a particular population. These haplotypes include *HLA* genes and also the intervening genes encoded on chromosome 6, many of which have immunological functions. Haplotype associations of HLA molecules differ in different populations.

Genetic diversity of HLA molecules helps to ensure that some members of a population can mount an immune response to any organism. While some individuals may be unable to eliminate a pathogen, diversity makes survival at population levels more likely. At an individual level, people who are heterozygous (expressing different maternal and paternal *HLA* alleles) can bind and present a greater repertoire of peptides to their T cells. It appears that progression to acquired immunodeficiency syndrome (AIDS) is slower in human immunodeficiency virus (HIV)-infected individuals who are heterozygous for HLA molecules, suggesting a possible survival advantage attributable to HLA diversity.

DISEASE ASSOCIATIONS

Particular HLA types have been associated with both disease susceptibility and resistance. Associations are relative rather than absolute, and therefore are rarely useful in establishing a diagnosis in individual patients. Apparent associations may reflect a true role of the HLA molecule or may be due to linkage between the *HLA* allele and a physically close disease related (non-*HLA*) gene. In the non-immunological sleep disorder narcolepsy, an apparent HLA association was explained by linkage disequilibrium between a mutated gene encoding a hypocretin receptor and particular *HLA* alleles.

Several non-*HLA* genes are encoded in the HLA region of chromosome 6, many of which affect the immune response. For example, the *TNF-α* gene is encoded in this region, and a functional polymorphism in this gene determines whether large or small amounts of TNF-α are produced. The high-producing *TNF-α* genotype is linked to HLA-DR3 and included in a haplotype associated with increased risk of autoimmunity. Determining whether an apparent HLA association is significant is complicated by the common occurrence of haplotypes. Demonstrating a true HLA effect usually requires the study of several populations where individual HLA molecules are found with different haplotype associations.

Table 1.9.1 HLA and disease associations

DISEASE	HLA ASSOCIATION	RELATIVE RISK[a]
Ankylosing spondylitis	B27	87.4
Rheumatoid disease	DR4	4.2
Diabetes (Type I)	DR4	6.4
Diabetes (Type I)	DR2	0.19
Dermatitis herpetiformis	DR3	15.9

Note: [a]Relative risk is the risk of disease in individuals expressing specific HLA type, divided by the risk in those who do no express this HLA antigen.

CROSS REFERENCES

Section 1.8   What the Immune System Recognises
Section 1.10   Antigen Presentation

Antigen Presentation

The protective function of T cells depends on their ability to detect cells that harbour or internalise pathogens. T cells do this by responding to pathogen-derived peptides bound to MHC molecules on cell surfaces. Antigens may be **endogenous** (derived from molecules inside the cell, including molecules derived from intracellular pathogens) or **exogenous** (occurring outside the cell, but taken up by the processing cell). The generation of peptides from antigens is known as antigen processing. Not surprisingly, different mechanisms are involved in processing endogenous and exogenous antigens. The display of these peptides on the cell surface is known as antigen presentation.

ANTIGEN PRESENTING CELLS

Pathogens and other exogenous antigens are internalised into the vesicular compartments of antigen presenting cells (APCs), by phagocytosis, endocytosis or macropinocytosis. APCs include professional APCs such as dendritic cells that specialise in stimulating a T cell response; non-professional APCs such as macrophages that can present antigen but have other primary functions and B cells that internalise antigen by receptor-mediated endocytosis of cognate antigen bound to their surface immunoglobulin (sIg).

MHC CLASS I AND CLASS II MOLECULES DELIVER PEPTIDES TO THE CELL SURFACE FROM DIFFERENT CELLULAR COMPARTMENTS WHERE THEY ARE RECOGNISED BY TWO DIFFERENT TYPES OF T CELL

MHC Class I molecules deliver peptides produced in the cytosol to the cell surface where they are recognised by CD8 cytotoxic T cells (Tcs). In this way cytotoxic T cells kill cells infected with viruses or bacteria residing in the cytosol.

MHC Class II molecules deliver peptides from the vesicular system to the cell surface where they are recognised by CD4 helper T cells. In this way, helper T cells detect pathogens and their products taken up from the extracellular environment into the vesicular compartment of cells and activate other cells to eliminate the pathogen.

ENDOGENOUS ANTIGEN PATHWAY – MHC CLASS I

Generally pathogen-derived peptides that bind MHC Class I molecules are derived from viruses that have infected host cells. Viruses take over the cell's biosynthetic mechanisms to make their own proteins, which are degraded and synthesised as part of normal cell protein turnover.

♦ Cytosolic protein degradation takes place in a multicatalytic protease complex called the proteosome (Figure 1.10.1).
♦ Degraded proteins are transported from the cytosol of a cell into the lumen of the endoplasmic reticulum (ER) via membrane transporter proteins (transporters associated with antigen processing or TAP-1 and TAP-2).
♦ In this compartment peptides bind to MHC Class I molecules. Peptide binding is an essential step in the assembly of MHC Class I molecules and this process involves a number of accessory proteins with chaperone-like functions.
♦ Peptide: MHC Class I complex is then transported to the cell surface where it can be recognised by cytotoxic T cells.

Some viruses have evolved ways to evade recognition by down-regulating the appearance of peptide:MHC complexes on the cell surface.

Figure 1.10.1 Endogenous antigen pathway – MHC Class I.

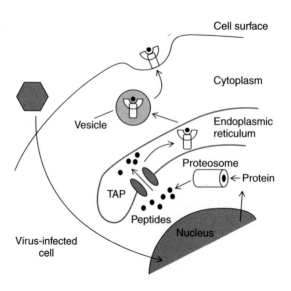

Figure 1.10.2 Exogenous antigen pathway – MHC Class II.

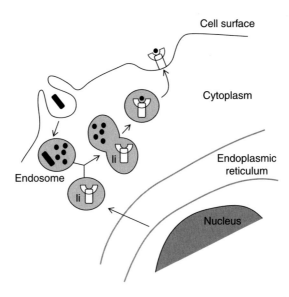

EXOGENOUS ANTIGEN PATHWAY – MHC CLASS II

Extracellular pathogens and other extracellular antigens that are internalised into endocytic vesicles (endosomes) of APCs are processed in the exogenous antigen pathway (Figure 1.10.2). The contents of endocytic vesicles are not accessible to cytosolic proteosomes.

- Protein degradation takes place in these vesicles which contain proteases.
- MHC Class II molecules are prevented from binding peptides in the ER by associating with the invariant chain (Ii), which also targets the molecule to endosomes. MHC Class II molecules reach the endocytic vesicles of macrophages, B cells and dendritic cells.
- When these endocytic vesicles fuse with peptide containing vesicles, the MHC molecules are loaded with peptides and transported to the cell surface where the peptide:MHC Class II complex can be recognised by helper T cells.

Initiation of an immune response requires activation of helper T cells by APCs with peptide bound to MHC Class II. APCs constantly take up antigen from their environment, and thus bacterial and viral antigens reach the endosomal compartment, even though this is not their normal site of infection. Additionally several pathogens including mycobacteria and *Leishmania* replicate in cellular vesicles of macrophages.

CROSS REFERENCES
Section 1.11   How Does the Immune System See Antigen?
Section 1.17   Helper T Cell Activation

How Does the Immune System See Antigen?

RECOGNITION MOLECULES OF THE INNATE IMMUNE RESPONSE

The innate immune response recognises microbes by the presence of molecular motifs, which are not present in mammalian cells, using pattern recognition molecules (PRMs). PRMs are constitutively expressed and allow the innate immune response to be constantly effective, as there is no delay required to rearrange microbe specific receptors. Important PRMs are outlined below. A summary of molecular targets of PRMs involved in the innate immune response was presented in Table 1.8.2.

Mannose receptor

The mannose receptor binds mannose in microbes and induces phagocytosis. Peptides from the microbe are processed and presented by macrophages, and can activate some T cell subtypes.

Toll receptors

Toll-like receptors (TLRs) are a family of closely related proteins that recognise several microbial motifs including peptidoglycan, teichoic acids (found on gram-positive bacteria), LPS (gram-negative bacteria), arabinomannans and glucans. Binding of ligand to TLRs induces expression of immunostimulatory molecules and cytokines important in initiation of the adaptive immune response.

CD14

CD14, found on macrophages, binds LPS, a unique bacterial surface structure found in cell walls of gram-negative bacteria, together with an adaptor protein. When LPS binds CD14, macrophages are activated facilitating destruction of the microbe and secretion of cytokines, triggering a wide variety of immune responses.

Scavenger receptors

These receptors are expressed by macrophages and recognise carbohydrates or lipids in bacterial and yeast cell walls.

RECOGNITION MOLECULES OF THE ADAPTIVE IMMUNE RESPONSE

In the adaptive immune response, lymphocytes have unique recognition structures that allow them to see antigen.

- B cell receptor (BCR)
- T cell receptor (TCR).

The BCR is surface bound immunoglobulin, and binds conformational epitopes. TCR binds linear epitopes, presented in grooves in MHC molecules. BCR, TCR and MHC proteins are all members of the immunoglobulin superfamily.

B cell receptor complex and B cell co-receptors

The BCR complex comprises BCR surface immunoglobulin (sIg) associated with two signaling molecules Igα and Igβ (Figure 1.11.1). Igα and Igβ are also required for assembly and expression of sIg. When antigen cross-links sIg, Igα and Igβ transduce activation signals into the B cell. Ligation of B cell co-receptors can enhance or inhibit signaling via the Ig–Igα/Igβ complex. Optimal activation requires additional signals from helper T cells. Activated B cells differentiate into plasma cells and secrete antibody.

Antibody–antigen interactions

The antigen-binding site of immunoglobulin molecules is composed of variable regions of both heavy and light chains. Antigen specificity of the immunoglobulin is determined by variation in the amino acid sequences of variable regions. Three segments are particularly variable – hypervariable (HV) regions 1–3. Hypervariable segments form surfaces complementary to the antigen: complementarity-determining regions (CDRs) 1–3. Variation in the amino acid sequences of CDRs creates different surface shapes. Antibodies bind epitopes with complementary shapes which fit tightly (Figure 1.11.1).

T cell receptor (TCR), the TCR complex and co-receptors

Most T cells have antigen receptors composed of α and β chains, each with variable and constant regions (V and C regions). A subpopulation of T cells, the function of which is poorly understood, express TCRs consisting of γ and δ chains. The TCR complex consists of the TCR associated with CD3 a signaling complex. CD4 or CD8 (co-receptors) play an important role in stabilising the interaction of TCR with MHC–peptide complex.

TCRs interact directly with both the antigenic peptide and some polymorphic regions of the MHC molecule presenting the peptide. CD4 or CD8 help to stabilise the TCR–peptide–MHC interaction which is of very low avidity. CD4 and CD8 distinguish two different functional sets of T cell. CD4 is expressed on helper T cells and binds a non-polymorphic region of MHC Class II molecules. This effectively restricts helper T cells to recognise peptides appropriately presented on MHC Class II molecules. In contrast, CD8 is expressed on cytotoxic T cells allowing recognition of peptides presented on MHC Class I molecules which is widely expressed.

Figure 1.11.1 The B cell receptor complex and its co-receptor complex. Antibody:antigen interaction.

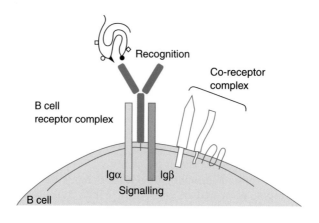

Figure 1.11.2 (a) T cell receptor complex and antigen:MHC binding. (b) Superantigen binds Vβ region of T cell receptor and MHC Class II molecule.

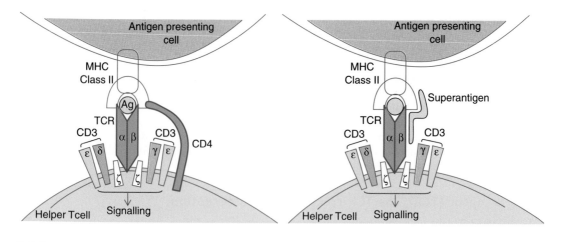

TCR–peptide–MHC interaction

TCRs recognise antigenic peptides bound to MHC molecules on cell surfaces (Figure 1.11.2(a)). This crucial interaction determines the antigen specificity of adaptive immune responses. Proteins are unfolded, processed into peptide fragments by intracellular proteases, and small peptides are presented in the groove of MHC molecules. Endogenous antigens, and viral proteins, associate with MHC Class I molecules, found on all nucleated cells. Antigens including those derived from pathogens internalised by endocytosis from extracellular fluid, associate with MHC Class II molecules, found on specialised APCs.

Superantigen

Classical antigens generate peptides that bind the peptide-binding groove of MHC Class II. In contrast superantigens bind directly to MHC without processing. Superantigens bind to relatively non-polymorphic portions of MHC Class II and the Vβ region of the TCR (Figure 1.11.2b). Each superantigen can bind a few families of Vβ gene segments, and therefore superantigens can stimulate 2–20% of all T cells. This type of response causes a massive production of CD4 T cell cytokines resulting in systemic toxicity and suppression of adaptive immunity.

Clinically important superantigens include Staphylococcal enterotoxins that cause food poisoning, and the toxic shock syndrome toxin (TSST).

CROSS REFERENCES

Section 1.8   What the Immune System Recognises
Section 1.9   Human Leucocyte Antigen (HLA) Molecules
Section 1.10   Antigen Presentation

Lymphocyte Maturation

Lymphocytes must recognise a huge diversity of antigens and must develop the functional capacity to play many roles in generating, enhancing and regulating specific immune responses. Each lymphocyte expresses *a single specificity of antigen receptor*. B and T cell maturation pathways share many common features but anatomical sites of maturation, and some molecular events in antigen receptor generation are distinct to each population. NK cells are another population of lymphocytes, which do not interact with antigens in a specific manner, and do not express rearranged antigen specific receptors.

The functions of lymphocytes are:

- Antibody production (specifically B cells)
- Cell-mediated inflammation (T cells)
- Regulation of other immune cell functions (T cell)
- Cytotoxicity (T cell and NK cells).

LYMPHOCYTE POPULATIONS

B lymphocytes

B cells recognise antigens through surface immunoglobulin (sIg). Terminally differentiated B cells, called plasma cells, produce and secrete antibodies, the specificity of which is identical to the sIg expressed by their B cell precursors. Following maturation in the bone marrow, most B cells that survive the selection process circulate through secondary lymphoid tissues. These are *conventional* or B-2 B cells.

B-1 B cells are a smaller subset of B cells, which produce a limited repertoire of low affinity and polyspecific antibodies reactive with common bacterial antigens. B-1 B cells may represent a primitive population whose function is intermediate between innate and specific immune responses.

T lymphocytes

T lymphocytes express T cell receptors (TCRs) and CD3. Most T lymphocytes express a TCR comprising α and β chains (αβ T cells) and also either CD4 or CD8, which direct the pattern of antigen interaction. Antigens recognised by αβ T cells are processed peptides, presented by host-derived MHC molecules. Factors influencing the pattern of T cell response include the pattern of innate immune activation, characteristics of the stimulating antigen, and type of antigen presentation.

αβ T cells

Two broad categories of αβ T cells are described as follows:

- Cytotoxic T cells (CTLs or Tcs) – usually express CD8 and recognise endogenous antigens (viruses, tumours).
- Helper T cells (Ths) usually express CD4. They respond to extracellular antigens including bacteria that are taken up into vesicles in the cells. Activation of helper T cells requires processing and presentation of antigen in association with MHC Class II molecules by professional APCs. These cells typically 'help' other cells of the immune system rather than having a direct effector function.

Helper T cells are in turn further sub-divided based on patterns of cytokine expression. The two extremes are:

- Th1 – produce IFN-γ and tumour necrosis factor that enhance macrophage function, cellular immunity, production of some antibody types and granulomatous inflammation.
- Th2 – enhance IgE-mediated responses through the action of IL-4 and IL-5.

Th1 and Th2 responses are for the most part mutually exclusive and suppressive of the other. Further T cell subpopulations are increasingly recognised, such as regulatory T cells – Tr – and Th3 that impose control on cell-mediated immune responses through the action of cytokines including IL-10 and TGF-β.

γδ T cells

γδ T cells express a TCR composed of γ- and δ-chains and are preferentially expressed in skin and at mucosal surfaces. Their antigen interactions are not as specific as those of αβ T cells. Diverse effector functions mirroring those of αβ T cells have been identified. These cells may represent a T cell equivalent of B-1 B cells.

Unconventional T cells

CD3+ T cells expressing unusual patterns of surface molecules common to conventional T cells and NK cells are called NK-T cells. Antigen recognition by NK-T cells extends beyond peptide fragments expressed by MHC molecules. The functional significance of this population is not fully understood.

NK cells

These can kill certain tumour targets and virus-infected cells. Early production of IL-12 by NK cells encountering viruses and intracellular bacteria skews the later specific immune responses towards a Th1-type response.

NK cells express activating receptors and inhibitory receptors, which interact with MHC Class I molecules, preventing uncontrolled activation of NK cells. If MHC expression is disturbed, as occurs in virus-infected or tumour-laden cells, inhibition is lost resulting in NK cell cytotoxicity.

THE DEVELOPMENT OF MATURE LYMPHOCYTE POPULATIONS

Haemopoietic stem cells (HSCs) differentiate into myeloid and lymphoid progenitor cells. Lymphoid-committed precursor cells mature in

♦   Bone marrow – where they receive signals that promote development into B cells

or

♦   Thymus – where T cells develop.

A small proportion of T cells, especially non-conventional ones like γδ T cells and NK-T cells may mature outside the thymus.

Lymphocytes mature by a series of sequential differentiation steps defined by patterns of molecular expression, especially antigen receptor or antigen receptor-associated molecules. The early phases of lymphocyte maturation occur independent of exposure to antigen. Once complete antigen receptors are expressed by developing lymphocytes, further survival and functional capacity requires interaction with antigen (Figure 1.12.1).

B lymphocyte maturation

B cells are generated throughout life in the bone marrow. Development stages are marked by the ordered rearrangement of immunoglobulin genes. The key stages and the important molecule expression patterns are highlighted.

♦   Pro-B cells – express B cell-specific molecules (CD19, surrogate light chain). Immunoglobulin genes are in germline configuration.
♦   Pre-B cells – express surface IgM heavy chain associated with surrogate light chain – pre-B receptor. Immunoglobulin genes are rearranged by enzymes encoded by *Recombinase Activating Genes* (RAG), and the IgM expressed originates from whichever chromosome successfully rearranged first. *RAG* gene expression is switched off, inhibiting rearrangement of immunoglobulin heavy chain genes on the other chromosome – allelic exclusion. Subsequent re-expression of *RAG* allows light chain immunoglobulin genes to rearrange. Kappa (κ) genes initially rearrange. If unsuccessful, the λ genes rearrange sequentially until a functional light chain is produced.
♦   Immature B cells – IgM+ IgD– immunoglobulin receptor expression allows these cells interact specifically with antigen. Further survival and differentiation is dependent on whether or not selection or activation signals are received through the BCR. This is discussed further in Section 1.14.

T lymphocyte maturation

T cells develop from thymic lymphoid progenitor cells. NK cells and NK-T cells also arise from thymic progenitors, but details of their development are unclear. As with B cells, stages of T cell maturation are marked by specific patterns of TCR and other molecule expression. The key stages are

♦   'Double-negative' cells – lack CD4 and CD8 expression. Most have not rearranged TCR gene segments. CD2 but not CD3 is expressed.
♦   'Double positive' cells – dually express CD4 and CD8. T cells only reach this stage if a successful TCR is made.

Figure 1.12.1 Lymphocyte maturation.

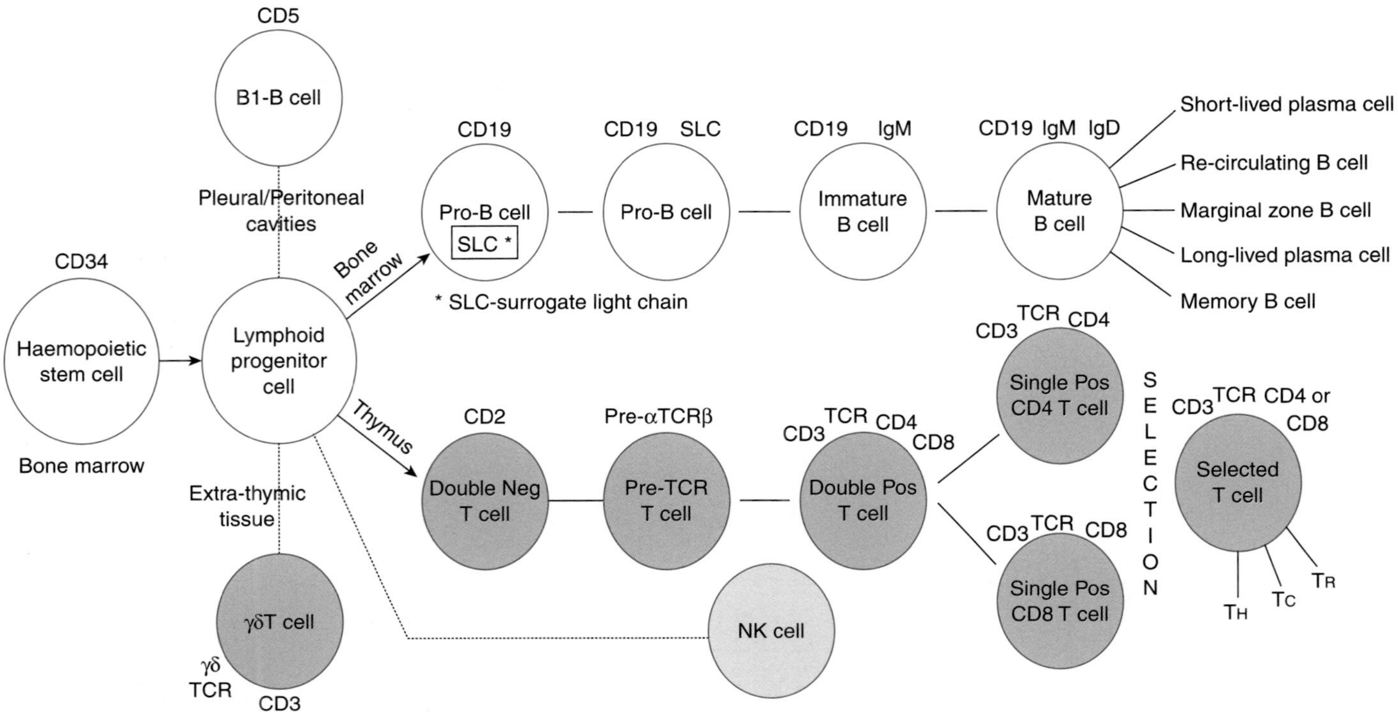

♦ Selected T cells – at this stage T cells are screened for ability to interact with host MHC – peptide complexes expressed on cortical epithelial cells and interdigitating dendritic cells. They also lose either CD4 or CD8 and become 'single positive' thymocytes. T cells must be able to recognise MHC for conventional T cell-mediated antigen recognition. Cells that pass this hurdle are positively selected for survival. T cells then undergo negative selection, where potentially autoreactive T cells are eliminated, an important safeguard against autoimmunity.

Negative selection in T cells is more rigorous than with B cells. A lack of T cell help will hold autoreactive B cells in check. Only about 1% of thymocytes mature and enter the peripheral pool.

Both $\alpha\beta$- and $\gamma\delta$-T cells are derived from the same early thymocyte precursor cell type. The type of TCR expressed – either TCR$\alpha\beta$ or TCR$\gamma\delta$ – depends on which of the TCR chains makes the first successful rearrangement. The same T cell cannot express both types of TCR. Successful rearrangement of TCRα disables δ-gene segments, and β and δ chains do not usually align correctly to form a functional TCR. Early in life, more T cells of the TCR$\gamma\delta$ lineage are produced, but subsequently TCR$\alpha\beta$-expressing T cells predominate. TCR$\gamma\delta$ cells often do not express either CD4 or CD8.

CROSS REFERENCES

Section 1.3   Cells and Organs of the Immune System
Section 1.11   How Does the Immune System See Antigen?
Section 1.14   B Cell Activation
Section 1.16   T Cell Receptor and Immune Repertoire

Immunoglobulin Structure

Antibodies, also called immunoglobulins (Ig), are glycoproteins, produced by plasma cells, that bind antigens with a relatively high specificity and affinity.

ANTIBODY STRUCTURE

Antibody molecules are comprised of two identical light chains and two identical heavy chains. Light chains may be kappa (κ) or lambda (λ) in type, but this does not affect antibody function.

The antibody isotype or class is determined by the heavy chain (μ, γ, α, ε or δ) giving rise to immunoglobulin M (IgM), immunoglobulin G (IgG), immunoglobulin A (IgA), immunoglobulin E (IgE) and immunoglobulin D (IgD), respectively. In addition to differences in the basic antibody unit, antibody isotypes differ in the number of units in a typical molecule – IgM is usually pentameric, IgA dimeric and both IgG and IgE monomeric (Figure 1.13.1). The five isotypes differ greatly in functional activity. IgG is subdivided into the subclasses IgG1, IgG2, IgG3 and IgG4 and IgA into IgA1 and IgA2 subclasses. Antibody subclasses differ in heavy chain amino acid sequences conferring functional differences (Section 1.15).

Variable and constant regions of heavy and light chains

Heavy and light chains have a variable region (composed of variable domains), and a constant region (composed of constant domains). Variable regions of heavy and light chains generate two identical antigen-binding sites, conferring specificity on the antibody. The heavy-chain constant region determines the antibody isotype and functional properties.

Functionally distinct fragments of the antibody molecule – Fc and Fab

Proteolytic cleavage by the enzyme papain cleaves immunoglobulin into two Fab fragments and one intact Fc fragment. The Fab fragment binds antigen and the Fc fragment contains constant domains.

Figure 1.13.1 Structure of immunoglobulin molecules.

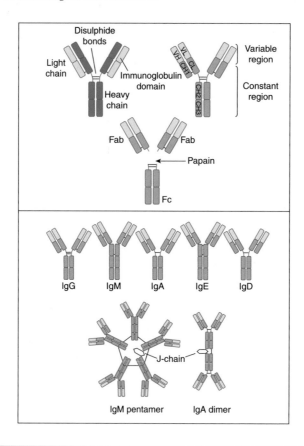

ALLOTYPES

Non-functional polymorphisms occur in genes encoding heavy chain constant regions giving rise to allotypes. Allotypes are differences between individuals' antibody molecules, comparable to different blood groups. There is no functional difference between antibodies of different allotypes.

IDIOTYPES

Idiotypes are unique antigenic determinants found in antigen-binding sites of antibodies. They result from different amino acid sequences in antigen-binding sites that determine the antibody specificity. Idiotypes are unique to antibodies produced by the same clone of B cells.

GENERATION OF DIVERSITY

The antibody response to an antigen is diverse, generating many different B cell clones each with its own unique specificity. An individual's collection of antibody specificities is called the antibody repertoire. Antibody diversity is generated during B cell development by random combination of gene segments from heavy-chain and light-chain gene groups (Figure 1.13.2).

There are three gene clusters encoding immunoglobulins:

♦ κ-chain clusters are found on chromosome 2
♦ λ-chain genes are found on chromosome 22
♦ Heavy-chain gene clusters are found on chromosome 14.

Variable and constant regions of immunoglobulin molecules are encoded by *V* gene segments and *C* gene segments, respectively.

Somatic recombination generates variable regions

The variable region of heavy and light chains is generated from separate *V* region gene segments by a process of DNA rearrangement known as somatic recombination. The heavy-chain V region gene segments include Variable (V_H), Diversity (D_H) and Joining (J_H), while the light chain contains variable (V_L) and joining segments (J_L).

V region recombination involves the 'VDJ recombinase' enzyme complex, which includes generic DNA cleavage and repair enzymes and lymphocyte-specific components. RAG-1 and RAG-2 are lymphocyte-specific enzymes, essential for VDJ recombination. VDJ recombination results in removal of intervening gene segments, permanently changing the genomic DNA in the B cell. The assembled variable regions of both heavy and light chains join to their respective constant regions after transcription, by RNA splicing. Heavy-chain C region genes have several gene segments, each encoding the constant region for a different antibody class (Cμ, Cγ, Cα, Cδ, Cε). κ chains have one *C* gene segment for its constant region, while λ chains have four *C* gene segments. Heavy chain genes undergo rearrangement before light chain genes.

Regulation of immunoglobulin gene rearrangement ensures that each B cell only expresses one rearranged heavy chain and one rearranged light chain. Therefore each B cell expresses millions of identical surface antibodies.

ANTIBODY DIVERSITY IS GENERATED BY FOUR PROCESSES, WHICH TOGETHER CREATE A VAST REPERTOIRE OF ANTIBODY SPECIFICITIES FROM A LIMITED NUMBER OF GENES

1   There are several different gene segments making up the variable regions of both heavy and light chains (Table 1.13.1). Different combinations of variable region gene segments recombining randomly generate considerable diversity in the antigen-binding site. This is known as combinatorial diversity.
2   Pairing of different heavy and light chains increases diversity.
3   During recombination, imprecise joining of gene segments results in insertion of additional nucleotides – known as junctional diversity.
4   Somatic hypermutation introduces point mutations into variable regions of rearranged heavy and light chain genes. This allows the antibody specificity to be changed after recombination occurs. Mutant antibody molecules may bind antigen better or less well than the original antibody. B cells expressing higher affinity antibody are selected and mature into antibody-secreting cells. Somatic hypermutation and selection of high affinity antibody gives rise to the physiological phenomenon of affinity maturation, whereby the affinity of antibodies produced improves as an immune response develops.

Figure 1.13.2 The production of immunoglobulin molecule heavy and light chains: somatic recombination, RNA splicing and production of protein. Rearrangement of κ light chain is used to illustrate the process, however, λ chain rearrangement follows identical steps.

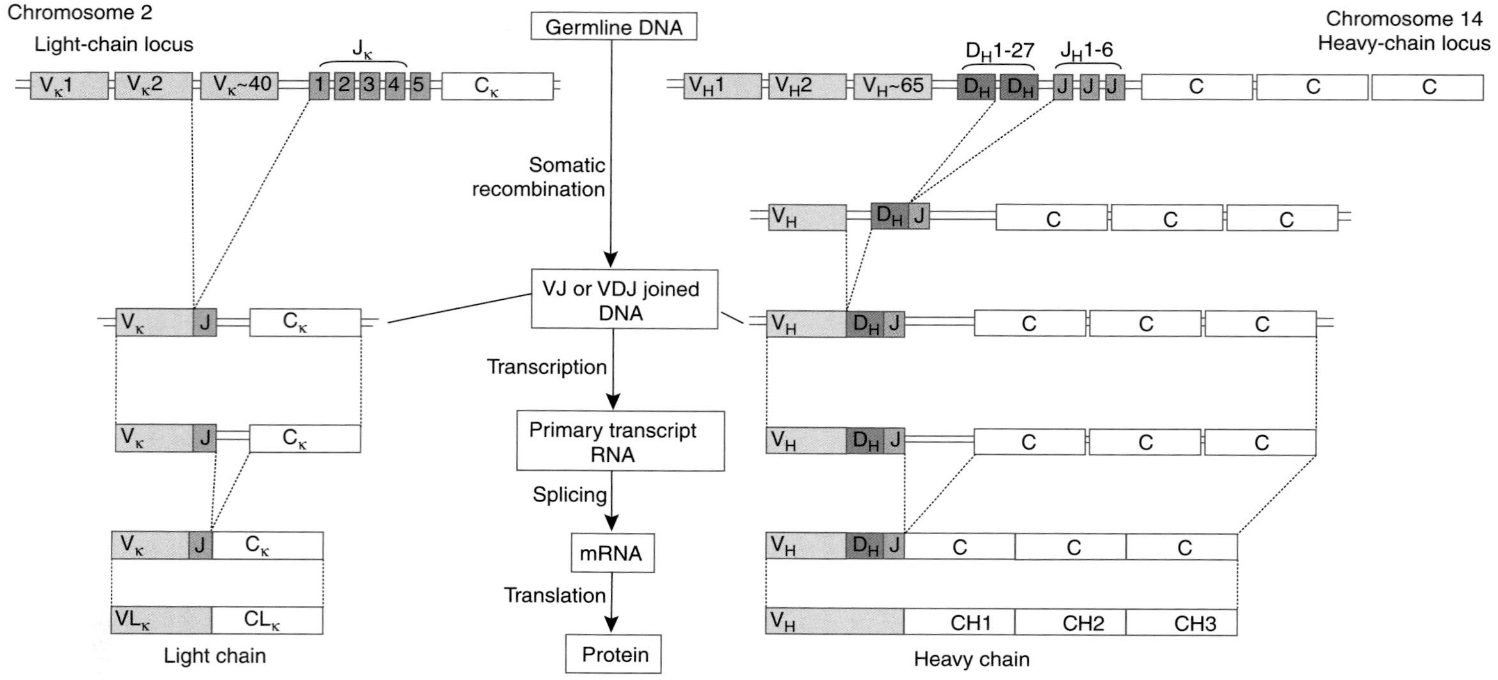

Table 1.13.1 Gene segments making up the variable regions of heavy and light chains

GENE SEGMENT	LIGHT CHAIN (κ)	LIGHT CHAIN (λ)	HEAVY CHAIN (H)
Variable (*V*)	40	30	65
Diversity (*D*)	0	0	27
Joining (*J*)	5	4	6

Figure 1.13.3 The B cell receptor complex and its co-receptor complex.

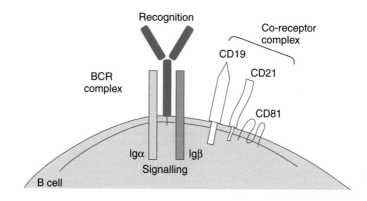

Rearrangement of gene segments occurs in developing B cells in bone marrow. Somatic hypermutation occurs in B cells in secondary lymphoid organs after functional antibody has been expressed.

THE B CELL RECEPTOR COMPLEX

Immunoglobulin was first discovered in plasma. However, before antibody can be secreted, immunoglobulin must function as the cell-surface antigen receptor, that is, the B cell receptor (BCR). Antigen binding to BCR activates B cells, leading to clonal expansion and differentiation into antibody-secreting plasma cells. B cells initially express transmembrane IgM and when activated differentiate into plasma cells. B cell activation usually requires specialised interactions with helper T cells that provide additional signals.

The BCR complex includes the antigen receptor, surface immunoglobulin, associated with two other polypeptides, Igα and Igβ. When sIg is crosslinked, these proteins transmit signals leading to B cell proliferation and differentiation. They are also required for the expression and assembly of immunoglobulin (Figure 1.13.3). B cell co-receptors (CD21, CD19 and CD81) play an important role in enhancing or inhibiting B cell activation. Activation of B cells and subsequent signalling events are described in more detail in Section 1.14.

CROSS REFERENCE
Section 1.14   B Cell Activation

B Cell Activation

B CELL SELECTION

B cells can interact with antigen once surface immunoglobulin is expressed. The type of responses initiated are influenced by

- B cell maturation stage
- Signal intensity through the antigen receptor.

The signal intensity also influences whether B cells become re-circulating follicular cells, marginal zone cells or B-1 B cells.

IgM+, IgD− immature B cells are exquisitely sensitive to antigen exposure (Figure 1.14.1). Antigen exposure can result in

- Clonal deletion – large concentrations of cross-linking antigen promotes cell death.
- Clonal anergy – cells remain viable but non-functioning following exposure to soluble antigen.
- Receptor editing – the immunoglobulin receptor alters. Continued *RAG* gene expression allows further immunoglobulin gene rearrangement. Following receptor editing, B cells which react with self antigen undergo clonal deletion, while those that do not react with self antigen persist. After the IgM+ IgD− stage, *RAG* expression is switched off and gene rearrangement ceases.

These responses reduce the chances of producing auto-reactive B cells. However, these processes are leaky and self-reactive B cells are usually present in the peripheral lymphocyte pool. Other mechanisms are required to keep these auto-reactive B cells in check (Section 1.21). B cells surviving these hurdles are called naïve (or 'virgin') newly produced B cells. IgM and IgD are co-expressed on their cell membranes.

B cells are produced so rapidly that the peripheral pool of mature B cells could be fully reconstituted with newly produced B cells every 4–5 days. Only a small minority (<10%) of newly produced B cells survive beyond a few days. Small numbers of newly produced B cells are recruited to the peripheral pool to replace dying mature B cells. Some cells interact

Figure 1.14.1 B cell selection.

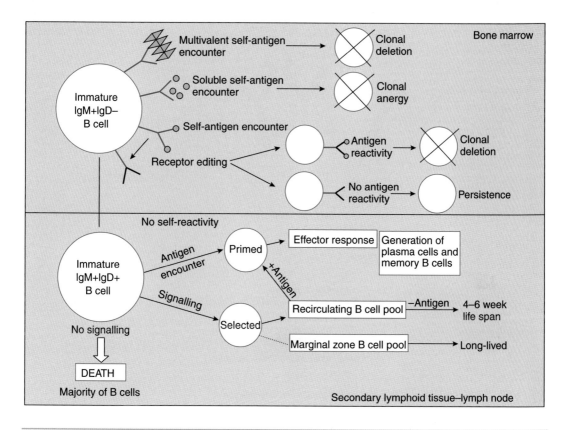

with antigen, proliferate and differentiate into antibody-producing plasma cells or memory B cells. Selection of virgin B cells involves signalling, possibly by self-antigens, via the antigen receptor. We do not yet understand how selection signals differ from activation signals. Variation in signalling strength appears to influence whether B cells become follicular-, marginal zone, or B-1 B cells. Re-circulating B cells can survive up to a few months.

B CELL ACTIVATION

The first signal

The BCR complex includes the immunoglobulin receptor and associated proteins on B cells (Figure 1.14.2(a)).

- Igα and Igβ (or CD79α and CD79β) maintain immunoglobulin receptor expression on the B cell surface and also transmit signals when antigen binds the immunoglobulin receptor.
- CD19, CD21 and CD81 (TAPA-1) alter the intensity of signalling generated on antigen binding.

Figure 1.14.2 (a) Signalling pathways initiated when antigen crosslinks B cell receptor. (b) T/B cell interactions.

(a)

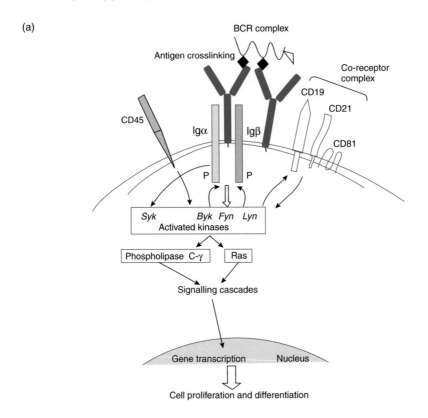

(b)

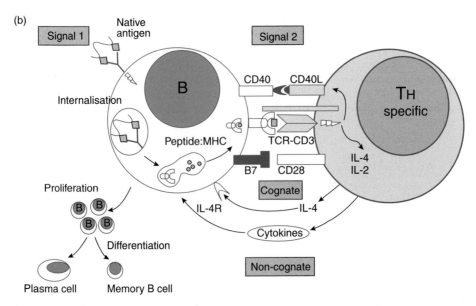

♦ Kinases (Fyn, Blk and Lyn) – enzymes that promote phosphorylation at target sites – associate with the immunoglobulin receptor and generate activation signals.

The signal generated on binding antigen (the primary signal) is usually not adequate to activate B cells to proliferate and differentiate.

The second signal

T cell help for B cell responses

Secondary signals usually delivered by antigen-specific T cells are typically required for B cell activation. Responses to most protein antigens are T dependent (TD). T cell dependence prevents self-reacting B cells from becoming functional. T cell influences on B cell immune responses include:

♦ Promotion of high affinity antibody production
♦ Induction of immunoglobulin isotype switching
♦ Enhancement of long-term memory responses.

Prior to antigen exposure, only about 1 in 100,000 lymphocytes are specific for a single conventional TD antigen. Secondary lymphoid organs concentrate rare antigen-specific B and T cells, increasing the chance of encounter. Inter-digitating dendritic cells 'trap' antigen-specific T cells re-circulating through the secondary lymphoid tissues and *prime* them for further antigen encounter. Meanwhile, antigen-specific B cells, on receiving the first antigen-specific signal move to the T cell zones under the control of several chemokines.

Antigen binding to the BCR mediates uptake of bound antigen into the B cell, processing into peptides and packaging with antigen-presenting MHC Class II molecules (Figure 1.14.2b). B cells express MHC Class II from the early stages of maturation.

Presentation of peptide with MHC Class II on the B cell surface brings antigen-specific T cells into close proximity with B cells responding to components of the same antigen. This is called linked recognition.

T cells provide 'help' to B cells through

♦ Cognate interaction – primed antigen-specific T cells help B cells to proliferate, and differentiate. The T cell interacting with B cell is specific for the same antigen. Interaction of CD40 expressed by B cells, with CD40 ligand (CD40L) expressed on antigen-specific activated T cells, drives B cell proliferation, antibody class switching and generation of memory responses. Deficiency of CD40L causes immunodeficiency – hyper IgM syndrome – characterised by failure of immunoglobulin class switching. Other B cell/T cell interactions are important in generating TD B cell responses, including B7/CD28.
♦ Non-cognate – reactions are not antigen-specific. Once activated through cognate interactions, B cells can respond to cytokines secreted by activated T cells. T cell cytokines affect B cell proliferation (IL-4), immunoglobulin class switching (IL-4, transforming growth factor-β (TGF-β) and IFN-γ), and differentiation into plasma cells (IL-6).

B cell proliferation hugely increases the frequency of antigen-specific cells over a few days. B cells do not proliferate indefinitely but rather differentiate, in a manner determined by the type of antigen, the type of T cell cognate interactions and the cytokine environment.

Activated B cells can differentiate into the following:

* Short-lived plasma cells – produce IgM predominantly.
* Follicular B cells – relocate from the T zone of secondary lymphoid tissues into the follicles where they establish a germinal centre reaction. Somatic hypermutation occurs in rapidly dividing germinal centre B cells (centroblasts). Variable regions of immunoglobulin genes are altered. Some B cells improve the affinity with which they bind antigen. This is a short-lived event in the immune response and cells that have undergone somatic hypermutation (centrocytes) subsequently require signals from antigen and T cells to survive. Only B cells that receive both these signals – that is, responsive to native antigen and not self-reactive – survive.

Some surviving centrocytes differentiate to become:

* Long-lived plasma cells – relocate to bone marrow and the lamina propria of the gut, or
* Memory B cells – colonise the marginal zones of secondary lymphoid tissues, responding with faster and bigger responses on second and subsequent exposures to antigen.

T INDEPENDENT B CELL ACTIVATION

The polysaccharide capsules of many pyogenic bacteria have distinct repeating structures. Antigen receptor binding of highly repetitive epitopes induces extensive cross-linking of the BCR complex and the B cell may be activated without additional signals. Activated complement and macrophage factors can also promote B cell activation. Antigens associated with lipopolysaccharide (e.g. gram-negative bacteria) are potent activators of complement and macrophages. If these factors can provide an adequate second signal to B cells during antigen-specific activation the requirement for T cells in B cell activation may be bypassed. Both LPS- and polysaccharide-based antigens are classed as T independent (TI) because T cells are not essential for B cells to make antibody responses.
  TI-type responses are either

* TI-1 – responses generated by LPS and similar antigens

or

* TI-2 – responses generated by polysaccharide antigens. Marginal zone B cells may preferentially respond to TI-2 antigens.

Different mechanisms allow both types of antigen to be TI. Although not essential, T cells can regulate B cell responses induced by TI antigens.

CROSS REFERENCES
Section 1.8   What the Immune System Recognises Section 1.12   Lymphocyte Maturation Section 1.13   Immunoglobulin Structure

REFERENCES

Maclennan, I. C. M. (1998) 'B cell receptor regulation of peripheral B cells', *Curr. Opin. Immunol.*, 10: 220–5.
Mond, J. J., Lees, A. and Snapper, C. M. (1995) 'T cell independent antigens type 2', *Annu. Rev. Immunol.*, 13: 655–92.

Immunoglobulin Function

Antibody binding to pathogen is not sufficient to kill the organism. The Fc portion of immunoglobulin (Ig) can recruit complement or phagocytes to kill the organism. In this way antibodies harness innate effector mechanisms to kill microbes. Antibody protects by

- Neutralising toxins
- Neutralising organisms
- Activating complement
- Opsonising organisms.

NEUTRALISING TOXINS

Toxins bind to receptors on cells, altering cell function. If antibody prevents interaction of toxin with receptor, cell function remains unaffected and the toxin is neutralised. Neutralisation is dependent on the antigen-binding domain only, and is not affected by the Fc portion of Ig (Figure 1.15.1).

NEUTRALISING ORGANISMS

To establish infection organisms must adhere to epithelial surfaces using a limited number of adhesion molecules. Antibodies that bind to key portions of these adhesion molecules prevent organisms binding to mucosae and subsequent infection. Neutralisation of organisms is only affected by the antigen-binding domain, and not by the Fc portion. However, the antibody isotype determines the ability of antibody to cross mucosal surfaces.

COMPLEMENT ACTIVATION

IgG and IgM activate complement via the classical pathway. This generates anaphylatoxins (C3a and C5a) that activate mast cells and attract neutrophils to the site of infection.

Figure 1.15.1 Antibody functions.

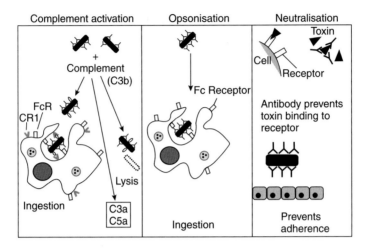

Deposition of C3 on the organism results in assembly of the membrane attack complex (MAC). In susceptible organisms, insertion of MAC causes leakage of cellular contents and lysis. Bacterial capsules may inhibit MAC assembly, conferring resistance to complement-mediated lysis. Complement activation requires the Fc portion of Ig, and the effectiveness of antibodies at activating complement varies with the isotype.

OPSONISATION

Opsonisation is the process whereby microbes and other cells are flagged for phagocytosis. Phagocytes (neutrophils and macrophages) ingest some organisms in the absence of antibody, however, this is relatively inefficient. Antibody-coated organisms are usually phagocytosed. The antibody acts as a bridge between the organism and Fc receptor on the phagocyte. Binding of Ig to the Fc receptor stimulates phagocytosis and the respiratory burst. Fc receptor activation renders the phagocyte competent to kill most pathogens. Opsonisation requires the Fc portion of the antibody molecule.

Complement (particularly C3b) deposition acts synergistically with antibody to greatly improve opsonisation. C3 fragments bind complement receptors on phagocytes, stimulating particle uptake and activation of neutrophils and macrophages. Co-stimulation of neutrophils through Fc and C3 receptors results in greatly enhanced activation.

ANTIBODY AFFINITY

Antibody affinity is the binding strength of an antibody-binding site to an antigen. High affinity results in tight binding and less chance of antibody dissociating from antigen. Different antibody molecules produced in response to the same antigen vary in their tightness of binding. Antibodies produced by a memory response have higher affinity than in a primary response.

ANTIBODY AVIDITY

An antibody's avidity is determined by the combined binding strength of all antigen-binding sites. More binding sites result in increased total binding strength or avidity of antibody binding to antigen.

IMMUNOGLOBULIN ISOTYPE AND FUNCTION

Antibody isotypes have functionally distinct properties, determined by the immunoglobulin constant regions. The constant region recruits cells and molecules to help destroy pathogens. Additionally, each antibody class has different biological activities, capable of dealing with different microbes at different sites (Table 1.15.1).

IgG

IgG is the most abundant antibody and is found in extracellular fluid. IgG crosses the placenta providing passive immunity that persists for 3–6 months after birth. IgG1, IgG2, IgG3 and IgG4 have slightly different sequences in their heavy chains and corresponding differences in their functions.

IgA

IgA is the main immunoglobulin in secretions (colostrum, saliva etc.) where it exists as a dimer. IgA is secreted locally by plasma cells in the mammary and salivary glands, and along the respiratory, gastrointestinal and genitourinary tracts. IgA is transported through

Table 1.15.1 Immunoglobulin isotype function and distribution

IMMUNOGLOBULIN	IgG	IgA	IgM	IgD	IgE
Molecular weight (kDa)	146	160	970	184	188
Functional activity					
Complement activation (classical path)	+++	–	+++	–	–
Complement activation (alternative path)	–	+	–	–	–
Neutralisation	++	++	+	–	–
Opsonisation	+++	+	–	–	–
Sensitisation for killing by NK cells	++	–	–	–	–
Sensitisation of mast cells	+	–	–	–	+++
Distribution					
Transports across epithelium	–	+++ dimer	+	–	–
Transports across placenta	+++	+/–	–	–	–
Diffusion into extravascular spaces	+++	++ monomer	+/–	–	+
Mean serum level (mg/ml) adults	13–15	2.1	1.5	0.04	3×10^{-5}
Half-life in serum (days)	21	6	10	3	2

the epithelial cells into the lumen. Secretory IgA contains a secretory component (SC) and a J-chain (joining chain) required for transepithelial transport and stability of the IgA molecule. IgA is the major component of the adaptive immune response at mucosal surfaces.

IgM

IgM is the first antibody produced by B cells. It is expressed on B cells as the B cell antigen receptor. Pentameric secreted IgM is also found in blood. IgM antibodies usually have low affinity antigen-binding sites, however, since IgM has 10 antigen binding sites per molecule, the overall binding avidity is high. This pentameric structure makes it very effective for activating the complement system.

IgD

IgD is present in low quantities in the circulation. The principal known function is as an antigen receptor on B cells. B cells can express both IgM and IgD, which have the same antigen specificity.

IgE

IgE is present in the serum in nanogram quantities. IgE plays an important role in protection from infection by parasites and in immediate hypersensitivity responses.

CROSS REFERENCES
Section 1.13   Immunoglobulin Structure
Section 1.5   Innate Immune Responses II – The Complement System

T Cell Receptor and Immune Repertoire

Cellular immunity is mediated through two subpopulations of T cells, helper T cells (THs) and cytotoxic T cells (TCs), distinguished by the cell markers CD4 and CD8, respectively. Helper T cells provide help for B cells, macrophages and other T cells, both by cell-to-cell contact, and by cytokine production. Cytotoxic T cells eliminate virus-infected cells and tumour cells, and may also reject transplants.

T CELL RECEPTOR

Antigen is recognised by the T cell receptor (TCR). Most T cells express a TCR formed from α- and β-chains. Both chains have variable and constant regions like the immunoglobulin molecule, and assembly of α- and β-chains combines their variable regions to form the antigen-binding site. A small population of peripheral T cells expresses a TCR that consists of γ- and δ-chains. In epithelial tissues most T cells express the γδ-TCR, however, γδ-T cells comprise only 1–5% of T cells in peripheral lymphoid tissue. The function of γδ-T cells is poorly understood.

TCR complex

The TCR cannot transmit signals to activate the T cell itself. The TCR-complex is composed of the TCR and a complex of proteins called CD3 that transduces signals into the T cell when its TCR binds to peptide: MHC. The CD3 complex of proteins is composed of a group of four separate polypeptides (γ, δ, ε, ξ). γ, δ and ε each have signalling motifs in their cytoplasmic domains (Figure 1.16.1a). CD3 proteins are required for TCR surface expression and deficiency in the γ or ε chains results in reduced numbers of TCRs. The TCR binds processed peptide, presented in the groove of an MHC molecule (Figure 1.16.1b).

Co-receptor molecules CD4 and CD8

Two other cell surface molecules play an important role in T cell activation. The CD4 molecule expressed on helper T cells, binds the non-polymorphic region of MHC Class II

Figure 1.16.1 (a) TCR complex and co-receptor. (b) TCR complex and antigen:MHC binding.

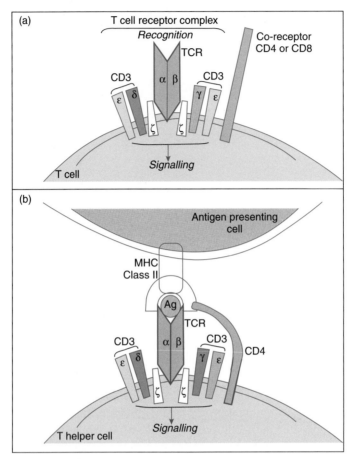

thereby restricting these T cells to recognising peptides presented on MHC II molecules, which are normally only expressed on antigen presenting cells (APCs). The CD8 molecule on cytotoxic T cells binds the non-polymorphic region of MHC Class I thereby restricting these T cells to recognising peptides presented on MHC I molecules, which are expressed on all nucleated cells (Figure 1.16.2). The presence of CD4 or CD8 results in a marked increase in the sensitivity of a T cell to antigen presented by MHC molecules.

GENERATION OF DIVERSITY – IMMUNE REPERTOIRE

The diversity of the cellular immune system results from generation of many different TCRs each with its own unique specificity. The complete collection of T cell specificities or T cell repertoire is generated during T cell development in the thymus, when a T cell randomly selects from its β and α chain (or δ and γ chain) gene groups. The diversity of the TCR is achieved by recombination of several gene segments in a similar way to that of immunoglobulin.

Figure 1.16.2 T cell restriction. CD8 and CD4 binds MHC Class I and Class II molecules, respectively.

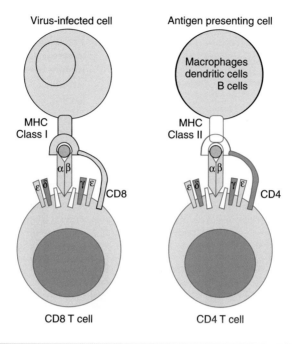

There are four gene groups or clusters that encode TCR chains:

- β and γ chain clusters are found on chromosome 7
- α and δ chain genes are found on chromosome 14.

β and α chains (or δ and γ chains) each consist of variable and constant domains. Variable and constant regions of TCRs are encoded by *V* gene segments and *C* gene segments, respectively.

Somatic recombination generates variable regions

During T cell development, the variable region of β or α chains (or δ and γ chains) is generated by rearrangement of separate *V* gene segments (Table 1.16.1) by a process known as somatic recombination. Multiple different *V* region gene segments are present in each gene cluster. Assembled variable regions (*V* regions) of the β or α chains are joined to the constant region (*C* region gene segments) after transcription, by RNA splicing.

The expression of a *V–C* gene product excludes further rearrangement events (allelic exclusion). The T cell becomes committed to the expression of a single V–C α chain, and a single V–C β chain. The α and β chain pair and both variable regions contribute to the antigen-binding site. The organisation of gene segments encoding TCR α and β chains is similar to that of the immunoglobulin gene segments. This process is summarised in Figure 1.16.3.

The process of gene rearrangement is similar for B cells and T cells and utilises the same enzymes. Defects in genes that control *V(D)J* recombination affect T cells and B cells equally. The structural diversity of TCRs is mainly attributable to combinatorial and

Table 1.16.1 Variable region gene segments

	VARIABLE REGION GENE SEGMENTS
β or δ chains	Variable (V_β or V_δ)
	Diversity (D_β or D_δ)
	Joining (J_β or J_δ)
α or γ chains	Variable (V_α or V_γ)
	Joining (J_α or J_γ)

Figure 1.16.3 T cell receptor α and β chain gene rearrangement.

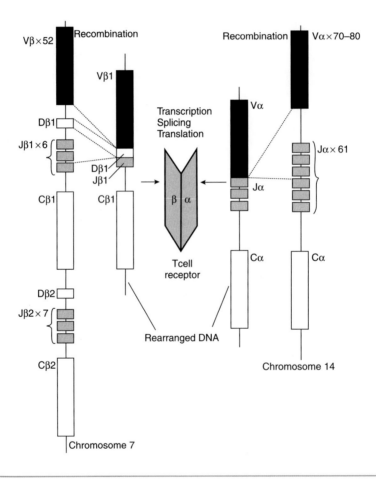

junctional diversity, however, T cells do not further increase diversity of rearranged *V*-regions by somatic hypermutation. As a consequence all the diversity in TCRs is generated during initial rearrangement and is focused on the antigen-binding region.

T cell precursors migrate from the bone marrow to the thymus where TCR rearrangement events result in the expression of an antigen-receptor. The T cell repertoire is shaped by

Table 1.16.2 Similarities and differences between BCR and TCR

BCR	TCR
Generation of diversity	
Somatic recombination of gene segments to generate variable regions	
Heavy chain – *V*, *D* and *J* gene segments	β-chains – *V*, *D* and *J* gene segments
Light chain – *V* and *J* gene segments	α-chains – *V* and *J* gene segments
BCR diversity increased by a somatic hypermutation	No somatic hypermutation
	All diversity generated during initial rearrangment events
Associated complex of invariant proteins required for signal transduction and surface expression	
Igα and Igβ	CD3 complex
Divalent	Monovalent
Immunoglobulin secreted upon B cell activation	TCR not secreted upon T cell activation
B cell effector functions depend on secreted immunoglobulins	T cell effector functions require cell–cell contact and are not mediated directly by the TCR.
Distinct constant region isotypes trigger distinct effector functions	TCR has fewer constant region genes
BCR recognises conformational epitopes of antigen alone	TCR recognises antigenic peptides complexed with MHC molecules

positive and negative selection (for more detail refer to Section 1.12). The resultant repertoire of T cells recognise peptides in the context of self-MHC but does not react subsequently with self antigens, in health.

COMPARISON OF TCR AND BCR

The TCR is structurally similar to the BCR; both receptors are encoded by homologous genes. The generation of diversity at the antigen binding sites involves broadly similar mechanisms of introducing diversity. Table 1.16.2 summarises similarities and differences between the BCR and the TCR.

CROSS REFERENCES

Section 1.17   Helper T Cell Activation
Section 1.9   Human Leucocyte Antigen (HLA) Molecules
Section 1.13   Immunoglobulin Structure
Section 1.12   Lymphocyte Maturation

Helper T Cell Activation

Mature, but antigen-naïve T cells recirculate between blood and lymphoid tissue until they encounter their specific antigen. On encountering their cognate peptide:MHC complex on the surface of an activated professional antigen presenting cell (APC) in lymphoid tissues, naïve T cells become activated, proliferate and differentiate. T cells are subdivided into cytotoxic T cells (Tcs) which are usually CD8+ and helper T cells (THs) which are usually CD4+. Helper T cells are further divided based on their profile of cytokine production.

Initial encounter with antigen initiates a primary immune response. Once activated, primed or memory T cells respond quickly and effectively to subsequent antigen exposure.

ACTIVATION OF NAÏVE T CELLS REQUIRES TWO SIGNALS

Signal 1   Engagement of T cell receptor
Signal 2   Engagement of co-stimulatory molecules

Naïve T cells recognise peptide:MHC complex on the surface of APCs, however, ligation of TCR and CD4 or CD8 is insufficient to activate naïve T cells. A second co-stimulatory signal is required. Dendritic cells are professional APCs that express MHC and co-stimulatory molecules required to activate naïve T cells. Non-professional APCs (B cells and macrophages) are capable of activating T cells previously primed by dendritic cells, including memory T cells. The interaction between peptide:MHC and TCR confers antigen specificity on the immune response. However, this interaction is of low avidity, and must be stabilised by pairs of adhesion molecules (such as LFA-1 and ICAM-1) and co-stimulatory molecules (Figure 1.17.1).

In lymphoid tissues, T cells bind transiently to APCs, sampling large numbers of peptide:MHC complexes. If the naïve T cell does not encounter specific antigen it dissociates from the APC and continues to recirculate. On recognising its peptide: MHC, signalling through the TCR increases the binding affinity of adhesion molecules, stabilising the antigen-specific T cell/APC interaction. In the presence of additional co-stimulation, the T cell is activated, proliferates and differentiates, producing armed effector T cells.

Figure 1.17.1 Interaction of naïve T cell with an APC.

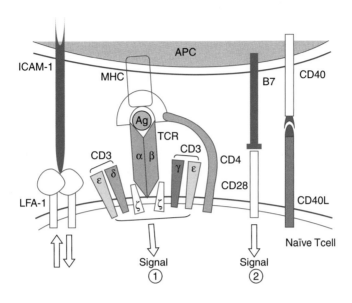

Co-stimulatory molecules

Activation of naïve T cells requires a co-stimulatory signal, usually delivered by the same APC that delivered the antigen-specific signal. Co-stimulatory molecules are upregulated on activated dendritic cells following ingestion of antigen and migration to lymphoid organs. APCs engage in a co-stimulatory dialogue with T cells involving several different pairs of molecules. This is initiated through binding of B7 molecules on activated APCs to CD28 on T cells. CD40 ligand expressed on the activated T cell binds CD40 on APCs providing further potent co-stimulation.

Antigen binding by TCR in the absence of co-stimulation induces anergy (T cell remains viable, but refractory to activation by antigen), or programmed cell death (apoptosis). As co-stimulatory molecules are not widely expressed, this helps to maintain self-tolerance in peripheral tissues.

T CELL ACTIVATION AND INTRACELLULAR SIGNALLING PATHWAYS

Activation of T cells by antigen together with co-stimulation results in sequential activation of enzymes and subsequent signalling cascades. These activation signals finally initiate transcription of genes and production of proteins that direct T cell proliferation and development of effector functions, including genes encoding IL-2 and the α-chain of the IL-2 receptor (Figure 1.17.2). When IL-2 binds the IL-2 receptor T cells proliferate, and then differentiate into armed effector T cells. Availability of potent immuno-suppressives that inhibit IL-2 production has greatly enhanced the success of clinical transplantation.

Figure 1.17.2 Intracellular signalling pathways of a T cell.

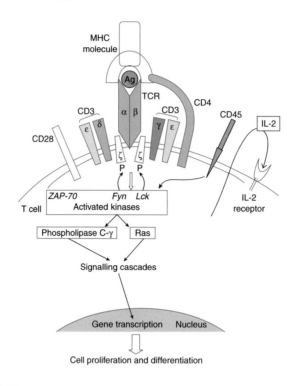

PROLIFERATING T CELLS DIFFERENTIATE INTO ARMED EFFECTOR CELLS THAT DO NOT REQUIRE CO-STIMULATION TO ACT

Once activated T cells differentiate into armed effector cells synthesising molecules required for specialised functions. CD8+ T cells become fully functional cytotoxic T cells (Tcs) while CD4+ cells become fully effective helper T cells (THs). Once differentiated, encounter with specific antigen results in immune attack without the need for further co-stimulation. Clearly cytotoxic T cells must be able to kill any virus-infected cell regardless of expression of co-stimulation molecules. CD4 T cells must be able to activate B cells and macrophages that have taken up antigen.

Interactions between effector T cells and target cells are initiated by transient interactions through adhesion molecules (LFA-1 and CD2). If TCR binds antigen the binding affinity increases, allowing enough time for effector T cells to release effector molecules locally on the target cell. Soluble cytokines and membrane-associated molecules act in combination to mediate T cell effector functions.

ACTIVATION AND DIFFERENTIATION OF NAÏVE CD4 T CELLS INTO TH1 OR TH2 CELLS DETERMINES THE CHARACTERISTICS OF THE SUBSEQUENT ADAPTIVE RESPONSE

Once activated, naïve CD4 T cells differentiate into helper T cells, which can be further differentiated based on the profile of cytokine production. Helper T cell cytokine production orchestrates the subsequent immune response. The functional fate of the helper CD4 T cell is decided during clonal expansion, however, the factors determining the type of helper T cell produced are unclear. Initial work classifying helper T cells, performed using cloned murine T cell lines demonstrated a clear division into two subtypes, TH1 or TH2 cells, with distinct cytokine production profiles. Human studies suggest that TH1 and TH2 cells are extreme ends of a spectrum, with many T cells having intermediate cytokine profiles, however, the paradigm remains useful. TH1 cells are essential for cell mediated immunity and also support production of some opsonising antibody isotypes. TH2 cells are essential for production of IgE and also support production of other antibody isotypes. TH1 cells suppress the development of TH2 cells and vice versa. T cell help is provided by

- Molecular interactions that occur during cell–cell contact
- Production of cytokines.

TH1 cells

- Activate macrophages that are infected by or have ingested pathogens.
- Secrete IFN-γ which activates macrophages, and lymphotoxin (LT-α or TNF-β) which activates macrophages and inhibits B cells.
- Express CD40L, which interacts with CD40 on macrophages sensitising the macrophage to IFN-γ.

TH2 cells

TH2 cells are required for IgE production and also contribute to production of other antibody isotypes. T cell help is required for B cells to produce antibody in response to T-dependent antigens, for isotype switching and affinity maturation of the antibody response. TH2 cells

- Produce cytokines involved in B cell proliferation and maturation – including IL-4, IL-5 and IL-6
- Express CD40L, which binds CD40 on B cells inducing B cell proliferation
- Secrete IL-10 which inhibits macrophages.

Both TH1 and TH2 cells produce IL-3 and GM-CSF which stimulate production of macrophages and granulocytes – important non-specific effector cells in both humoral and cell mediated immunity.

ACTIVATION OF MACROPHAGES BY ARMED CD4 TH1 CELLS

When macrophages ingest organisms, they form vesicles around the organisms. In the absence of help from TH1 cells, macrophages are relatively inefficient at killing these organisms. Resistant pathogens (e.g. *Mycobacteria*) can only be killed by activated macrophages. Macrophage activation requires both IFN-γ produced by the T cell and inter-action of macrophage CD40 with T cell CD40L (Figure 1.17.3). This process is CENTRAL to the host response to pathogens that proliferate in macrophage vesicles.

Activated macrophages upregulate expression of MHC Class II molecules, B7 molecules, CD40 and TNF receptors, thus increasing their effectiveness as APCs. TNF-α acts with IFN-γ in the induction of toxic oxygen radicals. Activated macrophages also secrete IL-12, which enhances differentiation of naïve CD4 T cells into TH1 effector cells.

Activated TH1 cells produce cytokines that activate the macrophage and coordinate the immune response to intravesicular pathogens. TH1 cells enhance recruitment of phagocytic cells to the site of infection. IL-3 and GM-CSF stimulate production of phagocytic cells in

Figure 1.17.3 TH1 CD4 cells activate macrophages to kill bacteria living in its vesicles.

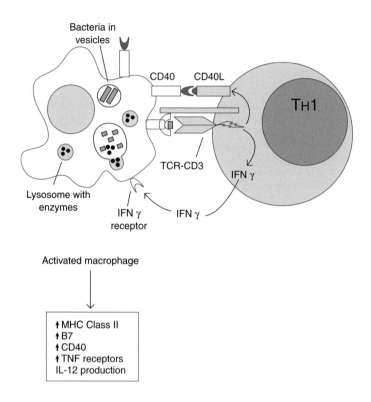

the bone marrow. TNF-α and TNF-β promotes adhesion of phagocytes to local vascular endothelium. Macrophage chemotactic factor-1 (MCP-1) attracts phagocytic cells to the site of infection.

Chronically infected macrophages lose the ability to kill intracellular bacteria. Fas ligand (FasL) expression or TNF-β produced by TH1 cells can kill these macrophages, releasing engulfed bacteria to be taken up and killed by other macrophages.

When antigen persists, for example, due to microbial resistance a chronic TH1 dominated cellular response ensues. This characteristically produces a central area of infected macrophages surrounded by activated lymphocytes, called a GRANULOMA.

Regulation of macrophage activation avoids damaging healthy tissue

Tight regulation of macrophage activity by TH1 cells allows specific and effective deployment of potent mechanisms of activated macrophages, while minimising local tissue damage. Control mechanisms include the following:

- T cell synthesis of IFN-γ limited by short half-life of mRNA encoding IFN-γ.
- Focal delivery of IFN-γ to point of contact of TH1 cell with macrophage limits effect to infected macrophage.
- Inhibition by cytokines including TGF-β, IL-4, IL-10, IL-13 which are produced by TH2 cells.

EFFECTOR T CELLS FALL INTO THREE FUNCTIONAL CATEGORIES

Protective immunity against pathogens in macrophage intracellular vesicles requires activated CD4 T cells. TH1 cells activate macrophages enabling them to kill these organisms.

Extracellular pathogens include bacteria and multicellular parasites. Sterilising immunity to bacteria relies on the humoral immune response, and T cell help is required for optimal antibody production. IgE production, requires help from TH2 cells, which provides some protection against multicellular parasites.

Intracellular pathogens multiplying in the cytoplasm activate cytotoxic T cells (TCs). Cytotoxic T cells kill infected target cells in minutes by releasing preformed proteins from their vesicles or inducing apoptosis (Figure 1.17.4). This is discussed in detail in Section 1.18.

Figure 1.17.4 Three main classes of effector T cell.

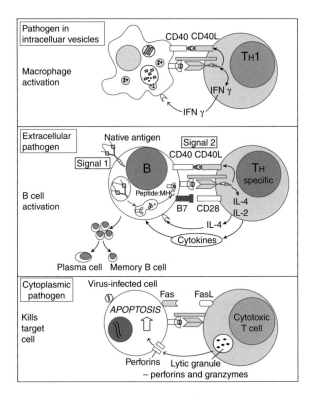

CROSS REFERENCES

Cytotoxic T Cells

Cell mediated immunity involves two separate populations of T cells: helper T cells (THs) and cytotoxic T cells (TCs). Viruses and some bacteria replicate in the cytoplasm of infected cells where they are inaccessible to antibodies. Cytotoxic T cells kill these infected cells either by inducing them to undergo programmed cell death (apoptosis) or by necrosis. Cytotoxic T cells also play a role in graft rejection and tumour immunity.

Apoptosis results in DNA fragmentation and destruction of the cell from within. Apoptotic cells are rapidly ingested and digested by phagocytes, allowing efficient removal of cells without an inflammatory response. Cell death by necrosis results in inflammation. These mechanisms prevent the release of infectious viruses to infect other healthy cells.

ACTIVATION OF NAÏVE CD8 T CELLS

Naïve CD8 T cells differentiate into cytotoxic T cells when they first encounter antigen (peptide:MHC) on the surface of antigen presenting cells (APCs) in lymphoid tissues (Figure 1.18.1). Proliferation and differentiation of cytotoxic T cells into armed effector cells depends on adequate co-stimulation and production of IL-2, in addition to TCR–peptide:MHC binding.

Dendritic cells, macrophages and B cells express both classes of MHC as well as the co-stimulatory cell-surface molecules required. The double requirement of co-stimulation and IL-2 production can be met in two ways:

- Dendritic cells, which have high co-stimulatory activity, can directly stimulate CD8+ T cells to synthesise IL-2, which drives their own proliferation and differentiation.
- During priming, helper T cells and naïve CD8 T cells recognise related antigens on the surface of the same APC. The helper T cell induces higher expression of co-stimulatory molecules on the APC, which in turn activates the CD8 T cell to make IL-2.

ACTIVATION OF ARMED EFFECTOR CYTOTOXIC T CELLS

Once a CD8 T cell has differentiated into an armed effector cytotoxic T cell, response to its specific antigen does not require co-stimulation. This makes sense, as cytotoxic T cells must

Figure 1.18.1 Activation of naïve CD8 T cells.

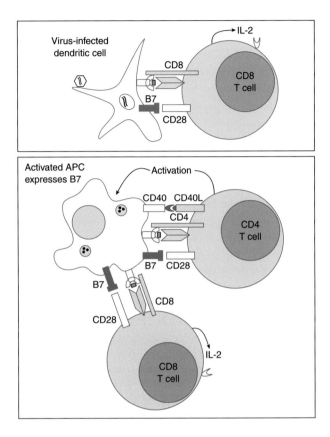

be able to act on any cell infected with a virus whether or not it can express co-stimulatory molecules.

Peptides derived from intracellular (cytoplasmic) microbes, are processed and presented bound to MHC Class I molecules on the cell surface, marking the cell for killing by cytotoxic T cells. Interactions between adhesion molecules on cytotoxic T cells and on the target cell allow the cytotoxic T cell to scan cell surfaces for the presence of specific peptide:MHC complexes. The TCR binds the peptide:MHC Class I complex. CD8 binds the non-polymorphic region of MHC Class I molecule.

CYTOTOXIC MECHANISMS OF ARMED EFFECTOR CYTOTOXIC T CELLS

Upon activation, cytotoxic T cells induce apoptosis or necrosis of a virus infected cell by two mechanisms (Figure 1.18.2).

Calcium dependent release of lytic granules

The granules of TCs contain effector proteins: perforin and proteases called granzymes. When TCs recognise antigen on a target cell, the lytic granules release effector molecules by a

Figure 1.18.2 Mechanisms of cytotoxicity in cytotoxic T cells.

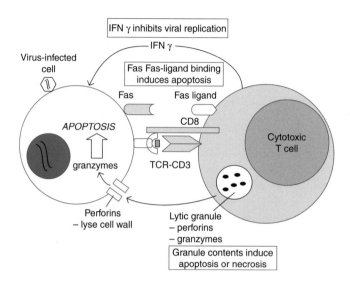

calcium-dependent mechanism. Perforins polymerise to form a pore through which the granzymes enter the target cell and can activate a cascade of enzymes inducing apoptosis. This mechanism may also result in cell death by necrosis. TCs can kill their targets rapidly because they store preformed cytotoxic proteins that reside in an inactive form in the lytic granules.

Fas ligand also induces apoptosis

Cytotoxic T cells (TCs) can also kill target cells in a perforin-independent manner. Infected nucleated cells upregulate Fas expression. Activated TCs upregulate their expression of FasL. Ligation of Fas on target cells by FasL activates caspases that induce apoptosis in the target cell.

Activated cytotoxic T cells release cytokines

In addition to releasing perforins and enzymes, cytotoxic T cells also produce immuno-stimulatory cytokines IFN-γ, TNF-α and TNF-β.

- IFN-γ upregulates the expression of MHC Class I molecules and slightly inhibits viral replication. IFN-γ also activates macrophages and recruits them to the site of infection as effector cells and as APCs.
- TNF-α and TNF-β synergise with IFN-γ in macrophage activation.

CROSS REFERENCES
Section 1.16   T Cell Receptor and Immune Repertoire Section 1.9   Human Leucocyte Antigen (HLA) Molecules

The Mucosal Immune System

The mucosal surfaces are particularly vulnerable to infection. The immune system must avoid responding to food antigens, while still detecting and killing pathogens. The MALT lining the gut is known as gut-associated lymphoid tissue or GALT and includes tonsils, adenoids and Peyer's patches.

PEYER'S PATCHES

Peyer's patches facilitate induction of immune responses in the small intestine. Specialised epithelial cells called M cells form a membrane overlying the lymphoid tissue and take up antigens from the gut lumen by endocytosis. Antigens are transported through M cells and delivered directly to APCs (dendritic cells) and lymphocytes of the mucosal immune system.

A DISTINCTIVE REPERTOIRE OF LYMPHOCYTES

There are small foci of lymphocytes and plasma cells scattered widely throughout the lamina propria of the gut wall. These are effector cells of the gut mucosal immune system and the T cells can be divided into conventional $\alpha\beta$-T cells and $\gamma\delta$-T cells.

Naïve lymphocytes leave the thymus and enter the mucosal immune system via the bloodstream. On encountering foreign antigens, lymphocytes are activated and traffic, via the lymphatics through mesenteric lymph nodes, to the thoracic duct and circulate in blood throughout the entire body. They re-enter mucosal tissues including other sites of MALT (respiratory and reproductive mucosa). Hence immune responses initiated in Peyer's patches are disseminated throughout mucosal sites. This pathway of lymphocyte trafficking is distinct from and parallel to that of lymphocytes in the rest of the lymphoid system.

SECRETORY IgA

The major antibody isotype present in the lumen of the gut is secretory polymeric IgA, synthesised by lamina propria plasma cells and transported into the gut lumen. Polymeric IgA binds mucus overlying the gut epithelium, acting as an antigen-specific barrier to pathogens and toxins.

MOST ANTIGENS PRESENTED TO THE MUCOSAL IMMUNE SYSTEM INDUCE TOLERANCE

The mucosal lymphoid system is exposed to many foreign antigens from foods and commensal bacteria to pathogenic microbes and parasites. Immune responses to food antigens are rarely detected. Feeding foreign antigens leads to specific, active unresponsiveness – known as oral tolerance. In contrast, pathogenic microorganisms induce strong TH1 responses.

The context in which peptide is presented to T cells of the mucosal immune system appears to determine whether tolerance or a powerful adaptive immune response ensues. In the absence of inflammation, presentation of peptides to T cells by MHC molecules on APCs occurs without adequate co-stimulation. However, pathogenic organisms induce inflammatory responses, which stimulate maturation and expression of co-stimulatory molecules on APCs. Subsequent antigen presentation favours development of a TH1 response.

CROSS REFERENCE

Section 2.18   Immune-mediated Gastrointestinal Disorders

Initiation of the Immune Response

When pathogens breach natural defences and overcome innate immunity, an adaptive immune response develops over several days, which as well as eliminating the organism usually, generates immunological memory and pathogen-specific protection in the future.

NON-SPECIFIC RESPONSES OF INNATE IMMUNITY ARE REQUIRED FOR INITIATION OF AN ADAPTIVE IMMUNE RESPONSE

Infection, and the responding innate immune system produce changes in the immediate environment, which are essential in initiating an adaptive immune response.

Macrophage activation-changes in vascular endothelium

Bacterial components, such as LPS, activate macrophages. Cytokines and chemokines released by activated macrophages initiate inflammation, enhancing adhesiveness of vascular endothelium. Neutrophils and then monocytes stick to blood vessel walls and migrate to the site of infection. Later, these changes in vascular adhesiveness permit the arrival of effector T cells.

Activation of professional APCs

Dendritic cells (DCs) take up antigen and are activated through innate immune receptors (CD14 and TLRs). DCs mature into potent APCs with increased expression of MHC Class II and co-stimulatory molecules and are carried in lymph away from infected tissue to secondary lymphoid tissues. Here DCs initiate an adaptive immune response by activating antigen-specific naïve T cells, which then divide and mature into effector cells that re-enter the circulation. Effector T cells leave blood vessels and migrate to the site of infection facilitated by the increased adhesiveness of blood vessels at sites of inflammation.

WHEN T CELLS ENCOUNTER ANTIGEN IN LYMPHOID TISSUES, AN ADAPTIVE IMMUNE RESPONSE IS INITIATED

The immune system includes several anatomically distinct compartments each capable of responding to pathogens in particular sites:

- Peripheral lymph nodes and spleen respond to antigens entering tissues or blood.
- Mucosa-associated immune system (MALT) responds to mucosal antigens.
- Two additional compartments are body cavities (peritoneum and pleura), and the skin.

Immune responses generated in one compartment are predominantly effective in that compartment. Lymphocyte homing receptors are adhesion molecules that bind ligands expressed within individual compartments.

Initiation of immune responses in lymph nodes illustrates the sequence of events common to all secondary lymphoid tissues (Figure 1.20.1). Activated DCs carry antigen to the lymphoid tissues. The architecture of peripheral lymphoid organs through which naïve T cells recirculate, optimises the chance of antigen-specific T cells encountering their cognate antigen on APCs.

Lymphocytes cross high endothelial venules

Lymphocytes enter lymphoid tissue from blood by crossing the walls of high endothelial venules (HEVs). Lymphocyte expression of L-selectin facilitates homing to lymphoid tissues, by binding GlyCAM-1 and CD34 on HEVs. Chemokines produced in lymph nodes induce lymphocyte expression of LFA-1, which binds endothelial ICAM-1 allowing lymphocytes to migrate across the endothelium.

Antigen recognition and non-recognition

T cells arriving in the T cell zone scan the surface of DCs for specific peptide:MHC complexes. If they do not recognise peptide:MHC complexes they leave the lymph node via the efferent lymphatic vessel and continue to recirculate.

When naïve T cells recognise peptide:MHC on DCs, LFA-1 is activated and the T cell adheres strongly to the DC. Binding to peptide:MHC and co-stimulatory molecules on the DC stimulates the T cell to proliferate and differentiate, producing armed antigen-specific effector T cells.

Lymphocyte re-circulation and recognition is efficient, enabling all antigen-specific naïve T cells to be trapped by antigen in one node within two days. Within days of antigen arrival, large numbers of activated effector T cells (helper or cytotoxic T cells) exit the lymph node via the efferent lymphatics.

DIFFERENTIATION OF CD4 T CELLS IS INFLUENCED BY THE CYTOKINE ENVIRONMENT

Interaction of different pathogens with dendritic cells, macrophages, NK cells and NK-T cells influences the cytokine environment early in the immune response, determining whether CD4 T cells differentiate into TH1 or TH2 cells and the subsequent type of immune response.

The early response to viruses and some intracellular bacteria includes secretion of IL-12 (DCs and macrophages) and IFN-γ (NK cells and CD8 T cells), which skew CD4 T cell differentiation towards TH1 cells. IFN-γ also inhibits the proliferation of TH2 cells.

Figure 1.20.1 Initiation of immune responses in a lymph node.

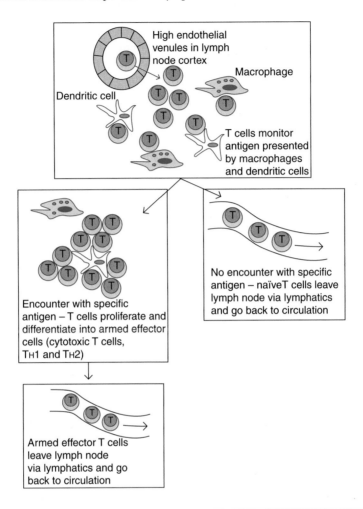

IL-4 and IL-6 promote differentiation of CD4 T cells into TH2 cells. IL-4 is produced by mast cells and some NK-T cells in response to parasitic worms or other pathogens. The exact mechanisms of these processes are not fully understood.

ARMED EFFECTOR T CELLS ARE GUIDED TO SITES OF INFECTION BY ADHESION MOLECULE EXPRESSION

Activation of naïve T cells takes several days during which their homing behaviour is altered. Armed effector cytotoxic CD8 T cells travel from lymphoid tissues to attack and destroy infected cells. Armed effector CD4 TH1 cells leave the lymphoid tissues to activate macrophages at the site of infection.

Most armed effector T cells replace L-selectin expression, which mediates homing to lymph nodes, with VLA-4 (an integrin which binds activated endothelium) expression.

Products of the innate immune response activate endothelium at sites of infection facilitating extravasation of VLA-4 expressing activated lymphocytes.

Differential adhesion molecules expression directs subsets of effector T cells to specific sites

Compartmentalisation of the immune system requires populations of lymphocytes to migrate through different lymphoid compartments and the different tissues they serve. This is achieved by selective expression of lymphocyte homing receptors that bind tissue-specific addressins.

- T cells that home to the lamina propria of the gut express LPAM-1 and L-selectin, which bind to MAdCAM-1 on vascular endothelium.
- T cells that home to the epithelium of the gut express αEβ7, which binds E-cadherin on epithelial cells.
- T cells that home to the skin express cutaneous lymphocyte antigen (CLA) and bind E-selectin.

Effector T cells that enter the tissue but do not recognise their antigen are rapidly lost. They either re-enter the bloodstream or undergo apoptosis.

ANTIBODY RESPONSES DEVELOP UNDER THE DIRECTION OF ARMED HELPER T CELLS IN THE LYMPHOID TISSUES

Humoral immune responses to protein antigens require help from antigen-specific T cells. They induce B cells to produce antibody, switch isotype and induce affinity maturation of the antibody. This involves surface contact between T and B cells (cognate interactions) and cytokine production both occurring in the lymphoid tissues. The migratory path of naïve antigen-binding B cells through lymphoid tissues brings them into contact with helper T cells, and T–B cell interaction allows B cells to proliferate, form germinal centres, and differentiate into plasma cells.

Interaction of naïve B cells with armed helper T cells in the T cell zone of peripheral lymphoid organs

- B cells bind specific antigen, receive signals from helper T cells and proliferate to form a primary focus.
- In the absence of T cell signals, B cells die within 24 hours.
- Some activated B cell blasts migrate to the medullary cords of lymph nodes, divide and differentiate into plasma cells that secrete antibody for a few days, before undergoing apoptosis.
- Other B cell blasts migrate into primary lymphoid follicles and proliferate rapidly to form a germinal centre. These B cells undergo isotype switching and affinity maturation before either becoming memory cells or leaving the germinal centre to become long-lived antibody producing plasma cells.

B cells leaving the germinal centres are called pre-plasma cells (10% leave, those remaining die) and migrate to bone marrow where they differentiate into plasma cells with a life span of months to years.

RESOLUTION OF AN INFECTION

When an infection is eliminated by the adaptive immune response, effector cells are removed by apoptosis and rapidly cleared by macrophages. Some effector cells are retained and generate memory B and T cells.

CROSS REFERENCES

Section 1.3   Cells and Organs of the Immune System
Section 1.4   Innate Immune Responses I
Section 1.17   Helper T Cell Activation
Section 1.14   B Cell Activation

Maintenance of the Immune Response

Effective adaptive immunity results in protective immunity and immunological memory. Vaccination produces protective immunity against a particular pathogen.

Immunological memory allows the immune system to respond more rapidly and effectively to pathogens previously encountered. Activation of naïve T and B cells in response to antigen is called a primary immune response. In addition to producing effector T and B cells, memory T and B cells are generated. These are long-lived specialised cells capable of an accelerated response to subsequent challenge by the same pathogen. Memory responses are secondary, tertiary and so on depending on the number of subsequent exposures to antigen. Memory lymphocytes play a prominent role in secondary responses with only a minor contribution from newly activated naïve lymphocytes (Figure 1.21.1).

MEMORY B CELLS

Secondary antibody responses produced by memory B cells differ from primary antibody responses. In primary responses, low affinity antibodies are produced by plasma cells derived from a large number of precursor B cells. The secondary response is generated from fewer high-affinity precursor B cells that have undergone clonal expansion.

Antigen-specific memory B cells differ quantitatively and qualitatively from naïve B cells

- After priming, there are 10- to 100-fold more memory B cells that can respond to antigen than naïve B cells.
- Memory B cells produce antibody of higher affinity than unprimed B cells.
- Most memory B cells have switched to IgG, IgA and IgE. The beginning of a secondary antibody response is characterised by the production of these isotypes.
- Memory B cells express higher levels of MHC Class II molecules. Increased affinity for antigen and increased MHC Class II expression facilitate antigen uptake and

Figure 1.21.1 Primary and secondary immune responses.

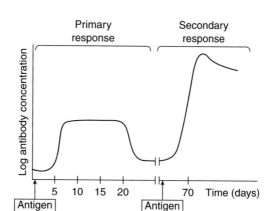

presentation. This allows memory B cells to interact with helper T cells more efficiently, at lower doses of antigen.

Memory B cells re-circulate through the same secondary lymphoid organs as naïve B cells, principally the follicles of the spleen, lymph nodes and Peyer's patches.

Increased antibody affinity (affinity maturation) in memory B cells

Memory B cells produce antibody of higher affinity than unprimed B cells and affinity continues to increase during secondary and subsequent antibody responses. This progressive increase in affinity involves two mechanisms.

Somatic hypermutation

Memory B cells migrate to follicles and become germinal centre B cells. They enter a second proliferative phase in which V domain DNA randomly mutates (termed somatic hypermutation) before these B cells differentiate into antibody-secreting plasma cells.

Germinal centre selection

Memory B cells making higher-affinity antibodies are selected for further clonal expansion and differentiation. In the secondary response antibody already produced is available to bind antigen marking it for phagocytes. Memory B cells with high affinity antigen-receptors (BCRs) compete with pre-existing antibody to bind antigen. As antigen becomes limiting only the highest affinity B cells receive activation signals through the BCR. Thus the affinity of the antibody produced rises progressively for the secondary and subsequent responses.

MEMORY T CELLS

The number of T cells reactive to a given antigen increases markedly after priming and then falls to a level 100- to 1000-fold higher than prior to priming. These long-lived memory

T cells have distinct surface molecule expression, response to stimuli, and expression of genes that control cell survival. Many of the cell-surface markers that distinguish memory T cells from naïve T cells are also shared with effector T cells. These molecules increase T cell adhesion to APCs and endothelial cells and increase sensitivity to antigen stimulation.

Memory CD8 T cells

Cyotoxic T cells programme target cells for lysis in about 5 minutes, however memory CD8 T cells need to be reactivated and require an induction period of 1–2 days to become cytotoxic.

Characteristics of memory CD8 T cells

- Increased expression of CD44 – activation marker
- Increased expression of Bcl-2 promoting survival (may be responsible for the long half-life of memory CD8 T cells)
- More sensitive to re-stimulation by antigen than naïve cells
- Rapid production of IFN-γ in response to re-stimulation.

Memory CD4 T cells

Memory CD4 T cells are long-lived cells that share characteristics similar to effector CD4 T cells, however, they require additional re-stimulation before acting on target cells. Significant changes in cell surface proteins on memory T cells compared to naïve T cells include:

- L-selectin is lost
- CD44 expression is increased
- CD45 isoform changes from CD45RA to CD45RO.

Changes in L-selectin and CD44 expression direct the migration of memory T cells from blood into tissues and then into lymphoid tissues. CD45RO associates with the TCR facilitating antigen recognition. This receptor complex transduces signals more effectively than the TCR-complex on naïve T cells. After re-exposure to antigen on an APC, memory T cells become armed effector T cells acquiring characteristics of TH1 or TH2 cells (secreting IL-4 and IL-5, or IFN-γ and TNF-β, respectively).

CROSS REFERENCES

Section 1.12   Lymphocyte Maturation
Section 4.11   Vaccination and Passive Immunisation

Control of the Immune Response

Regulation of the immune response is critical as uncontrolled responses may lead to autoimmune disease, allergy or immunopathology. Several factors contribute to immune regulation (Table 1.22.1).

Table 1.22.1 Key factors affecting the immune response

Antigen	Nature
	Polysaccharide antigens generate a predominantly IgM and IgG2 response
	Protein antigens produce cellular and humoral responses
	Particulate antigens produce stronger immune responses than soluble ones
	Dose
	Large doses of antigen induce tolerance
	Route of entry
	Polio vaccine given orally induces stronger antibody response than if given intramuscularly
Antibody	Modulation of the immune response
	Negative feedback by antigen-specific IgG
Cytokines	Cytokines released by T_H1 and T_H2 cells
	T_H1 cytokines essential for cellular immunity
	T_H2 cytokines favour antibody production
Genes	MHC genes control immune responses to specific antigens
	Non-MHC genes influence immune reponses
HPA axis	Glucocorticoids
	Neurotransmitters

ANTIGEN

Antigen initiates immune responses. Microbes are recognised by pattern recognition receptors of the innate immune response and antigen-specific receptors of the adaptive immune response.

Antigen is required to drive the immune response When antigen is removed, the immune response subsides. Once a pathogen is eliminated most armed effector T cells die and antibody levels decrease. The antigen that elicited the response is no longer present at levels required to sustain the response – a mechanism known as feedback inhibition.

The nature of the antigen is important The size, state (particulate or soluble), composition (protein or carbohydrate), dose and route of entry of antigen, affect the type and strength of immune response elicited.

The amount and sequence of peptide initiating the response influences differentiation of CD4 T cells into distinct effector subsets Large amounts of peptide, presented in high-density on APC surfaces stimulate TH1 responses, while low-density presentation elicits TH2 responses. Peptides that bind TCR strongly stimulate TH1 responses, while those binding weakly stimulate TH2 responses.

ANTIBODY

The presence of preformed antibody at the time of antigen exposure influences subsequent antibody formation.

IgM

The interaction of antigen–IgM–complement complexes with antigen-specific antibody (BCR) stimulates the B cell more efficiently than antigen alone.

IgG

Interaction of IgG–antigen complexes with antigen-specific B cells results in simultaneous binding of BCR and FcγRII and delivers a negative signal to the B cell. This feedback inhibition decreases the amount of antibody being produced.

Preformed antibodies inhibit host responses to antigens

Transfer of maternal IgG across the placenta during foetal development gives the infant maternal IgG-mediated humoral immunity at birth. As long as maternal antibody persists in the infant's circulation it binds and removes antigen. This provides passive protection but slows development of endogenous immunity.

GENETIC CONTROL

Many genes are involved in immune regulation including genes encoding cytokines, receptors and signalling proteins, as well as MHC molecules. An individual's MHC molecules (HLA type) determines the repertoire of peptides to which they can respond.

HELPER T CELLS

The type of immune response generated depends on the nature of the antigen, how it is presented, and the type of cytokines produced by CD4 helper T cells. TH1 cells are crucial for activating macrophages while TH2 cells are the most effective activators of B cells. These two subsets crossregulate each other:

◆ IL-10 and TGF-β, TH2 cell products, inhibit development of TH1 cells.
◆ IFN-γ, a TH1 cell product, prevents activation of TH2 cells.

If a particular CD4 T cell subset is activated first it can suppress the development of the other subset. However, under many circumstances, there is a mixed TH1 and TH2 response.

TH3 CELLS AND TR1 CELLS

The development of regulatory T cells in the mucosal immune system induces tolerance, actively suppressing antigen-specific responses following antigen re-challenge:

◆ TH3 cells produce IL-4, IL-10 and TGF-β on stimulation with antigen.
◆ TR1 cells produce TGF-β in an IL-10 dependent manner.

Figure 1.22.1 Neuroendocrine influences on the immune system.

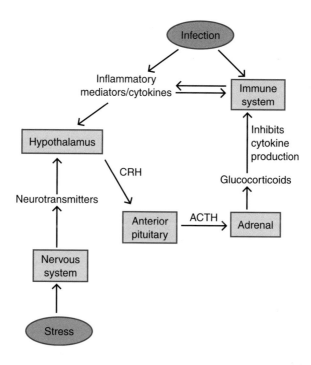

This pattern of cytokine secretion in response to antigen-specific stimulation inhibits the development of TH1 responses and is associated with low levels of antibody and absent inflammatory T cell responses.

NEUROENDOCRINE SYSTEM: THE HPA AXIS

The hypothalamus/pituitary/adrenal axis (HPA) controls the immune system through the release of mediators such as corticotrophin-releasing hormone (CRH), opioids, catecholamines and glucocorticoids. Cytokines such as IL-1, IL-6 and TNF-α directly affect the HPA inducing the production of glucocorticoids (Figure 1.22.1 and Table 1.22.1).

Glucocorticoids – downregulate immune responses

- Reduces numbers of circulating lymphocytes, monocytes and eosinophils
- Dampens cell-mediated immunity by inhibiting release of pro-inflammatory cytokines
- Reduces antigen presentation
- Inhibits mast cell function.

CROSS REFERENCES	
Section 1.8	What the Immune System Recognises
Section 1.13	Immunoglobulin Structure
Section 1.17	Helper T Cell Activation
Section 1.9	Human Leucocyte Antigen (HLA) Molecules

Ontogeny of the Immune Response

The 'normal' immune system in infants and young children is immature, and children are predisposed to infectious diseases. Exposure to a massive range of foreign antigens occurring in the normal post-natal environment is essential for immune maturation. In addition, microbial encounter in infancy influences lifelong immune response patterns.

IN UTERO DEVELOPMENT

Immune cells are produced from the first trimester of pregnancy. The main sites are:

- Yolk sac initially
- Liver and spleen – active haemopoietic sites until birth
- Bone marrow – predominant site from the second trimester and remains so for life.

Intra-uterine infection stimulates antigen-specific antibody production. While functional, the prenatal immune response is suboptimal. Infections that are typically mild in the immunocompetent child or adult (rubella, toxoplasmosis, cytomegalovirus (CMV)) can cause overwhelming illnesses in the foetus. Impaired antigen presentation, altered cytokine production and limited lymphocyte proliferation compared with adults are just some of the factors underlying this susceptibility.

Transplacental transfer of maternal IgG (but not IgM) occurs progressively from the early second trimester through to birth. Maternal antibody provides passive immunity until 3–6 months after birth. Endogenous antibody production takes over at this time. Premature infants are usually antibody-deficient in early life because of restricted transplacental antibody transfer.

INFANCY – A PERIOD OF PHYSIOLOGICAL IMMUNODEFICIENCY

All key immune response components are present at birth, but optimal concentrations and functional capacities are only achieved after further post-natal development. The age at which immune competence is reached varies for individual components.

- ◆ Natural defences and innate responses are not fully functional in neonates. Deficiencies are particularly relevant in premature infants. Anti-microbial chemicals (e.g. lactoferrin, complement proteins etc.) are not expressed at adult levels until some time after birth. Skin and mucous membrane barriers are less efficient.

- ◆ Commensal microbial colonisation in the early post-natal period is a critical factor in protection (or predisposition) to gastrointestinal infections. Operative delivery and artificial feeding increase colonisation with disease-causing gastrointestinal microbes.

- ◆ Breast-feeding confers protection against infection. Breast milk IgA and specific anti-microbial enzymes like lactoferrin, and cytokines such as TNF-α mediate this protection.

- ◆ Cell-mediated immunity – there are many quantitative and qualitative differences in newborn T lymphocytes and APCs compared with adult cells. In practical terms full-term, healthy infants are adequately protected against most viral and other intracellular organisms commonly encountered.

- ◆ Antibody-mediated immunity – suboptimal antibody predisposes to infection in early life. Pyogenic infection is a major cause of morbidity and mortality in children <5 years. Four million children die annually, mainly in developing countries, as a result of pneumococcal infection alone. Meningococcal infection is particularly prevalent in this age-group. Viral infections, although typically trivial, impact hugely on well-being of young children.

  — A physiological trough in immunoglobulin levels ('transient hypogammaglobulinaemia of infancy') and predisposition to infection occurs normally at 3–6 months. This is due to falling maternal Ig levels and poor endogenous production.

  — Initially, antibody production is mainly of IgM isotype with adult concentrations reached by about 12 months.

  — IgG production is poor until the latter half of the first year. Near-adult concentrations of IgG are not reached until the second year.

  — Endogenous IgA production is slow and may only reach adult levels by 10 years of age.

- ◆ The response to particular antigenic structures (e.g. proteins, lipopolysaccharides, polysaccharides) is age-dependent.

  — Production of antibodies against protein-based antigens is T-dependent (TD). Adequate T cell help is available from birth. Response to challenge with TD antigens is intact and protein-based vaccines (diphtheria, tetanus, pertussis and polio) are effective from early infancy.

  — Both lipopolysaccharide- and polysaccharide-based antigens induce antibody production without T cell help – T-independent (TI) responses. TI-1 responses to LPS-based antigens (universally expressed by gram negative bacteria) are intact even before birth.

  — The onset of antibody responsiveness to polysaccharide, or TI-2 antigens is delayed. Limited TI-2 responses are detectable from 6 months of age, with adequate responsiveness reached by 5 years. Pyogenic bacteria surrounded by polysaccharide capsules are resistant to destruction in the absence of antibodies. Poor antibody responsiveness underlies frequent infection with these organisms at this stage of life.

  — Polysaccharide – protein conjugate vaccines (e.g. HiB, MenC conjugates) are effective in infant immunisation programmes. Vaccine protein conjugates stimulate T cell responses to 'help' polysaccharide-specific B cells produce antibodies. Pure polysaccharide vaccines are ineffective in children less than 2 years.

THE INFANT MICRO-ENVIRONMENT – SHAPING IMMUNE RESPONSIVENESS

At birth, cytokine responses generated by activated T cells are naturally skewed towards a TH2-type pattern. There is growing evidence that *microbial encounters* early in life are essential in re-directing infant T cells towards TH1 or TH3-regulated cytokine patterns. High levels of LPS, intracellular infections and some viral infections appear to be particularly important in stimulating TH1 and TR responses. The very hygienic environments in which western children are raised limits exposure to infective stimuli and is believed to contribute to the growing prevalence of TH2-mediated allergy. Manipulation of the infant microenvironment such that TH2 responses are regulated has huge potential in relation to allergy prevention. This is an area of intense research interest currently.

THE AGEING IMMUNE SYSTEM

Variable alterations in immune function are reported in the elderly. These variations underlie some important disease predispositions seen in this population. The impact of confounding illnesses on results of immune parameters cannot be disregarded. Well-conducted studies are needed to identify the precise impact of age rather than disease on elderly immune functioning.

Infections caused by pathogenic microbes such as influenza and *Streptococcus pneumoniae* are major causes of morbidity and mortality in the elderly. Effective vaccines are available for both infections, but responsiveness in the elderly is diminished in comparison with younger individuals. Despite this, benefits of vaccination programmes in the elderly are proven and should be encouraged, especially in frail and debilitated patients.

Numerical and functional defects in T and NK cells and impaired immune surveillance may be important in higher rates of malignancies seen in the elderly. Certain haematological malignancies such as multiple myeloma (MM) and chronic lymphocytic leukaemia (CLL) are especially prevalent in older people. Secondary antibody deficiency disorders predisposing to recurring pyogenic infections are common in these disorders.

Immune dysregulation with higher baseline inflammatory mediators but impaired responsiveness to microbial challenge are seen and partly explain the propensity to overwhelming sepsis syndromes in the elderly.

Auto-antibody production, especially low affinity IgM antibodies, occur with increased frequency with increasing age. Autoimmune diseases do not occur with increasing frequency though. Careful interpretation and correlation of autoimmune serology results in the elderly is critical.

The roles of the immune system in the pathogenesis of Alzheimer's disease and atherosclerosis are areas of intensive research. Immunomodulation may become an important additional therapeutic approach in these major causes of morbidity and mortality in the Western world.

CROSS REFERENCES

Immune Responses to Infection

Preceeding sections have described individual elements of the immune response. This section describes the immune response to viral, bacterial and mycobacterial infection. The purpose is to integrate information learned in the preceding sections.

VIRAL INFECTION

Viruses enter the body, gaining access to cells following adhesion to the cell surface. Once in the cell cytoplasm, the virus hijacks the host cells' protein synthesis machinery to produce viral proteins. The virus then assembles particles that can bud from the cell surface, and infect more cells. Viruses have a short extracellular phase in their life cycle, however, usually the virus is in the cytoplasm. Viral proteins are subject to protein degradation by proteosomes, and similarly to self-peptides, viral peptides are transported to the endoplasmic reticulum, incorporated into MHC Class I molecules and displayed on the cell surface.

Thus in order to cause infection, a virus must

- Enter the body
- Adhere to and enter host cells
- Produce viable viruses capable of infecting other cells.

Viral infection of a cell may lead to cell lysis, syncytium formation and occasionally to tumour formation. The course of a viral infection and the host immune response will be considered using influenza as an example.

Influenza is spread by inhaled droplets, containing viable virus. The first challenge faced by the virus is to adhere to the respiratory epithelium. The host's first line of defence is the mucociliary elevator, which traps the virus in mucus, while cilia waft the mucus to the oropharynx to be expectorated or swallowed. If the host has previously encountered the same strain of influenza, neutralising antibodies, particularly IgA, present in respiratory secretions may prevent adhesion of the virus to respiratory epithelial cells.

Viral neuraminidase reduces the viscosity of mucus, and in the absence of antibodies may allow the virus to bind to and enter respiratory epithelial cells. Once the virus has entered the cell, Type I IFNs (IFN-α and -β) are produced by infected cells. Influenza replicates very rapidly within the cell, however, replication is slowed down by these IFNs. Additionally IFNs have a paracrine effect on neighbouring cells, inhibiting viral entry and reducing protein synthesis making it difficult for the infecting virus to replicate.

Some viruses cause a reduction in HLA Class I expression on the surface of cells in an attempt to become invisible to the hosts T cells. NK cells are normally held in check by the presence of host HLA Class I on cells, and reduced HLA Class I expression may lead to killing of the infected host cell by NK cells. IFNs also enhance NK cell activity. NK cells produce IFN-γ, which activates T cells and biases differentiation towards a TH1 response.

Injury of respiratory epithelium causes an inflammatory response resulting in an influx of neutrophils, monocytes and T cells. Uptake of virus particles or proteins facilitates antigen presentation by resident dendritic cells or macrophages (APCs). In a primary immune response the dendritic cells normally migrate to the draining lymph nodes. Intact antigen is also carried in lymph. Lymph node structure increases the chance of antigen-bearing APCs meeting their cognate T and B cells. T cell activation leads to clonal expansion and differentiation of cytotoxic T cells and helper T cells. B cells are also activated and mature into plasma cells, producing antibody.

Antigen-specific T cells and antibody exit the lymph node in the blood stream. T cells activated by mucosal antigen are programmed to home to mucosal sites. Additionally the presence of inflammation at the site of infection delivers more antibody and lymphocytes to the site. Peptide-specific cytotoxic T cells kill infected cells. Antibody may limit the ability of budding virus to enter other uninfected cells, and also plays a role in preventing future infection by the same virus.

Once the virally infected cells are killed, symptoms rapidly resolve and inflammation resolves slowly. It takes approximately 4 weeks for the ciliated respiratory epithelium to normalise completely, and during this time the host is more vulnerable to bacterial infection. This secondary bacterial infection causes death in vulnerable subjects during influenza epidemics (Figure 1.24.1).

Figure 1.24.1 Overview of immune responses to infections.

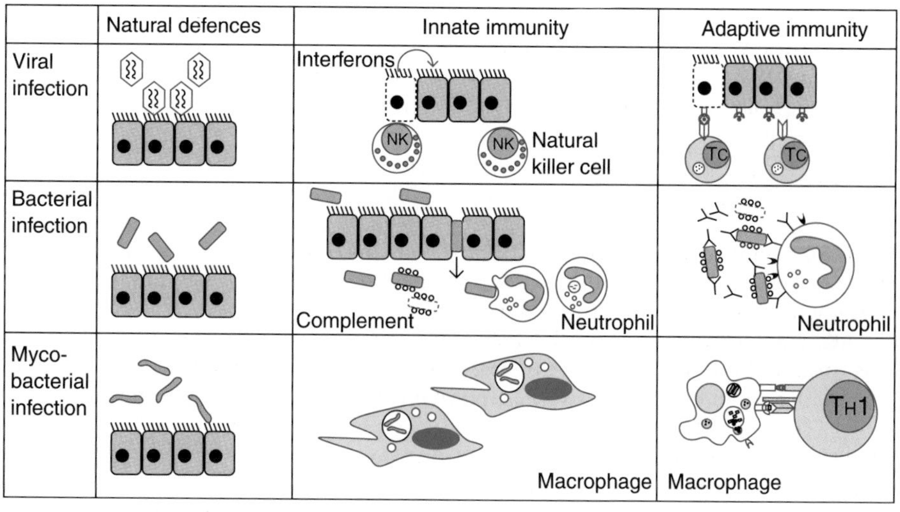

BACTERIAL INFECTION

Bacteria must also bypass the body's natural defences to cause infection. This may result from ineffective mucociliary function, obstruction of urinary flow or breaches in skin integrity. Once natural defences are breached, bacteria usually remain in the extracellular compartment. The innate immune response includes activation of complement (by the alternative pathway). However, bacterial capsules inhibit complement deposition, allowing encapsulated bacteria to evade complement activity. Bacteria can be phagocytosed by neutrophils and macrophages, however, this system is inefficient in the absence of opsonisation. Natural opsonins such as C reactive protein and mannan binding lectin bind some bacteria. MBL activates complement via the lectin pathway and also independently opsonises organisms.

As bacteria proliferate and die, bacterial antigens are released and carried in lymph to the lymph nodes. Intact antigen and APCs that have ingested antigen, travel to the draining lymph node. Both T and B cells are activated. T cell help is essential for B cells to undergo affinity maturation and isotype switching. Antibody may be produced locally or after plasma cells have migrated to the bone marrow. Antibody enters the blood stream, and delivery of antibody as well as complement and inflammatory cells is enhanced by inflammation at the site of infection.

Antibody binding to bacteria activates complement via the powerful classical pathway, and this may result in lysis of susceptible bacteria. Antibody also opsonises bacteria, facilitating bacterial ingestion by phagocytic cells. Antibody and complement act synergistically as opsonins. Ingestion of bacteria by healthy phagocytic cells results in bacterial killing and digestion.

Antibody reduces the risk of future infection by the same bacterium, as neutralising antibody prevents bacterial adhesion to cells, and preformed antibody may kill a small innoculum of bacteria before clinically apparent infection occurs.

MYCOBACTERIAL INFECTION

There are over 60 species of mycobacterium known, the majority of which do not cause disease in humans. *Mycobacterium tuberculosis* and *Mycobacterium leprae* cause tuberculosis (TB) and leprosy, respectively.

Usually *M. tuberculosis* enters the body via the respiratory tract, although gastrointestinal TB may also be seen. Once inhaled, mycobacteria may be cleared by the mucociliary elevator. However, if mycobacteria gain access to the lung, they are taken up by macrophages through recognition of mycobacterial lipoproteins by Toll-like receptors (TLRs). Within the phagosome the mycobacterium is relatively resistant to lysis because of a waxy protective capsule, as well as its ability to inhibit fusion of lysosomes with the phagosome. Failure of lysosome fusion prevents acidification of the phagosome and inhibits killing of the mycobacterium. Thus the innate immune response is relatively ineffective at killing *M. tuberculosis*. However, cells of the innate immune response play a pivotal role in activating the adaptive response.

Macrophages secrete IL-12 and present antigen, eliciting a TH1 response. TH1 cells produce IFN-γ and TNF-α, further activating macrophages and enhancing the macrophages ability to kill mycobacteria. TH1 induced macrophage maturation results in granulomatous inflammation, and the infection is usually sealed off. The centre of granulomata may become hypoxic and undergo necrosis (termed "caseous necrosis"). It is common for some mycobacteria to persist for years or decades within granulomata, while the host remains in good health. However, mycobacterial infection may become reactivated, usually within the lungs, if macrophage function is even moderately inhibited – for example by steroid treatment, malnutrition or other immunosuppressive therapy. More profound immunosuppression with TNF-α blockade, HIV, or potent immunosuppression may allow widespread reactivation, which spreads beyond the lungs. This demonstrates that an on-going TH1 driven response is essential to maintain lifelong control of a tuberculous lesion.

In order to cause infection all organisms must bypass the body's natural defences. Once a pathogen enters the body, the innate immune response immediately aims to control an infection. The adaptive immune response is slower but more effective in eliminating infection. The type of pathogen determines which elements of the innate and adaptive immune responses contribute to sterilising immunity. Cells of the innate immune response frequently activate the adaptive response. Additionally the adaptive immune response can harness many of the effector mechanisms of the innate response.

How Organisms Evade the Immune System

Organisms that overcome natural defences enter body tissues and face a battle with the innate and adaptive immune responses. Organisms that win this battle (some of the time) are pathogens that cause disease. Successful pathogens frequently evade the immune response (Figure 1.25.1). Strategies include hiding, camouflage, decoys, evading key immune effector mechanisms and disabling the attacking immune response.

Organisms divide rapidly – often within hours – and therefore genetic variation can occur extremely rapidly. The immune system, which can generate diversity and select appropriate clones rapidly, must keep pace with changes in organisms if the host is to eliminate the pathogen. Immunological memory greatly increases the effectiveness of the adaptive immune response; however, organisms frequently change key molecules to bypass the memory response. Other strategies aim to overcome specific protective mechanisms.

HIDING FROM THE IMMUNE SYSTEM

Organisms can 'hide' from the immune system by entering a latent phase, often within cells of an immunologically privileged site. For example, herpes viruses can remain latent for life within nerve cells. Cytomegalovirus 'hides' by taking up host antigen, appearing as self to the immune system. Several viruses downregulate expression of HLA (MHC) molecules, reducing the ability of the infected cell to present viral peptide:MHC complexes to T cells.

Some organisms camouflage themselves by closely mimicking human antigens, to which the host is tolerant. These organisms include some *Streptococcus* species (which express antigens cross reactive to heart, brain and joints). An effective immune response to such organisms carries a risk of inducing autoimmunity.

EVADING MEMORY BY VARIATION AND DIVERSITY

The adaptive immune response is highly specific and changing even one amino acid in an immunodominant molecule may allow an organism to evade the memory response. When

Figure 1.25.1 Common mechanisms used by pathogens to evade the immune response.

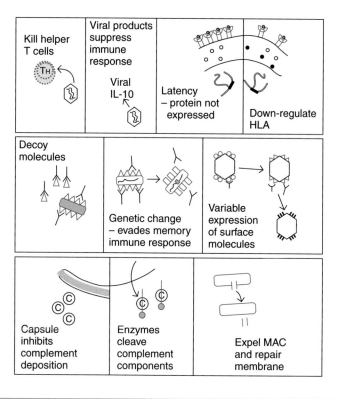

this change is compatible with survival of the organism, the pathogen gains an advantage. The rapid evolution of the influenza virus necessitates annual preparation of influenza vaccine from components of the current strains.

Variation in the influenza virus may be subtle, which is termed antigenic drift or more dramatic, which is termed antigenic shift. Antigenic drift is a constant, ongoing process resulting from mutations often in key adhesion molecules. Once neutralising antibodies to 'virus type A' have been developed this virus subtype cannot adhere to respiratory epithelium. However, if a mutation occurs giving rise to 'virus type B' the neutralising antibodies are no longer effective, and 'virus type B' can then infect people with effective immunity to 'virus type A'. Antigenic shift occurs when a subject is infected with two related viruses simultaneously – for example, human and avian influenza viruses. If exchange of genetic material between the viruses occurs, a dramatic change in the makeup of both viruses results. If the new virus is still capable of infecting humans it will spread rapidly, as few if any of the population will have effective immunity. This is frequently the basis for influenza epidemics and pandemics (epidemics which spread around the world).

Organisms also evade the secondary immune response by the presence of multiple serotypes each varying only slightly. For example over 50 serotypes of *Streptococcus pneumoniae* are described. Previous infection with Type I only provides protection from reinfection by Type I and not the 50+ other serotypes.

Organisms may also vary expression of different antigens at different stages of their life-cycle – thus by the time effective immunity develops to antigens present in the original infecting organism, these antigens may no longer be present. In malaria infection, many antibodies that bind the sporozoite (which infects the liver) will not bind the merozoites, which infect the red blood cells.

The surface of *Trypanosoma brucei* (which causes sleeping sickness) is made up of identical molecules of variable surface glycoprotein (VSG). The trypanosome has approximately 1000 different types of VSG encoded in its genetic material. When effective immunity to the first type of VSG develops, the organism switches to expression of a different VSG that the immune system cannot recognise – effectively changing its coat.

DECOY MOLECULES

Several immune mechanisms are effective within a short distance only – thus activating the immune system some distance from the organism is ineffective and wastes the immune system's recources. *Plasmodium falciparum*, which causes a severe form of malaria, releases large amounts of decoy protein. This mops up large amounts of antibody, leaving less to bind organisms. Complement activation when the antibody binds the decoy molecule is ineffective, as complement activity is spatially limited.

EVASION OF KEY DEFENCE MECHANISMS

Several organisms can inhibit key immune functions that may be effective in their disposal. Encapsulated bacteria, such as *S. pneumoniae* have a gelatinous capsule that prevents effective phagocytosis by phagocytic cells. Antibodies overcome this by binding to Fc receptors on phagocytes, however, these organisms cause repeated infection in patients with hypogammaglobulinaemia.

Other bacteria have a variety of mechanisms, which can inhibit complement deposition:

- Gram positive organisms have a thick capsule which resists complement deposition.
- *Pseudomonas* can cleave C3a and C5a, anaphylatoxins which attract neutrophils to the site of infection.
- *Leishmania* can expel the formed membrane attack complex from its surface.

DISABLING THE IMMUNE SYSTEM

HIV very effectively disables the immune system, as it destroys CD4+ helper T cells. However, other organisms disable components of the immune system in a variety of ways:

- Epstein–Barr Virus (EBV) produces a viral IL-10, which downregulates cellular immune responses.
- Adenovirus inhibits IFN release.
- *Staphylococcus aureus* produces toxins which can kill phagocytic cells.

Organisms have developed several mechanisms to evade the immune response. The immune system often overcomes these escape mechanisms and frequently other components of the immune response can compensate where a specific function is inhibited. Investigation of pathogen escape mechanisms has helped us understand how the human immune system functions, and the relative importance of different components of the immune response.

CROSS REFERENCES
Section 1.5   Innate Immune Responses II – The Complement System
Section 1.11   How Does the Immune System See Antigen?

Consequences of an Immune Response

Evolution of the immune system has facilitated the elimination of pathogens, however this usually generates an inflammatory response. Inflammation contributes to tissue injury, may become chronic and can cause scarring and long-term damage to organs. Additionally the immune response to an infection can cause immunopathology, even inducing autoimmunity. Occasionally the immune response is triggered by inappropriate stimuli such as self-antigens or non-pathogenic substances (allergens such as pollens or foods). Possible outcomes of an immune response are shown in Figure 1.26.1.

The immune response to infection is characterised by acute inflammation. When the immune response is effective the organism may be eliminated, allowing resolution of inflammation and restoration of health. Usually recovery is complete and the affected organ is not damaged. For example, *S. pneumoniae* pneumonia causes severe pulmonary inflammation, but complete resolution is usually seen. Even in the pre-antibiotic era, the majority of patients who survived had no residual lung damage. A successful immune response that clears the infection may be associated with some residual scarring. For example, infection with pyogenic organisms may be localised by the immune response giving rise to a localised abscess. This can burst and discharge, but usually some scarring will result.

Despite the immune response a large innoculum of a virulent organism may result in fulminant infection and death. Patients may also die of the effects of acute inflammation in response to infection – for example, in acute epiglottitis when the inflamed epiglottis can obstruct the airway.

The immune response may be unable to eliminate the organism, particularly in infections with organisms that reside in vesicles within cells, such as mycobacteria. When the organism cannot be eliminated chronic inflammation ensues. This allows the infection to be controlled, however, this is at the expense of ongoing tissue injury. Chronic inflammation is associated with ongoing fibrosis and repair at the site of inflammation. Ongoing fibrosis results in scarring and tissue damage. If the chronic inflammatory response is suppressed the infection may reactivate. Initiation of steroid therapy in patients who have inactive tuberculosis may result in reactivation of their infection.

Immunopathology (damage to tissues or organs due to the action of the immune system) can result from the immune response to infection. The damage caused by the immune system may be greater than that caused by the organism itself. For example, hepatitis B is

Figure 1.26.1 Consequences of an immune response.

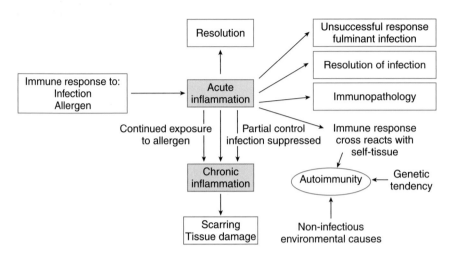

a non-cytolytic virus and does not kill liver cells. However, a vigorous immune response to the virus results in liver injury, chronic inflammation and eventually scarring and cirrhosis.

Antibodies formed as part of the humoral immune response may also contribute to tissue injury. When antibodies bind bacterial antigens immune complexes form and can get trapped in tissues causing inflammation (Type III hypersensitivity; see Section 1.29). Common examples include complications of subacute bacterial endocarditis, and post-streptococcal glomerulonephritis.

The immune response to a pathogen can also induce true autoimmunity. If pathogens express antigens that are closely related to self-antigens, the immune response to the pathogen may cross-react with self-tissues. The ensuing autoimmune reaction may persist even after elimination of the pathogen. Rheumatic fever may follow infection with strains of *Streptococci* and is due to molecular mimicry between the organism and antigens expressed in joints, skin, brain and heart.

Immune responses to allergens result in a particular type of acute inflammatory response characterised by marked oedema initially and a late eosinophilic infiltrate. Continued exposure to the allergen results in chronic inflammation that can result in scarring and permanent structural change in affected organs.

Autoimmune responses frequently cause chronic inflammation and if untreated usually result in scarring and organ damage. Occasionally autoimmune disease may be characterised by acute inflammation in the early stages, however, this usually is only detected clinically in severe autoimmune responses that rapidly damage tissues.

CROSS REFERENCES

Section 1.7   Inflammation
Section 1.29   Hypersensitivity
Section 2.25   Hypersensitivity Induced by Pathogens
Section 2.21   Immune-mediated Renal Disease
Section 1.28   Autoimmunity
Section 1.30   Atopy and Allergic Inflammation

Host Defence Against Tumours

Malignant tumours (or cancers) are characterised by uncontrolled cell division, and they can invade into adjacent tissues and spread to distant sites. Malignant cells usually have multiple DNA mutations, which remove normal controls on cell division and survival, allowing proliferation of the abnormal cells. Malignant cells can be carried by lymph or blood to distant sites where they establish new foci of cancerous growth, a mode of spreading called metastasis.

Chemical and physical agents that damage DNA, increasing the mutation rate, are called mutagens. Carcinogens are mutagens associated with cancer. Prolonged exposure to carcinogens, including some chemicals, ultraviolet light and radiation increase the risk of malignant transformation or cancer.

Viruses that can induce malignant transformation of cells are called oncoviruses. Oncoviruses frequently encode proteins that interfere with mechanisms for regulating cell division, impairing control of proliferation in infected cells, for example, EBV is associated with B cell malignancies.

Mutations in two main classes of gene contribute to malignant transformation:

*   Proto-oncogenes – involved in initiation and execution of cell division.
*   Tumour suppressor genes – encode proteins that prevent unwanted proliferation of mutant cells, for example, *p53* is expressed in response to DNA damage and results in apoptosis.

TUMOUR ANTIGENS

Transformed cells have genomic differences that distinguish them from other cells. Some mutations in tumour cells produce antigenic changes on the tumour cell surface that may be recognised by the immune system – tumour antigens.

*   Tumour specific antigens (TSA) are present on tumour cells and not on normal cells. TSAs can derive from viral proteins.

♦ Tumour associated antigens (TAA) are expressed on tumour cells and on normal cells. TAAs can derive from proteins produced in larger amounts by tumour cell, for example, proteins involved in cell division. They are also derived from the re-expression of proteins normally only expressed on embryonic cells, for example, carcinoembryonic antigen (CEA).

IMMUNE SURVEILLANCE

The primary defence against cancer is well-controlled cell division. Mechanisms that have evolved to ensure this include DNA repair systems and mechanisms that prevent the survival of cells with badly damaged DNA. When malignant transformation occurs, the immune system may be able to eliminate the abnormal cells before a tumour becomes established.

Figure 1.27.1 Anti-tumour immune responses.

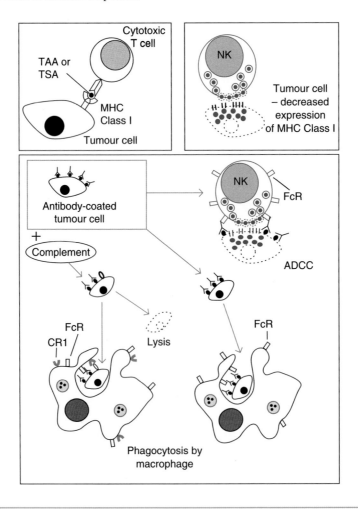

Immune surveillance describes the immune system's ability to detect tumour cells and destroy them. Immunodeficient patients have an increased tumour incidence, however, most tumours occur despite normal immune function. Most tumour types that occur with increased frequency in immunodeficiency are virus-associated tumours. Therefore, while immune surveillance is critical for control of virus-induced tumours, the immune system has limited ability to respond to other tumours.

Effector mechanisms

Anti-tumour immune responses may develop in the same way as immune responses against pathogens or foreign antigens.

◆ Tumour antigens (TSAs and TAAs) are presented as peptides bound to MHC Class I molecules, making tumour cells targets for cytotoxic CD8 T cells.
◆ Changes in tumour-cell surface also produce tumour antigens recognised by B cells and antibodies.
◆ NK cells kill tumour cells not expressing sufficient MHC Class I molecules.
◆ Antibody coated tumour cells may be killed by complement activation, by macrophages and PMNs via phagocytosis and/or by antibody dependent cellular cytotoxicity (ADCC).

Although some tumour specific CD8 cytotoxic T cells and antibodies can be detected in cancer patients, cancers are rarely controlled or eliminated by the immune response (Figure 1.27.1). This is probably because *most* tumours do not make distinctive antigenic proteins and do not express co-stimulatory molecules necessary to initiate an adaptive immune response.

Figure 1.27.2 Tumour evasion of immune responses.

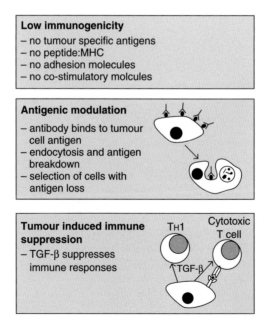

Low immunogenicity
– no tumour specific antigens
– no peptide:MHC
– no adhesion molecules
– no co-stimulatory molcules

Antigenic modulation
– antibody binds to tumour cell antigen
– endocytosis and antigen breakdown
– selection of cells with antigen loss

Tumour induced immune suppression
– TGF-β suppresses immune responses

TH1

Cytotoxic T cell

TGF-β

TUMOUR MECHANISMS OF ESCAPE

Tumours have other ways of avoiding or suppressing the immune responses.

Low immunogenicity   Most tumours do not express novel proteins that can activate the immune system. Others have suppressed MHC molecule expression. Tumour cells expressing little or no MHC Class I on their surface can avoid recognition by cytotoxic T cells. Tumour cells rarely express adhesion and co-stimulatory molecules, required to activate naïve T cells.

Antigenic modulation   Some tumour cells initially express antigens which generate an immune response. Tumour antigens are lost from the cell surface by antibody-induced internalisation. This permits tumour cells lacking the antigen to evade FcR bearing effector cells.

Selection for tumour antigen negative variants   As tumours grow, their cells acquire different mutations, which may generate mutants that do not express tumour antigens. Cytotoxic T cell responses kill cells presenting tumour antigens, thus selecting for variant tumour cells that do not express the antigen.

Tumour-induced immune suppression   Tumours release TGF-β or IL-10, which have immunosuppressive properties. TGF-β suppresses inflammatory T cell responses and cell mediated immunity needed to control tumour growth and may even directly enhance tumour growth (Figure 1.27.2). IL-10 reduces dendritic cell development and activity. Tumour cells sometimes express FasL, which binds Fas on T cells resulting in apoptosis.

Autoimmunity

A healthy immune system mounts effective immune responses against pathogens, but does not attack normal tissues. Tolerance describes the lack of immune response to antigen(s). Self-tolerance, the lack of response to self-antigens, is an essential attribute of the healthy immune system. A breakdown of self-tolerance may lead to autoimmune disease.

Autoimmune reactivity must be distinguished from autoimmune disease. Autoimmune reactivity is common, particularly in women and older people. Autoimmune reactivity means that autoantibodies and/or autoreactive T cells are present, without detectable organ dysfunction or inflammation. Autoimmune disease is present when there is (or has been) inflammation, usually associated with organ dysfunction, driven by the immune system in the absence of external stimuli.

Organ-specific autoimmune diseases occur when the autoantigen is expressed in a particular organ, which is the sole target of the immune response. Examples include autoimmune thyroid disease and myasthenia gravis. Non-organ specific autoimmune disease occurs when the autoantigen(s) are not tissue-specific, and the immune response can damage several organs. Examples include systemic lupus erythematosus and rheumatoid disease.

TOLERANCE – A BRIEF REMINDER!

The mechanisms involved in maintaining tolerance are described in previous sections. Self-tolerance is primarily maintained at the level of T cells, however, mechanisms of deleting and inactivating autoreactive B cells have been described.

T cell tolerance is divided into central tolerance (thymic deletion of autoreactive T cells) and peripheral tolerance, which includes mechanisms that delete, inactivate or regulate T cells after exit from the thymus. Central tolerance is a 'leaky process' with occasional autoreactive T cells escaping negative selection even in healthy individuals. In patients who are genetically predisposed to autoimmune disease, thymic selection may be defective, with reduced expression of self-peptide or inability of those individuals' MHC molecules to present peptides that are present. Defective negative selection may reduce the number of

111

autoreactive T cells deleted in the thymus and consequently increased numbers of autoreactive T cells migrate to the periphery.

Autoreactive T cells in the periphery are generally controlled by mechanisms of peripheral tolerance, including

Lack of co-stimulation   Naïve T cells respond to antigenic peptide presented in the context of MHC Class II molecules, together with co-stimulatory signals delivered by CD40, and the B7 family of molecules. Tissues normally express MHC Class I, but expression of MHC Class II may be induced. However, co-stimulatory molecules are not present. When a naïve T cell encounters peptide in the absence of co-stimulation it becomes anergic (remains viable but fails to respond).

Regulatory T cells   Several T cell subsets which play a regulatory role have been described in recent years. Specific markers for regulatory cells have not yet been validated. Regulatory T cells usually express activation markers, and many secrete TGF-β with or without IL-10.

Autoreactive T cells may not cause tissue damage if antigen is expressed only in an immunologically privileged site. Immunological privilege may be due to physical sequestration of the antigen (the lens of the eye is non-vascularised and T cells have no access). Additionally, expression of Fas results in apoptosis of activated T cells. For example, only activated T cells, which express FasL, can cross the intact blood–brain barrier. Expression of Fas by glial cells causes apoptosis of these cells via the Fas programmed cell death pathway.

B cells cannot mature and produce high affinity antibodies without T cell help, and therefore T cell tolerance prevents production of high affinity IgG autoantibodies. Additionally some autoreactive B cells are deleted in the bone marrow, and may also be anergised in the periphery. However, the importance of these B cell tolerance mechanisms in preventing autoimmune disease is not well established.

AUTOIMMUNITY

Autoimmune reactivity may be seen in healthy individuals, usually limited to low affinity IgM autoantibodies produced by the B-1 subset of B cells. B-1 cells produce antibodies without genetic recombination and do not show affinity maturation or isotype switching. Such antibodies are rarely associated with disease, with the exception of rheumatoid factor.

Autoimmune disease is associated with pathogenic T cells or high affinity (usually IgG) autoantibodies, resulting from a breakdown of T cell tolerance. Well-documented mechanisms whereby T cell tolerance is broken include (Figure 1.28.1):

- Molecular mimicry (Rheumatic fever)
- Release of sequestered antigen (Sympathetic ophthalmitis)
- Presentation of altered self (Drug-induced lupus)
- Polyclonal activation of the immune system (Kawasaki syndrome)
- Tissues become competent to present antigen.

Molecular mimicry

Some organisms have antigens which are sufficiently different to self to elicit an immune response, but sufficiently similar to self for cross-reactivity to occur. For example, infection with some types of *Streptococcus* can lead to development of rheumatic fever (see Section 2.14). Antibodies and T cells directed against the streptococcus cross-react with self-tissue, leading to inflammation in joints, heart and brain, in the absence of the

Figure 1.28.1 Autoimmunity arises from many mechanisms.

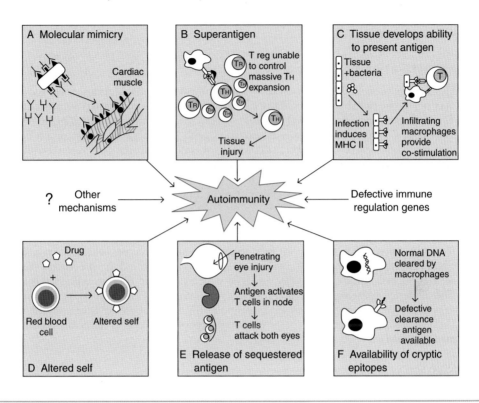

organism. Antibody binding to tissues can be prevented by adsorption with *Streptococcus*, proving the presence of true cross-reactivity.

Release of sequestered antigen

Some antigens are not seen by the immune system, such as proteins present in parts of the eye. As peptides from these proteins are not expressed in the thymus, T cells capable of reacting to them are not deleted. Following a penetrating eye injury, physical separation of the immune system from the eye is bypassed. Development of an immune response to these tissues may damage the uninjured eye. This is called sympathetic ophthalmitis and prevention of this devastating cause of blindness requires rapid enucleating of the injured eye or potent immunosuppression to prevent development of the autoimmune response.

A related mechanism is the availability of cryptic epitopes to activate the immune system. DNA from necrotic cells is normally cleared extremely rapidly, and therefore usually does not elicit an immune response. If this clearance mechanism is defective, these cryptic antigens are present in increased quantities for prolonged periods and can stimulate an immune response.

Altered self

Binding of a hapten to a self-molecule can alter the self-molecule sufficiently to bypass tolerance and elicit an immune response. This occurs in penicillin-induced haemolytic anaemia. Usually the immune response switches off once the hapten is no longer available (i.e. penicillin is stopped and metabolised). However, occasionally the immune response includes antibodies capable of binding to carrier protein alone, and true autoimmune disease may result.

Polyclonal activation of T cells

Superantigens result in activation of whole families of T cells, and this powerful activation may overcome the ability of regulatory T cells to control the occasional autoreactive T cells. Toxic shock syndrome is caused by a *Staphylococcal* superantigen activating 30–40% of an individual's T cells, and has been associated with a number of autoimmune diseases in patients who survive the original disease. Kawasaki syndrome is a vasculitic illness that mainly affects children; this disorder frequently follows infection with *Staphylococcus* or *Streptococcus*. It is thought to result from release of autoreactive T cells from regulatory control, facilitated by massive T cell activation induced by bacterial superantigens.

Tissues may acquire the ability to present antigen competently

Infection of a tissue results in recruitment of macrophages, which may provide the cytokines and co-stimulatory molecules normally not found in the tissue. Expression of MHC Class II may be induced on cells which normally do not express this molecule. The presence of self-peptide in HLA Class II molecules on cells in peripheral tissues, together with macrophage-derived co-stimulation may initiate an autoimmune response. Viral infection of pancreatic islets is thought to play a role in inducing type I diabetes mellitus (DM).

CROSS REFERENCES

Hypersensitivity

Hypersensitivity reactions occur when the immune system mounts an excessive response to a stimulus. This includes an excessive response to an infectious agent or a response to self-antigen resulting in autoimmune disease. More commonly, hypersensitivity refers to reactions against non-pathogenic environmental stimuli, such as house dust mite, pollens, foods and drugs.

Gell and Coombs originally classified hypersensitivity reactions in the 1960s, based on the immunological mechanisms involved. This classification remains a very useful framework for considering many aspects of immunopathology.

Many of the examples shown in Table 1.29.1 are predominantly due to a single type of hypersensitivity mechanism. In several diseases, more than one type of hypersensitivity mechanism may be involved, and different manifestations of the same disease may be due to different mechanisms. Joint destruction in rheumatoid disease is predominantly T cell mediated; however, rheumatoid vasculitis is immune complex mediated. Extrinsic allergic alveolitis (EAA) is a chronic lung disease caused by hypersensitivity to a variety of inhaled antigens. Common examples of EAA include farmers' lung (due to hypersensitivity to *Micropolyspora faeni* spores), and pigeon fanciers' lung (hypersensitivity to proteins in pigeon droppings). However, hypersensitivity to a long list of antigens have been implicated in this disorder. Most patients have precipitating antibodies to the offending antigen, which led to the theory that EAA was due to Type III hypersensitivity with immune complex formation in the lung when inhaled antigen complexed with precipitating antibody. However, histology of affected lungs showed granulomatous inflammation, indicating the involvement of T cells (Type IV hypersensitivity). Type IV hypersensitivity is now thought to be the major cause of lung damage in EAA.

Most types of immunopathology can be classified according to the above scheme, however in some disorders other mechanisms of tissue damage may occur. The mechanism of tissue damage in ANCA-associated vasculitis probably involves Type IV hypersensitivity, however additional novel mechanisms may be present. Similarly cytokine release syndromes induced by pathogens (toxic shock syndrome) or drugs (OKT3) represent additional mechanisms of tissue injury (Figure 1.29.1).

Table 1.29.1 Classification of hypersensitivity reactions

TYPE AND MECHANISM	ENVIRONMENTAL STIMULI	SELF ANTIGENS	INFECTIOUS TRIGGERS
Type I: Immediate hypersensitivity	House dust mite Cat dander Foods (peanut) Drugs	None known	Schistosomiasis
Type II: Antibody-mediated cytotoxicity	Drug-induced immune haemolytic anaemia	Goodpasture's syndrome, Myasthenia gravis, Graves' disease	Infection-induced haemolytic anaemia, Rheumatic fever
Type III: Immune complex deposition	Serum sickness	Systemic lupus erythematosus	Post-infectious glomerulonephritis, Hepatitis C
Type IV: Delayed hypersensitivity (cellular)	Contact hypersensitivity, for example, Nickel	Rheumatoid arthritis, Hashimoto's thyroiditis	Hepatitis B, Tuberculoid leprosy

TYPE 1 HYPERSENSITIVITY

Type I hypersensitivity results in rapid clinical manifestations, and underlies many disorders widely recognised as 'allergies' such as hay fever and asthma. In individuals predisposed to Type I hypersensitivity, antigen exposure leads to IgE production. IgE binds Fc receptors on mast cells, packed with granules containing histamine and other preformed mediators. IgE cross-linking by allergen causes degranulation of mast cells and rapid release of mediators (Figure 1.29.1). This type of reaction is discussed in more detail in the subsequent sections.

TYPE II HYPERSENSITIVITY

Type II hypersensitivity is caused by cytotoxic antibodies binding to components of cells or tissues or antigen/hapten which has become intimately associated with cells. Usually IgG is involved and complement activation follows. Anaphylatoxins are produced and attract inflammatory cells to the site of antibody binding. In Goodpasture's disease antibodies to glomerular basement membrane (GBM) bind to basement membrane in kidney and lung. Bound antibody cannot be removed by phagocytosis and intense inflammation results.

Antibodies may bind and affect the function of key molecules on a cell as in myasthenia gravis where antibodies bind to acetylcholine receptors at the motor end plate, reducing the ability of nerve impulses to activate muscles. Antibodies may activate cells; in Graves' disease antibodies bind to the TSH receptor and induce thyroxine production leading to hyperthyroidism.

TYPE III HYPERSENSITIVITY

Type III hypersensitivity results from formation or deposition of immune complexes (ICs) in tissues. ICs may be formed in the blood and trapped in tissues, or may be formed in situ if soluble antigen binds autoantibody. When antigen binds antibody, complement is activated and neutrophils and other inflammatory cells are attracted. Phagocytic cells ingest the ICs, however, when the capacity to clear complexes is exceeded, inflammation may occur.

Figure 1.29.1 Mechanisms of hypersensitivity.

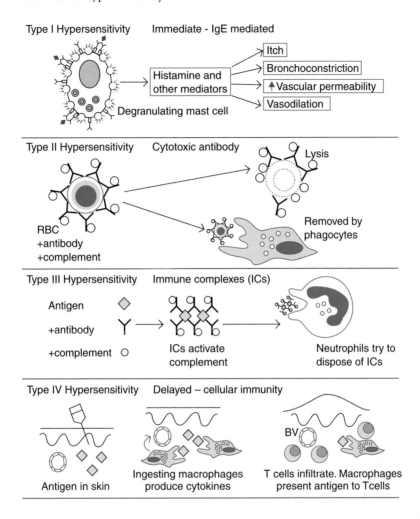

Immune complex formation occurs in healthy individuals during infections and even after eating. However, in health immune complexes are cleared and do not cause inflammation. Antibody binding to antigen activates complement, and C3 cleavage products become incorporated into the immune complex lattice. C3 fragments bind to C3 receptors on red blood cells (RBCs), which then carry the immune complexes. RBCs move in the centre of blood vessels due to laminar flow of blood, and hence immune complexes are not normally in contact with blood vessel walls. In the spleen, phagocytic cells remove and ingest the immune complexes without damaging the RBCs. However, immune complexes may cause disease when this system is overwhelmed by excessive production, or when the capacity to dispose of immune complexes is reduced by complement deficiency or reduced numbers of complement receptors. Additionally immune complexes formed *in situ* depend on the clearance capacity of local macrophages. If the capacity of resident macrophages is exceeded, inflammation results.

TYPE IV HYPERSENSITIVITY

Type IV hypersensitivity is due to activation of cellular immunity and the onset of clinical manifestations is typically delayed by 48–72 hours. Antigen is taken up by antigen presenting cells (APCs), which then migrate to regional lymph nodes. Following antigen processing, APCs present antigen to responsive T cells, which proliferate and mature. Antigen specific TH1 cells then migrate to the periphery and when they encounter antigen are further stimulated. They secrete IFN-γ which activates macrophages, and both T cells and macrophages contribute to the inflammatory process. When antigen is persistent, this process can result in granulomatous inflammation.

The Gell and Coombs classification of hypersensitivity is a useful framework to use when considering many aspects of immunopathology, however, more than one mechanism may be relevant to a single disease. Additionally other methods of tissue injury may occur.

CROSS REFERENCE

Sections 2.1–2.6   Describe several types of allergic diseases

---

Atopy and Allergic Inflammation

Atopy is a predisposition to generate IgE-mediated responses to environmental allergens. Atopy has a significant genetic component, inheritance being polygenic. When both parents are atopic over 50% of their children will also be atopic, however, 10% of children of non-atopic parents are atopic. The prevalance of atopy has increased rapidly, even within a single generation. This implies significant environmental influences.

Allergy describes an inappropriate immune response to a non-pathogenic antigen. The term allergy is often used synonymously to describe atopic reactions. Allergy is a broader term including all mechanisms of hypersensitivity. However, as atopic reactions are extremely common, and other types of allergic reactions are rare, most allergic reactions are atopic.

Production of IgE frequently leads to Type I hypersensitivity reactions. Clinically this type of immune response is associated with asthma, eczema, rhinitis, urticaria, angioedema and anaphylaxis. Clinical manifestations of atopic inflammation will be discussed in Sections 2.1 to 2.5. This section will explain mechanisms underlying this form of inflammation (Figure 1.30.1).

PHASE I – SENSITISATION

On initial exposure to allergen, no clinical manifestations occur. Antigen is presented to the immune system and TH2 cells are produced. TH2 cells promote production of IgE, rather than other types of antibody. IgE binds to high-affinity IgE receptor on mast cells. Mast cells contain granules packed with histamine, tryptase and other inflammatory mediators and when stimulated produce leukotrienes and a number of cytokines.

PHASE II – EXPOSURE AND EARLY PHASE

Once mast cells are coated with allergen-specific IgE, reactions may occur on subsequent allergen exposure. Cross-linking of surface-bound IgE activates the mast cell, leading to

Figure 1.30.1 Antigen cross-linking of surface bound IgE on mast cell causes degranulation and release of histamine.

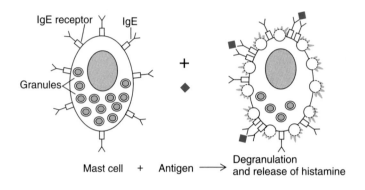

Figure 1.30.2 Late phase of atopic inflammation is characterised by eosinophil dominated inflammation.

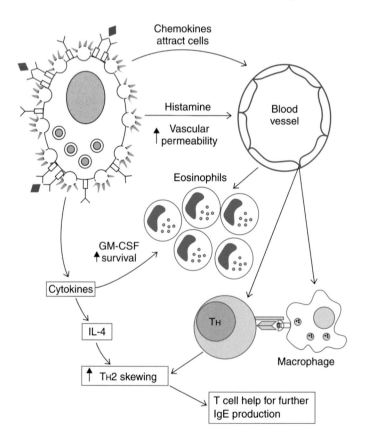

rapid degranulation (Figure 1.30.1). Histamine and leukotrienes are prominent early mediators and cause vasodilatation, increased vascular permeability, itch and bronchoconstriction. Vasodilatation causes swelling of tissues, erythema of skin and if generalised, hypotension. Increased vascular permeability in the skin causes wheals seen in an urticarial reaction, and angioedema when subcutaneous tissues are involved. In the airway, mucosal oedema contributes to airway narrowing in acute asthma.

PHASE III – LATE PHASE OF ATOPIC INFLAMMATION

Leukotrienes and cytokines produced by the mast cells attract monocytes, eosinophils and T cells to the site of inflammation. By 6–12 hours a mixed inflammatory response with abundant eosinophils is seen at the site of allergen exposure. Eosinophil products prolong the inflammatory response. The IL-4 rich environment predisposes to further TH2 cell development and subsequent IgE production. After repetitive exposure to an allergen, the inflammatory late phase of the response may become chronic. Once this occurs, histamine plays a minor role, with eosinophils playing a major role in tissue injury (Figure 1.30.2). Tissue remodelling may occur, leading to irreversible changes.

Clinically, the late phase of the inflammatory response causes recurrence of symptoms, often with a severity comparable to the initial symptoms. Thus a patient who responds to treatment initially for an acute asthmatic attack may deteriorate significantly a few hours later, if appropriate treatment is not given.

CROSS REFERENCE

Sections 2.1–2.5   Describe atopic diseases

Self Assessment

Section 1

State which of the following are true or false

1. In relation to the innate immune response
   a. Pathogens and infected cells are recognised by pattern recognition molecules, which are constitutively expressed.
   b. Phagocytosis is an important defence mechanism against viral infections.
   c. In health, NK cells are held in check by signalling through inhibitory receptors.
   d. Clinically significant opsonins are all products of the adaptive immune response.
   e. Effector mechanisms are distinct from those used by the adaptive immune response.

2. In relation to the adaptive immune response
   a. Lymphocytes recognise pathogens using highly specific antigen receptors, formed by gene rearrangement.
   b. The primary response is slow, however, subsequent responses are more rapid and more effective due to the phenomenon of immunological memory.
   c. Macrophages and dendritic cells are the only cell types which present antigen to helper T cells.
   d. Secondary lymphoid organs have a specialised structure which facilitates antigen trapping and optimises the chance of antigen meeting appropriate lymphocytes.
   e. Lymphocyte migration from the circulation is a multi-stage process initiated by rolling, mediated by selectin adhesion molecules.

3. The complement system
   a. Interacts with antibody, MBL and bacterial surfaces.
   b. When activated can rapidly lyse mammalian cells.
   c. Plays a role in transporting and solubilising immune complexes.
   d. C3b, C4b and C5b are potent chemoattractants.
   e. When activated, complement components are labile, and act for a short time over a short distance.

4. The acute phase response
   a. Is specific for infection.
   b. Results in increased production of transport proteins.
   c. Does not alter levels of complement components.
   d. CRP rises within 6–12 hours of an inflammatory stimulus.
   e. IL-6 stimulates production of acute phase reactants including CRP.

5. In relation to inflammation
   a. Acute inflammation alters endothelial function, enhancing anticoagulant function and increasing adhesion molecule expression.
   b. Granulomata formation is dependent on TNF-α and interferon-γ, and requires the presence of TH1 cells.
   c. Chronic inflammation may persist for years, but rarely results in scarring.
   d. Allergic inflammation results from histamine release from mast cells and influx of neutrophils.
   e. The inflammatory response stimulates maturation of APCs and enhances activation of the immune system.

6. In relation to immune recognition
   a. Epitopes are the specific parts of antigens which elicit an adaptive immune response.
   b. T and B cell epitopes are identical.

    c.   T cell help is required for all antibody responses.

    d.   NK cells respond to reduced expression of MHC Class I.

    e.   Macrophages use pattern recognition molecules to distinguish motifs found on prokaryotic cells from mammalian cells.

7. In relation to HLA molecules
   a. Class I molecules are expressed on all nucleated cells and platelets, and play a physiological role in presenting peptides from intracytoplasmic pathogens to cytotoxic T cells.
   b. HLA molecules are inherited as haplotypes from both parents and are expressed in a co-dominant fashion.
   c. The genes encoding HLA molecules are expressed at diverse loci in the genome.
   d. Class II molecules are expressed on a limited repertoire of antigen presenting cells (APCs) in health, but may be induced on other cell types during episodes of inflammation.
   e. The diversity of the HLA system contributes to population survival from infectious disease.

8. In relation to antigen presentation
   a. Peptides produced in the cytoplasm are actively transported into the endoplasmic reticulum in a process involving polymorphic TAP proteins.
   b. APCs take up antigen from outside the cell, digest it and load it onto MHC Class II molecules for presentation to helper T cells.
   c. Naïve T cells can be equally well activated by dendritic cells, macrophages and B cells.
   d. Peptides presented in the context of MHC Class I molecules can activate cytotoxic T cells.
   e. Superantigens bind relatively conserved portions of MHC Class II and TCR and activate whole families of T cells.

9. Immunoglobulins
   a. Use the idiotype, which is encoded by three hypervariable regions to bind antigen.
   b. May be expressed on the surfaces of B cells, where they act as an antigen receptor, or secreted by plasma cells.
   c. Both IgG and IgM activate complement and can cross the placenta.
   d. Serum concentrations of each immunoglobulin isotype are similar to the concentrations seen in extravascular fluid and on mucosal surfaces.
   e. As the immune response progresses the affinity of antibody increases, due to somatic hypermutation and selection of B cell clones with high affinity surface immunoglobulin.

10. B cells
    a. Must interact with helper T cells both by surface contact involving CD40 and CD40L and cytokines to undergo class switching.
    b. Can present antigen, particularly antigen bound by their surface immunoglobulin, to T cells.
    c. Can respond to some antigens without T cell help, but require T cell help to respond to proteins.
    d. Surface immunoglobulin is expressed at all stages of B cell differentiation.
    e. Long-lived plasma cells which play an important role in B cell memory remain in the lymph node following activation.

11. The T cell receptor
    a. Is formed by somatic recombination of gene segments, a process involving many enzymes also involved in immunoglobulin gene rearrangement.
    b. Undergoes somatic hypermutation to increase receptor diversity.
    c. Most T cells express TCR comprising $\alpha\beta$ TCRs, however a minority express $\gamma\delta$ TCRs.
    d. Binds to both peptide and MHC molecule.
    e. Is itself able to transmit activation signals.

12. In relation to helper T cells
    a. Naïve T cells can be activated by a signal delivered through the TCR if this is sufficiently strong, but require co-stimulation with weak signals.
    b. Activated T cells continue to require co-stimulation, comparable to that required by naïve T cells.
    c. CD40L and CD28 are important co-stimulatory molecules expressed on activated T cells.
    d. The profile of cytokines produced by helper T cells determines the type of immune response which will ensue.
    e. TH1 cell activation of macrophages is the key effector function involved in fighting mycobacterial infection.

13. Cytotoxic T cells
    a. Express CD8 which binds to a relatively invariant part of the MHC Class I molecule, and are the principal effector mechanism of defence against viruses.

b. Kill their targets by causing necrosis.
c. Can produce IL-2 which acts in an auto- and paracrine fashion to enhance their own proliferation.
d. Cannot produce cytokines other than IL-2.
e. Have granules in their cytoplasm, which contain perforin and proteases used to kill target cells.

14. In the initiation of the immune response
   a. Cytokines produced by cells of the innate immune response influence T cell differentiation and the subsequent type of immune response seen.
   b. Presentation of antigen to the mucosal immune system usually induces tolerance to the antigen.
   c. Recirculating naïve lymphocytes which fail to encounter antigen in a lymph node may recirculate to other lymphoid organs.
   d. Addressins are adhesion molecules which direct lymphocytes to particular areas.
   e. Antigen presented to the mucosal immune system together with an inflammatory stimulus is likely to induce a powerful immune response.

15. In relation to maintenance and regulation of the immune response
   a. Memory T and B cells are the cellular basis of immunological memory, and vaccines aim to exploit this characteristic of the immune response.
   b. Memory B cells do not undergo any further somatic hypermutation.
   c. The presence of preformed antibody may inhibit the development of an immune response.
   d. Regulatory T cells produce IL-10 and TGF-β, and play a role in peripheral tolerance.
   e. The type of antigen and route of entry do not affect the subsequent immune response.

16. In relation to ontogeny of the immune system
   a. Immune function in neonates is similar, regardless of gestational age.
   b. The immune response to polysaccharides is very poor before the age of 2 years and may not mature until 5 years.
   c. Infants have a tendency to make TH2 responses, but exposure to infection may skew the immune response more towards TH1 responses.
   d. Maternal antibody provides good passive immunity for the first year of life.
   e. The lymphocyte count in infants is similar to adults, but the T cells are not fully functional.

Section 2

Match the organism from the list on the left with the evasive strategy which each one typically uses from the list on the right. Each item on the right may be used more than once or not at all.

1.	EBV	a.	Expel formed membrane attack complex
2.	Influenza	b.	Inhibit phagocytosis
3.	Encapsulated bacteria	c.	Remain in latent state
4.	Herpes viruses	d.	Frequent genetic change
5.	Leishmania	e.	Produce immunosuppressive substances

Match the disease from the list on the left with the mechanism of autoimmunity thought to be involved from the list on the right.

6.	Rheumatic fever	a.	Release of sequestered antigen
7.	Sympathetic ophthalmia	b.	Superantigen stimulation of T cells
8.	Drug-induced lupus	c.	Infection of tissue allowing competent antigen stimulation
9.	Kawasaki syndrome	d.	Molecular mimicry
10.	Type I diabetes mellitus	e.	Altered self breaks tolerance

Match the type of immune response from the list on the left with the most appropriate description of the mechanism involved from the list on the right. Each item on the right may be used more than once or not at all.

11.	Type I hypersensitivity	a.	Cytotoxic antibody
12.	Type II hypersensitivity	b.	Cellular immune response
13.	Type III hypersensitivity	c.	IgE activates mast cells
14.	Type IV hypersensitivity	d.	TH1 activation of macrophages
15.	Granuloma formation	e.	Immune complex deposition
		f.	Antibody activates cells

Match the type of cytokine from the list on the left with the most appropriate action from the list on the right. Each item on the right may be used more than once or not at all.

16.	IL-2	a.	Essential for IgE production
17.	IFN-γ	b.	Neutrophil chemoattractant
18.	IL-8	c.	Lymphocyte proliferation
19.	IL-12	d.	Macrophage activation
20.	IL-4	e.	Promotes TH1 response, activates NK cells
		f.	Induces the acute phase response

Section 1 – Answers

1a. True.
1b. False – plays little role in viral infections.
1c. True.
1d. False – complement and MBL are important opsonins of the innate system.
1e. False – many innate effector mechanisms are harnessed by the adaptive immune response.

2a. True.
2b. True.
2c. False – B cells are also very effective APCs.
2d. True.
2e. True.

3a. True.
3b. False – rarely lyses nucleated cells, because of the presence of protective complement regulatory proteins and the ability of cells to repair the membrane.
3c. True.
3d. False – C3a, C4a and C5a are chemoattractants.
3e. True.

4a. False – occurs following any inflammatory stimulus.
4b. False – reduces production of most transport proteins, and favours the production of protective proteins.
4c. False – complement production increases. This may mask complement consumption which is followed to monitor immune complex diseases.
4d. True.
4e. True.

5a. False – procoagulant rather than anticoagulant function is enhanced.
5b. True.
5c. False – typically results in progressive scarring.
5d. False – mast cell degranulation is followed by influx of eosinophils, which differentiates allergic inflammation from more typical acute inflammation.
5e. True.

6a. True.
6b. False – T cell epitopes are short linear peptides, while B cell epitopes are conformational and may involve discontinuous pieces of the amino acid sequence.
6c. False – there are two classes of thymus independent antigens.
6d. True.
6e. True.

7a. True.
7b. True.
7c. False – genes are clustered on chromosome 6.
7d. True.
7e. True.

8a. True.
8b. True.
8c. False – usually require dendritic cells, unlike primed or memory T cells.
8d. True.
8e. True.

9a. True.
9b. True.
9c. False – IgM cannot cross the placenta. The presence of pathogen specific IgM implies that the baby has made antibody, rather than acquiring antibody passively, indicating exposure to the pathogen.
9d. False – IgM restricted to intravascular space with little in extracellular fluid, IgA increased at mucosal surfaces relative to serum level.
9e. True.

10a. True.
10b. True.
10c. True.
10d. False – sIg is not expressed by early B cell precursors, or by plasma cells.
10e. False – most relocate to bone marrow or lamina propria.

11a. True.
11b. False – this process only occurs in immunoglobulin formation.
11c. True.
11d. True – this interaction confers specificity on the immune response. The requirement for binding to the MHC is the basis of MHC restriction of T cell responses.
11e. False – The TCR itself has a short cytoplasmic tail and cannot itself transmit signals. Other molecules in the TCR complex are required for signal activation.

12a. False – costimulation is required regardless of how strong the TCR signal is.
12b. False – once activated, T cells can be activated without or with minimal co-stimulation.
12c. True.
12d. True.
12e. True.

13a. True.
13b. False – usually induce apoptosis, either by activating the Fas pathway or granzyme activation of caspases within the target cell.
13c. True.
13d. False – can produce IFN-γ and TNF-α etc.
13e. True.

14a. True.
14b. True.
14c. True.
14d. True.
14e. True.

15a. True.
15b. False – memory B cells undergo a further round of somatic hypermutation and affinity maturation as the antibody response continues.
15c. True – this is why many infant vaccinations are delayed until the level of maternal antibody has reduced.
15d. True.
15e. False – these factors do affect the immune response.

16a. False – premature babies have further impairment of immune function.
16b. True.
16c. True.
16d. False – usually eliminated between 3 and 6 months.
16e. False – normal lymphocyte count in children is about twice that in adults.

Section 2 – Answers

1e;   2d;   3b;   4c;   5a;   6d;   7a;   8e;   9b;   10c;
11c; 12a; 13e; 14b; 15d; 16c; 17d; 18b; 19e; 20a.

PART 2

CLINICAL IMMUNOLOGY

INTRODUCTION

This part describes many immunological conditions commonly encountered in practice. These include allergic disorders, immunodeficiencies, autoimmune disorders, transplantation and lymphoproliferative disorders. This is not intended to be a comprehensive textbook of medicine – it provides brief outlines of conditions particularly focussing on immunological aspects of the disease. Case histories are included, as well as self-assessment questions.

GENERAL REFERENCES FOR PART 2

Chapel, H., Haeney, M., Misbah, S. and Snowden, N. (1999) *Essentials of Clinical Immunology*, 4th edn, Oxford, Blackwell Science.

Primary immunodeficiency diseases. Report of an IUIS scientific group. (1999) *Clin. Exp. Immunol.*, 118 (Suppl. 1): 1–28.

Clinical Manifestations of Atopy

Atopy is a genetic predisposition to produce IgE in response to antigen. An IgE response to allergens is necessary, but not sufficient to produce clinical manifestations of atopy. Not everyone who is atopic develops atopic disease, as environmental influences are also important. Sensitisation to a single allergen can occur, but the majority of atopic individuals become sensitised to multiple allergens. Asthma, rhinitis and eczema comprise the so-called 'atopic triad'.

In utero, the developing immune system is biased towards TH2 responses. In non-atopic individuals this rapidly switches to predominantly TH1-type responses, while atopic children continue to develop TH2 responses for a prolonged or indefinite period. The reasons for this are poorly understood.

EPIDEMIOLOGY

Atopy is common, and the incidence is rising. A family history is a significant risk factor for the development of atopy. Approximately 60% of children with two atopic parents and 40% of those with one atopic parent develop atopic disease. However, 10% of children in families where neither parent is atopic also develop atopic disease.

Environmental factors in early childhood appear to greatly influence whether atopic disease will develop. Children with older siblings, or attending nurseries appear less prone to developing atopic diseases, possibly due to increased exposure to infection early in life. It has been suggested that better hygiene with decreased infection rates contributes to the increased prevalence of allergy – the so-called 'hygiene hypothesis'. Other environmental factors thought to contribute include early exposure to allergens (house dust mite and pet dander as well as outdoor allergens), dietary allergens (particularly highly allergenic foods such as milk, egg, nuts and fish), and pollution including cigarette smoke.

Approximately 15% of children in Western countries suffer from asthma, 15% have rhinitis, and 10% have eczema. Epidemiological studies record a significantly increased prevalence of asthma over the last three decades.

CLINICAL MANIFESTATIONS

The classic atopic triad consists of asthma, eczema and rhinitis, but atopic individuals also have an increased incidence of urticaria, angioedema and anaphylaxis. The following sections describe many atopic disorders; however, a brief outline of rhinitis and eczema is included in this section.

Rhinitis

Rhinitis means inflammation of the nasal airways. This may result in sneezing, itch, congestion, nasal blockage, disturbed smell and taste and occasionally nasal polyps. Allergic rhinitis is commonly accompanied by conjunctivitis. Rhinitis may be infective, allergic or non-allergic (Table 2.1.1).

The diagnosis of rhinitis is based on history. Clinical examination excludes nasal polyps or a deviated septum as the cause of obstruction. Skin prick tests (SPTs) or measurement of allergen-specific IgE to common aeroallergens is useful.

Treatment consists of:

- Allergen avoidance, where possible.
- Topical nasal steroids, using a spray or drops. Nasal steroid sprays are ineffective if the nasal airway is obstructed. However, once patency is restored using nose drops, sprays are a more convenient maintenance therapy.
- Non-sedating antihistamine may be added if required.

Allergen immunotherapy appears to be effective for allergic rhinitis caused by mites, pollen or animal dander. It is very time-consuming for the patient and clinical staff, and may be reserved for when allergen avoidance is impossible and pharmacotherapy has failed.

When rhinitis fails to respond to appropriate therapy, the diagnosis should be reviewed, particularly when nasal obstruction is the prominent symptom. Nasopharyngeal tumours, Wegener's granulomatosus, nasal polyps, deviated septum, adenitis and the presence of a foreign body should be excluded.

Table 2.1.1 Rhinitis: causes and clinical features

CAUSE	TYPES	COMMENTS
Infective	Viral Bacterial	Symptoms self-limiting, may be associated with sinusitis. Occasionally purulent discharge (e.g. 'common cold')
Allergic	Seasonal	Symptoms over summer months. Commonly pollen allergy
	Perennial	Symptoms all year. Common allergens include house dust mite, cat and other pets, and occasionally moulds
Non-allergic	Rhinitis medicamentosa	Chronic nasal obstruction due to overuse of sympathomimetic decongestants
	Eosinophilic Vasomotor Other	Chronic symptoms. Pathogenesis poorly understood. Usually respond to similar therapy as allergic rhinitis

Atopic eczema/dermatitis

Atopic eczema/dermatitis (AD) is a chronic inflammatory skin disorder affecting approximately 10% of children. There is considerable geographical variation in prevalence, with highest rates in Northern Europe and Australia. Approximately 40% of individuals with AD will have associated rhinitis and/or asthma, however, these atopic manifestations may appear later.

AD usually begins in early childhood, and the majority of children outgrow it, although a small number experience recurrence during adolescence (Figure 2.1.1). It is rare to see new onset AD in adults, and most adults who have AD have had the disease since childhood.

SPTs are positive in the majority of patients with AD, but allergens identified correlate poorly with symptoms. Allergen challenges have a better predictive value, and therefore putative allergens identified by SPT should be evaluated by food avoidance and challenge. Food allergy plays a role in approximately one third of AD patients, usually those with early onset of severe disease. The majority of positive food challenges involve egg, milk, wheat, soya and peanut. In adults, contact sensitivity may play a role in some patients with AD, and patch tests may be useful in assessing such allergens. Children with AD are at increased risk of infection, which may lead to an exacerbation of inflammation.

Figure 2.1.1 Typical distributions of eczema in adults and infants. Severe eczema may be generalised at any age.

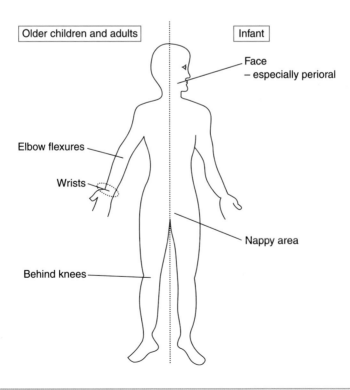

Treatment of AD includes:

- Avoidance of allergens and irritants
- Emollients to ensure skin is constantly well moisturised
- Topical steroids for exacerbations
- Antibiotics for infection
- More potent topical and systemic immunomodulatory therapies are available for severe disease.

CROSS REFERENCES

Section 1.30   Atopy and Allergic Inflammation
Section 2.2   Asthma
Section 3.14   Allergy and Hypersensitivity
Section 4.13   Management of Acute Allergic Reactions

REFERENCE

British Society for Allergy and Clinical Immunology ENT Sub-Committee. Rhinitis – Management Guidelines (2000) Dunitz, London, UK.

Asthma

Asthma is a lung disease, characterised by reversible airway obstruction, airway inflammation and airway hyper-responsiveness to allergens and irritants. Asthma is frequently due to atopy, however, other causes account for 20–30% of cases. This section focuses on atopic asthma, although there are similarities with other types (Table 2.2.1).

PATHOGENESIS

Genetic factors play a role in determining both atopic tendency and predisposition to asthma. However, environmental factors also play a significant role.

Table 2.2.1 Types of asthma

TYPE OF ASTHMA	FEATURES
Atopic	Associated with atopic disorders. High serum IgE and sensitisation to common aeroallergens
Occupational asthma	Sensitisation to specific allergen, associated with work/hobby. Symptoms initially exposure-related, may become chronic
Aspirin-sensitive asthma	Asthma often severe and brittle. Associated with rhinitis and nasal polyps. Responds well to desensitisation
Intrinsic	Mechanism poorly understood. Early or late onset. Frequent eosinophilia and sinusitis. No allergen sensitisation
Asthmatic component of other lung disease	Chronic obstructive pulmonary disease, bronchiectasis
Associated with vasculitis	Churg–Strauss syndrome – late onset asthma. Marked eosinophilia. Precedes vasculitis by years

Airways obstruction in asthma is due to:

◆ Contraction of airway smooth muscle
◆ Inflammation of airway mucosa
◆ Hypersecretion of mucus.

Inflammatory mediators (histamine, leukotrienes, bradykinin and prostaglandins) and neural influences cause contraction of airway smooth muscle. Airway inflammation follows with eosinophil and TH2 lymphocyte infiltration. Inflammation increases the ratio of mucus-producing cells to ciliated cells in the airway. Increased mucus production coupled with decreased mucus clearance by ciliated cells causes accumulation of mucus in the airway, which may become plugged during severe attacks. Chronic bronchospasm eventually leads to hypertrophy of bronchial smooth muscle. Chronic inflammation leads to airway remodelling with thickening of the basement membrane and fibrosis. Long-term control of asthma is critically dependent on controlling airway mucosal inflammation (Figures 2.2.1 and 2.2.2).

EPIDEMIOLOGY

The prevalence of asthma is rising, with approximately 15% of children and 5–10% of adults affected. While awareness is increased, it is generally accepted that the true prevalence is rising. Prevalence has increased within one generation, which cannot be explained by genetic factors, implying a significant environmental component. Recent studies in Leipzig have shown that Westernisation of lifestyle is associated with a significant increase in childhood asthma.

Figure 2.2.1 Early and late phase of the allergic response to allergen challenge.

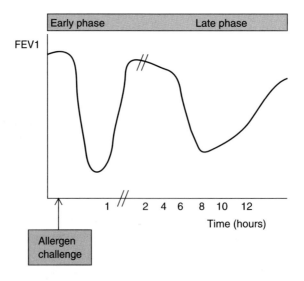

Figure 2.2.2 Changes in the asthmatic airway. Inhaled steroids are required to reverse inflammation.

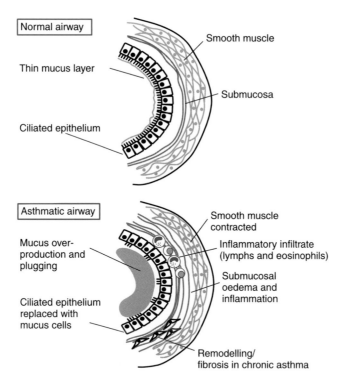

CLINICAL PRESENTATIONS

Asthma classically presents with episodic wheeze, breathlessness and cough. Symptoms usually show diurnal variation with 'morning tightness' – maximal wheeze and cough early in the morning, improving as the day goes on.

Mild asthmatics may be apparently symptom-free for days or weeks. Generally, however, there is mild airway inflammation even when symptom-free, with further inflammation triggered by infection or increased allergen exposure. In more severe disease symptoms are present most days, but vary in intensity.

In 'cough variant' asthma episodic or chronic dry cough is the only complaint. Exercise commonly precipitates wheeze or cough as the associated cooling and drying irritates the airway mucosa. However, particularly in children, exercise-induced wheeze may be the only symptom.

DIAGNOSIS

Asthma should be considered in patients with a history of cough and wheeze. Physical examination may be normal or wheeze may be audible on auscultation. Spirometry demonstrating airflow obstruction with >15% reversibility is diagnostic. Peak flow monitoring showing >20% variability is also suggestive of asthma.

If no variability is evident, bronchial provocation testing with histamine may demonstrate airway hyperreactivity. When exercise-induced asthma is suspected, comparing peak flows before and after 6–10 minutes of running may establish the diagnosis.

Measurement of IgE as well as SPT to determine specific allergies is of value.

TREATMENT OF ASTHMA

Treatment of asthma is aimed at:

* Controlling airway inflammation
* Alleviating symptoms.

When specific allergens are identified, allergen avoidance may make asthma easier to control. However, allergen avoidance is demanding for the patient and often expensive to maintain. Unfortunately partial allergen avoidance is rarely beneficial.

Short-acting β_2 agonists relax airway smooth muscle and relieve symptoms. They may be used alone to treat mild intermittent asthma. Mild persistent asthma is usually treated with regular inhaled steroids, with a short-acting β_2 agonist as required. As disease becomes more severe prophylactic treatment is stepped up with:

* High dose inhaled steroids
* Long-acting β_2 agonists
* Leukotriene antagonists.

In severe asthma, sustained release theophylline and even oral steroids may be required to control airway inflammation. Short-acting β_2 agonists and also anti-cholinergic drugs are added as required to control symptoms.

CROSS REFERENCES

Section 1.30   Atopy and Allergic Inflammation
Section 4.13   Management of Acute Allergic Reactions

REFERENCE

British Guidelines on the Management of Asthma (February, 2003) *Thorax*, 58(2) (Suppl. 1): il–94.

Urticaria and Angioedema

Urticaria is a rash characterised by itchy, well-demarcated erythematous papules. Lesions vary in size and each lesion lasts for a few hours. Angioedema is swelling of subcutaneous or submucosal tissues resulting from increased vascular permeability. Angioedema commonly occurs on the face, and when the larynx is involved respiratory difficulty may result. Angioedema in peripheral tissues, although uncomfortable is not dangerous.

Acute urticaria/angioedema appears quickly (usually over minutes) and resolves within hours. Several episodes may occur, and if these continue for more than 6 weeks, the condition is classified as chronic.

PATHOGENESIS

Urticaria and angioedema result from similar mechanisms – the clinical difference results from the location of vascular changes. Urticaria results from mast cell activation and increased vascular permeability in skin, while angioedema results from increased vascular permeability in the subcutaneous tissues.

Mast cells are packed with granules containing histamine, heparin and tryptase, and when activated produce leukotrienes and cytokines. IgE binds to high affinity IgE receptors highly expressed on mast cell surfaces. Cross-linking of IgE, chemical and physical stimuli, and complement components can trigger mast cells to rapidly release histamine and other inflammatory mediators. This results in vasodilation (which causes redness), increased vascular permeability (leading to wheal formation), and nerve ending irritation (causing itch). In about 30% of patients with chronic urticaria an autoantibody is present which binds the IgE receptor, directly triggering mast cell degranulation.

Angioedema (without urticaria) can also occur in patients with excessive complement activation due to C1 inhibitor deficiency. The mechanism of angioedema is not fully understood, but bradykinin and thrombin are thought to be involved. Patients get subcutaneous and submucosal angioedema that may result in respiratory difficulty and severe abdominal pain. C1 inhibitor deficiency may be hereditary (due to deficiency or dysfunction of protein) or acquired (autoimmune, malignancy-associated) (Table 2.3.1).

Table 2.3.1 Types of C1 inhibitor deficiency

TYPE	MECHANISM	COMMENTS
Hereditary angioedema, Type 1	Impaired production of C1 inhibitor. Protein produced is functional	Autosomal dominant. Symptoms often begin during teens
Hereditary angioedema, Type 2	Normal or high level of C1 inhibitor. Protein is unable to function	
Acquired angioedema, Type 1	Consumption of C1 inhibitor, usually in patients with B cell lymphoproliferative disease (often occult)	Occurs at any age. May precede diagnosis of lymphoma
Acquired angioedema, Type 2	Autoantibody to C1 inhibitor, allows C1s to cleave C1 inhibitor	Associated with lymphoproliferative disease and connective tissue disease

ACUTE URTICARIA – AETIOLOGY AND INVESTIGATIONS

Acute urticaria and angioedema (Figure 2.3.1) may be due to:

- Allergy
- Sensitivity to non-steroidal anti-inflammatory drugs
- Infections
- Idiopathic.

A thorough history of food and medications, occupational/hobby exposures, insect bites/stings and exposure to latex, chemicals, cosmetics and detergents is essential. Previous uneventful exposure does not exclude a causal role, however, uneventful exposure since the episode of angioedema and urticaria makes a causal role unlikely (Table 2.3.2). Selected skin tests or measurement of allergen-specific IgE are usually performed. Occasionally challenge tests may be required to confirm or eliminate a suspected allergen.

CHRONIC URTICARIA AND ANGIOEDEMA

Chronic urticaria and angioedema appear indistinguishable from their acute counterparts, however, while individual lesions last less than 24 hours, the rash persists for several weeks. Causes of chronic urticaria differ from acute urticaria – in particular food allergy is rarely identified. A higher proportion of patients with chronic urticaria have idiopathic disease. Causes of chronic urticaria/angioedema include:

- Idiopathic.
- Physical causes – dermographism (induction of wheals on skin by physical stimulus – e.g. scratching), cold, cholinergic, heat, solar, aquagenic and delayed pressure urticaria.
- Autoimmune (antibody to IgE receptor).
- Food and food additives – salicylates in fruit and vegetables, azo-dyes, benzoates, inadvertent exposure to foods causing acute urticaria.

Figure 2.3.1 Mast cell activation from many causes results in urticaria or angioedema, depending on vessel location.

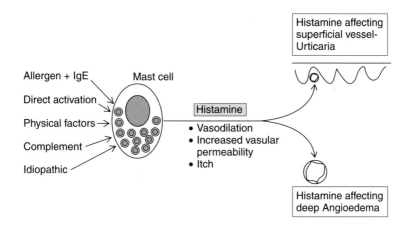

Table 2.3.2 Causes and mechanisms of acute urticaria and angioedema

CAUSE	EXAMPLE	MECHANISM
Food	Nuts, seafood, milk, egg, soya	IgE
Drug	Antibiotics, anaesthetic agents	IgE
Blood products and biologicals	Antisera, monoclonal antibodies, vaccines, desensitisation vaccines	IgE and ? other antibodies
NSAID sensitivity	Aspirin, Ibuprofen and other NSAIDs ? salicylates in food	Prostaglandins and leukotrienes
ACE antagonists	Captopril	Inhibit bradykinin metabolism
Opiates	Morphine, codeine	Direct release of
Radio-contrast agents	Hypertonic radiopaque contrast	histamine from mast cells
Insect stings	Allergy to bee and wasp venom	IgE
Latex	Contact, inhalation of glove powder	IgE
Infection	Parasites (e.g. roundworm, scabies). Also bacteria and viruses	Unknown
Idiopathic		Unknown

- ◆ Drugs – aspirin and other NSAIDs, ACE inhibitors and receptor antagonists, codeine-based analgesics.
- ◆ Urticarial vasculitis – some associated with connective tissue disease or other vasculitic syndromes.
- ◆ Chemicals including cosmetics and detergents.
- ◆ Infections.

- Thyroid disease.
- Malignancy – lymphoma.
- Autoantibody to IgE receptor.

Urticarial vasculitis typically causes lesions lasting more than 24 hours that often bruise or become haemorrhagic. Typically in urticarial vasculitis systemic features are present, response to antihistamines is poor and an acute phase response occurs. C1 inhibitor deficiency causes chronic angioedema without urticaria. IgE mediated allergy is a rare cause of chronic urticaria and extensive allergy investigations is unrewarding.

When the history suggests a physical urticaria, appropriate challenge may allow confirmation. More than one physical cause may be relevant in an individual patient. A history suggestive of food, chemicals, drugs or contact urticaria can be confirmed with challenges, SPTs or patch tests as appropriate and specific avoidance measures advised. When no cause is apparent from the history, physical examination and baseline investigations including FBC, ESR, CRP, thyroid function, complement levels, ANA and ANCA should be undertaken. Antihistamines may control the symptoms. Skin biopsy may be useful in difficult cases.

TREATMENT

Treatment of urticaria and angioedema includes:

- Avoidance of any precipitating or exacerbating factors identified.
- Antihistamines – non-sedating, long-acting agent with rapid onset of action. Addition of H2 antagonists is often useful.
- Occasionally steroids may be required to treat severe acute urticaria.
- Angioedema associated with respiratory compromise should be treated with adrenaline. Patients at risk of such episodes should be taught to use an adrenaline self-injector. Drugs which are contraindicated in combination with adrenaline (e.g. amitryptyline) or which inhibit the action of adrenaline (β-blockers) should be avoided.
- Immunomodulatory therapies may be useful in specific circumstances – for example, IgE receptor autoimmunity.
- Patients with chronic urticaria have significant impairment of their quality of life, however, the majority of patients with chronic urticaria will ultimately settle.

CROSS REFERENCES

Section 1.30   Atopy and Allergic Inflammation
Section 3.14   Allergy and Hypersensitivity
Section 4.13   Management of Acute Allergic Reactions

Food Allergy

Adverse reactions to food are common, occurring in 20–30% of the population, however, true food allergy affects only about 2%, being more common in children than adults.

Adverse reactions to food may be classified as:

- Food aversion – to a specific food or most foods in anorexia nervosa.
- Food intolerance – non-immunological reaction to food including lactose intolerance, sensitivity to pharmacologically active components of food (monoamines in cheese; salicylates in some fruits and broccoli), and sensitivity due to metabolic disorders.
- Non-IgE immunological reactions to food – coeliac disease.
- IgE mediated allergy.

Patients rarely distinguish between an allergy and intolerance. However, symptoms are often dose-related in food intolerance and effects are not life-threatening. IgE reactions to even minute quantities of allergen can provoke reactions which may be life threatening.

IMMUNOLOGICAL ASPECTS

Food is normally digested into amino acids, sugars and peptides, which are no longer immunogenic. Traces of intact proteins cross the normal gastrointestinal tract, normally resulting in production of small amounts of IgG antibodies. Mucosal IgA inhibits absorption and immune responses to food proteins. In childhood, gut permeability is increased and IgA responses sub-optimal. These factors may contribute to the increased prevalence of food allergy in infancy and early childhood. Atopic individuals respond to absorbed protein by production of IgE, which may lead to allergic manifestations.

CLINICAL FEATURES

Allergic reactions to food commonly involve the skin and gastrointestinal tract, although all organs may be involved. Common features include:

- Acute urticaria and angioedema – occurring within minutes to hours after ingesting the food, and the history frequently suggests the diagnosis. Food allergy rarely causes chronic urticaria (2–5%).
- Gastrointestinal symptoms – nausea, vomiting, abdominal pain and diarrhoea, often accompanied by more typical allergic features. In children symptoms may cause failure to thrive.
- Anaphylaxis – common foods implicated include peanuts, tree nuts, shellfish, fish, eggs and milk, although any food may cause anaphylactic reactions. Minute quantities of food – for example, food fried in peanut oil or contamination of a meal by cooking utensils may cause severe reactions. Infection, exercise following the meal, alcohol, or NSAIDs can increase reaction severity.
- Respiratory symptoms – wheeze, breathlessness, and cough may occur, usually as part of an anaphylactic reaction. Food allergy rarely causes isolated respiratory symptoms. Rarely in patients with asthma, occult food allergy contributes to the severity of symptoms.
- Atopic eczema is related to food sensitivity in approximately one-third of cases (severely affected young children, most commonly). Exclusion diets improve the eczema, but have major nutritional and social consequences. Both IgE and delayed cellular mechanisms may be involved.
- Oral allergy syndrome causes perioral rash, numbness and pruritus of the lips, tongue, and oropharyngeal mucosa and swelling of lips. Cross-reactions between fresh fruits and pollen are usually responsible. Progression to a systemic reaction is very unusual.

Food allergies are often blamed for a myriad of symptoms such as fatigue, migraine and childhood behavioural disorders. Allergy does not cause these symptoms, although pharmacologically active amines in some foods may contribute to migraine. While it appears prudent to avoid a food that causes significant symptoms, allergy tests (evaluating IgE related pathology) are not helpful. It is important to encourage patients to critically re-evaluate nutritionally inadequate exclusion diets.

INVESTIGATION OF FOOD ALLERGY

The history usually produces a shortlist of foods related to symptoms. SPT and/or specific IgE measurement is useful to confirm sensitisation (see Section 3.14). When symptoms are frequent, a detailed symptom and food diary may provide valuable clues.

Food avoidance and challenge are used in several situations. To establish whether food allergy is playing a role in chronic/frequent symptoms a 'few food' or elemental diet may be used for a short period. If symptoms disappear, gradual food reintroduction adding two foods every 5–7 days is subsequently undertaken. Should symptoms recur, the foods are eliminated and reintroduced one at a time. This procedure can be used to identify both food allergy and intolerances.

Food challenge can be open or double-blind placebo-controlled food challenge (DBPCFC). The DBPCFC is the gold standard in food allergy diagnosis. Placebo or suspect foods are given in a double-blind manner and symptoms recorded. DBPCFC is important when there are no objective signs during a reaction. When objective signs occur, an open challenge is usually satisfactory.

TREATMENT

Treatment of food allergies requires avoidance. Elimination diets have major social and nutritional consequences and are only recommended for severe or dangerous allergies. Patient education is critical, as minute quantities of food may cause symptoms. Patients must check labels, and clarify all ingredients when dining out. Many restaurants purchase components of meals making it difficult to correctly establish whether a meal is free of a particular ingredient.

Even the most conscientious patients will make errors, therefore an emergency plan with a fast acting antihistamine, and if appropriate adrenaline, must be implemented.

Any patient requiring elimination of a staple food should have input from a dietician both for detailed education in allergen avoidance and to ensure nutritional adequacy. This is especially important in children.

CROSS REFERENCES

Section 3.14   Allergy and Hypersensitivity
Section 4.13   Management of Acute Allergic Reactions

Anaphylaxis

Anaphylaxis is a severe allergic reaction that includes at least one life-threatening feature – hypotension, bronchospasm or laryngeal oedema. Anaphylactic shock means hypotension due to allergy, usually occurring with other allergic features. Anaphylaxis is due to IgE mediated mast cell activation. Clinically indistinguishable reactions occur when mast cells are triggered by mechanisms other than IgE cross-linking – these are called anaphylactoid reactions.

WHAT CAUSES ANAPHYLACTIC REACTIONS?

Anaphylaxis can result from allergen entering the body by any route. In extreme cases, smelling or touching the offending agent may trigger a reaction. Common precipitants include:

- Drugs – penicillins, cephalosporins, anaesthetic agents including local anaesthetics
- Foods – especially peanuts, tree nuts, fish, shellfish, egg, milk and soya
- Venoms – including bee and wasp
- Latex.

Mechanisms involved in anaphylactoid reactions include:

- Complement activation – immunoglobulin and colloid infusions
- Hypertonic solutions activating mast cells – X-ray contrast media
- Unknown – non-steroidal anti-inflammatory agents.

WHAT IMMUNOLOGICAL MECHANISMS ARE INVOLVED?

The final common pathway of anaphylactic and anaphylactoid reactions is mast cell activation. Release of histamine and other inflammatory mediators (including tryptase, chymase, heparin) causes the early phase of allergic reactions. Once triggered, mast cells synthesise prostaglandins, leukotrienes and cytokines involved in late phase responses. Because the immediate response is due to release of preformed mediators, the onset of anaphylaxis is within minutes of exposure to the allergen.

CLINICAL FEATURES

Anaphylaxis frequently affects many organ systems. Prominent symptoms and signs include:

- Skin – flushing (due to vasodilation), itch, urticaria and angioedema
- Upper airways – sneezing and laryngeal oedema
- Lung – bronchospasm (contraction of bronchial smooth muscle, mucus production and oedema of airway mucosa)
- Heart – tachycardia and arrhythmias
- Cardiovascular – hypotension (vasodilation and increased vascular permeability)
- Gut – nausea, vomiting, cramps, diarrhoea (spasm of GI muscle)
- Nervous system – anxiety, dizziness, loss of consciousness.

INVESTIGATIONS

A full and accurate history of all foods/drugs and exposures prior to the reaction is essential. Exposure is usually within a few hours and often minutes of the reaction. It is also important to identify any exacerbating factors that may have been present including:

- Infection
- Exercise
- Alcohol
- Non-steroidal agents
- β-blockers and ACE inhibitors.

Further investigations of allergic reactions are described in Section 3.14.
  Investigations are divided into:

- Tests differentiating anaphylaxis from other disorders

    — Mast cell tryptase
    — Urinary methylhistamines.

- Tests to identify the allergen responsible

    — SPTs or intradermal skin testing
    — Allergen specific IgE.

Full investigation of the cause of the reaction is not undertaken until the patient has recovered. If history and straightforward investigations fail to identify the cause, provocation testing may be required (see Section 3.14).

TREATMENT

Immediate treatment requires adrenaline as well as antihistamines and corticosteroids. Long-term management of patients includes education about allergen avoidance and emergency self-administration of adrenaline. It is also essential to ensure that asthma is maintained under good control, as poorly controlled asthma is a major risk factor for mortality in future attacks (see Section 4.13).

Desensitisation to the allergen is possible in some situations (e.g. venom allergy) where avoidance of allergen is not possible and appropriate preparations are available. Desensitising protocols have been described for some drugs, but these procedures are labour-intensive and carry a risk of provoking anaphylaxis. Hence, desensitisation is usually reserved for patients where there is no alternative therapy available.

Case 2.5.1 Nut allergy

A 16-year-old girl was brought to A&E after developing a severe asthma attack while eating in a Thai restaurant. On admission she had severe bronchospasm, and was hypotensive (BP 90/50 mmHg). She had angioedema of the lips, and oropharynx and stridor was present. A diagnosis of anaphylaxis was made and she was immediately treated with intramuscular adrenaline, intravenous antihistamine and hydrocortisone. Nebulised β2-agonists and oxygen were also administered. She began to improve, and 15 minutes later her blood pressure was 120/60 mmHg, however, inspiratory stridor was still present. A second dose of adrenaline was administered with further improvement.

She was admitted to hospital for further assessment and management. On review, she reported that she had stopped eating nuts some months ago as they caused an unpleasant tingling sensation in her mouth. She had a past history of eczema, and had asthma since the age of 5. She used inhaled steroids regularly but also needed daily rescue inhalers, indicating suboptimal control of her asthma. Skin prick tests showed positive reactions to peanuts, walnuts and almonds as well as house dust mite. A diagnosis of anaphylaxis secondary to nut allergy was made. The patient was given advice about nut avoidance, and was taught how to use a self-administered epinephrine pen. The importance of achieving good control of her asthma was stressed, and she was advised to wear a Medic-Alert pendant. Follow up in the Allergy clinic was arranged.

Cross reference

Section 4.13   Management of Acute Allergic Reactions

CROSS REFERENCES

Section 1.30   Atopy and Allergic Inflammation
Section 3.14   Allergy and Hypersensitivity
Section 4.13   Management of Acute Allergic Reactions

REFERENCE

Pumphrey, R. S. (2000) 'Lessons for management of anaphylaxis from a study of fatal reactions', *Clin. Exp. Allergy*, Aug 30(8): 1144–50.

Other Types of Hypersensitivity Reactions

Atopy is the basis of most allergic disorders (discussed in the preceding units), however other types of hypersensitivity can also give rise to allergic reactions. In this section, allergy due to Type II, Type III and Type IV hypersensitivity will be discussed (Figure 2.6.1).

TYPE II HYPERSENSITIVITY – CYTOTOXIC ANTIBODY

Type II hypersensitivity results from binding of cytotoxic antibody to cells or tissue components. Drug-induced haemolytic anaemia often results from this mechanism.

Penicillin acts as a hapten, binding red blood cells to form altered self. The penicillin/cell complex may stimulate antibody formation. On subsequent exposure to penicillin, antibody binds to the hapten–red blood cell complexes and complement activation causes cell lysis. Antibody-coated red blood cells are also ingested by macrophages of the reticulo-endothelial system.

Usually penicillin-induced haemolytic anaemia settles spontaneously when the drug is stopped. Occasionally antibodies are produced which bind red blood cells in the absence of the drug, resulting in true autoimmune haemolytic anaemia – self-tolerance has been broken. Haemolytic anaemia that persists after stopping the drug is treated in the same way as idiopathic autoimmune haemolytic anaemia (Section 2.16).

TYPE III HYPERSENSITIVITY – IMMUNE COMPLEX DEPOSITION

Type III hypersensitivity is due to immune complex deposition in tissues. Immune complexes may be formed in the tissue, or deposited in tissue when immune complex formation exceeds the body's capacity to safely dispose of the complexes (see Section 1.28). Immune complexes may be deposited in any vascular bed but are most commonly deposited in organs with high blood flow such as the kidney and skin.

Allergic reactions to heterologous serum such as anti-thymocyte globulin (ATG) are frequently due to Type III hypersensitivity. ATG is produced in rabbit or horse, and depletes

Figure 2.6.1 Mechanisms involved in Types II, III and IV hypersensitivity reactions.

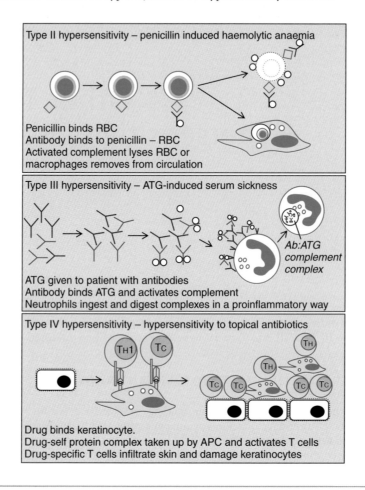

T cells. It is a potent immunosuppressive agent. Some patients make antibodies against the foreign protein that they have received, despite concurrent potent immunosuppression. After 8–14 days of treatment or during a second course of ATG, these patients are at risk of developing serum sickness – an immune complex disease. Typical clinical features include a vasculitic skin rash, polyarticular arthritis and mild glomerulonephritis due to immune complex deposition in the skin, joints and glomeruli respectively. Patients are often systemically unwell with fatigue, myalgia and pyrexia, and an acute phase response reflects generalised inflammation.

TYPE IV HYPERSENSITIVITY – DELAYED HYPERSENSITIVITY

Type IV hypersensitivity results from activation of the cellular immune response. As it takes 48–72 hours for naïve T cells to be activated, proliferate and respond, this type of reaction is slow in onset – hence the term delayed type hypersensitivity.

This type of sensitivity can occur in response to antibiotic or local anaesthetic containing creams. Many drugs are small molecules and act as haptens. Applied topically, drugs bind to keratinocytes leading to altered self. Hapten and carrier molecule are taken up by Langerhan's cells, which then migrate to the draining lymph nodes. Antigen presenting cells (APCs) may then activate cognate T cells, which proliferate and mature, and subsequently home to the skin. Migration of T cells to the skin, which are reactive to allergen, results in inflammation while the hapten is present.

This type of sensitivity is not detected by SPTs, which only detect IgE mediated allergies. However, patch testing may confirm the diagnosis. Patch testing involves applying suspected allergens to the skin under small chambers held in place by an adhesive strip. Inflammation detected at 48 hours or as late as 96 hours indicates sensitivity.

CROSS REFERENCES

Section 1.29   Hypersensitivity
Section 2.16   Immune-mediated Haematological Conditions
Section 2.20   Immune-mediated Skin Disease
Section 4.6   Targeted Cell Depletion

Immunodeficiency

Exquisite predisposition to infections is a characteristic feature of immunodeficiency disorders. Autoimmune or malignant conditions also occur. A multitude of factors can predispose to an immunodeficient state. Immunodeficiency disorders should be considered in patients presenting with repeated, recurrent, severe or unusual infections. A suggestive or definite family history also warrants attention given that many primary immuno-deficiency conditions have a genetic basis. Organ damage secondary to infection (e.g. deafness, bronchiectasis) may indicate underlying immunodeficiency.

CLASSIFICATION OF IMMUNODEFICIENCY DISORDERS

Classification according to aetiology – primary or secondary

Primary immunodeficiency – intrinsic dysfunction of one or more components of the immune system. Some causes of primary immune dysfunction are:

- Genetic

    — X-linked agammaglobulinaemia (Bruton's)
    — Hyper-IgM syndrome (X-linked and autosomal recessive forms)
    — SCID subgroups (X-linked commonest)
    — Chronic granulomatous disease (X-linked; autosomal)
    — Complement deficiencies
    — Some IgG subclass deficiencies
    — Metabolic disorders (ADA and PNP deficiencies).

- Maturational

    — Transient hypogammaglobulinaemia of infancy
    — Specific antibody deficiency.

- ◆ Undefined/multifactorial

  - — Common variable immunodeficiency (CVID)
  - — Specific antibody deficiencies.

Many primary immunodeficiencies come to light in early childhood but others, including some recently recognised subtle defects, present at any time through to old age. They are life-long conditions unless successfully managed using curative therapies. Bone marrow transplantation and gene therapy are now a reality in primary immunodeficiency practice. Evidence-based therapies are available that improve outcome even if cure is not achieved in some of these disorders. Individual conditions are rare, but they remain nonetheless an important group of disorders to diagnose and treat effectively. Failure to do so results in significant morbidity and mortality.

Secondary immunodeficiency – dysfunction of one or more immune components occurring as result of another process.
  Causes include:

- ◆ Infections – most notably that associated with HIV, also occurs with measles, CMV and EBV infections.
- ◆ Haematological malignancies – multiple myeloma; chronic lymphocytic leukaemia; lymphoma; treatment for these disorders.
- ◆ Renal disease – nephrotic syndrome; uraemia.
- ◆ Cancer therapies – chemotherapy and radiotherapy; some immune therapies (monoclonal antibodies).
- ◆ Drugs – corticosteroids; other immunosuppressants; cytokine inhibitors; anticonvulsants; excessive alcohol intake.
- ◆ Poor nutritional status – primary malnutrition; cachexia secondary to other diseases.
- ◆ Surgery and trauma – major procedures; burns; multi-organ failure.
- ◆ Extremes of age – prematurity and very elderly.
- ◆ Protein-losing states – nephrotic syndrome; protein-losing enteropathy (reduction in immunoglobulin levels often dramatic, although clinical problems with infection are rare).

Many secondary immunodeficiencies involve defects in multiple immune pathways. Each defect may be subtle in isolation but in combination they predispose to very significant infection risk. Secondary immunodeficiency is a major problem worldwide. Globally, malnutrition and the HIV epidemic are major factors. Growing numbers of immuno-compromised patients arise secondary to ever-increasing use of intensive chemo- and radio-therapies in treatment of malignant diseases, immunosuppressive therapies in autoimmune and transplant settings and major surgical and other interventions.

Classification according to immune defect

An alternative approach is to classify immunodeficiency in terms of which limb of the immune system is predominantly deficient. The following categories are widely used:

- ◆ Innate defect

  - — Complement deficiency
  - — Neutrophil deficiency.

- ◆ Specific defect (B cell/T cell)

  - — Antibody (B cell) deficiency
  - — T lymphocyte deficiency.

One or more pathways may function inadequately. Specific clinical characteristics are associated with defective functioning of each of these pathways. The following are useful pointers in pin-pointing the type of defect in patients with suspected immunodeficiency.

- *Age at onset* – major primary T cell defects become apparent soon after birth (days to weeks). If untreated death results within the first two years of life usually. Antibody defects typically occur after maternal antibody starts to decline (3–6 months).
- *Type of infection* – antibody-deficient patients typically are predisposed to pyogenic bacterial infection of the upper and lower respiratory tract. Complement deficiencies predispose especially to recurrent neisserial infections (meningococcal septicaemia and meningitis). Neutrophil disorders predispose to bacterial and fungal infections of the skin and deep-seated organs depending on the severity. T cell deficits predispose to all types of infection but especially opportunistic infections (e.g. atypical mycobacteria and other intracellular bacteria; disseminated viral infections; *Pneumocystis carinii* pneumonia).
- *Pattern of infection* – what qualifies as 'excessive' depends on the age of the patient, the living environment and the past infection and immunisation history. Infants and toddlers in day-care facilities have a high incidence of mild viral infections (maybe as many as 15 in the first year). Development of an infection after appropriate immunisation is highly suspicious of impaired immunity. As a general guideline one major infection (e.g. pneumonia, septicaemia, meningitis, arthritis) and a number of minor infections or two major infections in a year is enough to warrant assessment of immune function.
- *Associated features* – many primary immunodeficiencies are associated with distinctive disorders in other systems (e.g. thrombocytopaenia, small platelet size and eczema in Wiskott–Aldrich syndrome; eczema in Omenn-type SCID; dwarfism; dysmorphic face, cleft lip and palate, hypocalcaemia and cardiac abnormalities in DiGeorge syndrome). Failure to thrive in infants and young children often accompanies significant immunocompromise. Assessment for such features is an essential part of the assessment in patients with suspected immunodeficiency.

CROSS REFERENCES

Section 1.2	Overview of Defence Mechanisms
Section 1.24	Immune Responses to Infection
Sections 2.8–2.11	Further information on immunodeficiencies
Section 3.11	Immunodeficiency

REFERENCE

Primary immunodeficiency diseases. Report of an IUIS scientific group. (1999) *Clin. Exp. Immunol.*, 118 (Suppl. 1): 1–28.

Defects in Antibody-mediated Immunity

CLASSIFICATION

Antibody-deficiency disorders (hypogammaglobulinaemia) may be classified as:

◆ Primary hypogammaglobulinaemia – resulting from an intrinsic disturbance of humoral (antibody-producing) immunity.
◆ Secondary hypogammaglobulinaemia – where another disorder leads to antibody deficiency.

Hypogammaglobulinaemia is the most common primary immunodeficiency, with an estimated prevalence of 1 per 25,000 of the population. Secondary defects are more common.

Primary antibody deficiency disorders can present at any age. The most common form – CVID – is usually diagnosed after the age of 6 years and in some as late as 70 years. Regardless of the cause, even the most severe primary disorders of antibody production usually do not become apparent until about 3–6 months after birth, when protective maternal antibody becomes depleted.

CLINICAL PRESENTATION

Clinical presentation is varied, ranging from absence of symptoms through to major susceptibility to infections. Features of dysregulated immunity (autoimmunity and malignancy) occur less commonly. Patients are susceptible to repeated and sometimes severe infections particularly with encapsulated bacteria (*Streptococcus pneumoniae*, encapsulated *Haemophilus influenzae*, and *Neisseriae* spp). Susceptibility to other classes of microorganisms is not a major feature, with some exceptions. *Giardia lamblia* infection causing diarrhoea and malabsorption is well-described. Atypical bacterial infections in unusual sites – for example *Mycoplasma* arthritis and *Ureaplasma* UTIs also occur. Disseminated paralytic polio is described in a small number of antibody-deficient patients previously immunised with live polio vaccine. Chronic CNS enteroviral infection, causing a gradual decline in neurological function associated with myositis, is a rare but important condition in some severe antibody deficiencies. Opportunistic infections are rarely seen.

Respiratory tract infections, both upper (middle ear, sinus, throat infections) and lower (bronchitis and pneumonia) occur in most patients. Skin infections (boils and abscesses), gut infections, central nervous system infections (meningitis), and joint infections also occur. Structural damage from repeated infections may result in bronchiectasis, deafness, chronic sinusitis and arthritis, particularly if diagnosis is delayed. Failure to thrive is common.

Primary antibody deficiency disorders

Disorders are broadly categorised as genetic or acquired. Genetic defects account for only 10% of cases, but have provided important insights into B cell function. Genetic defects tend to be severe with early onset. The main defects are highlighted in Table 2.8.1. A number of other rare defects have recently been characterised.

Secondary antibody deficiency disorders

Conditions associated with secondary antibody deficiency are many (Table 2.8.2). Onset may be at any age, dependent on the type of underlying disease. Antibody deficiency may or may not be clinically evident.

INVESTIGATION

A clinical immunologist should review all patients with known or suspected antibody deficiency. The following investigations are required:

- Total IgG, IgA and IgM compared with values in age-matched normal controls.
- Serum and urine electrophoresis to exclude underlying lymphoproliferative conditions.
- IgG subclasses, even if IgG levels normal.
- Specific antibody levels as a baseline and following immunisation if initial levels are low.
- Immunophenotypic analysis of peripheral blood measuring B and T cell numbers and subsets, and occasionally CD40 ligand expression. Functional analyses of lymphocytes *in vitro* are rarely required to make a diagnosis.
- Specialist laboratories can identify specific protein deficiencies and genetic mutations in selected cases. The tests undertaken will be directed by the clinical and laboratory findings.
- Assessment of active infection and/or damage in susceptible organs is important. Culture, polymerase chain reaction (PCR) testing, computer tomography (CT) scanning of chest and sinuses, endoscopic sinus examination and pulmonary function testing are undertaken in selected cases.
- Full blood counts and baseline liver biochemistry should be performed. There are many different reasons why abnormalities may arise depending on the condition (e.g. cytopaenias in CVID, sclerosing cholangitis in hyper-IgM) and the treatment received (IVIg-related hepatitis).

Table 2.8.1 Primary antibody deficiencies

DISEASE	AETIOLOGY	CHARACTERISTIC CLINICAL FEATURES	CHARACTERISTIC LABORATORY FEATURES
X-linked agamma-globulinaemia Bruton's agamma-globulinaemia	B cell tyrosine kinase (btk) mutation on X chromosome	Males affected, transmitted by females Symptoms usually begin in second half of first year of life Giardiasis Live attenuated Polio vaccine induced paralysis is a risk Chronic CNS enteroviral infection a rare complication	Mature B cells absent Impaired production of all antibody isotypes
Hyper-IgM deficiency	CD40 ligand deficiency	Males affected. Extremely rare female hyper – IgM identified with different molecular basis Opportunistic infections (e.g. *Pneumocystis carinii*, *Cryptosporidiosis*) occur in addition to pyogenic bacterial infections Autoimmune and malignant haematological conditions occur	Mature T and B cells Impaired T/B cell interaction CD40L expression impaired; occasionally, expression is normal but function is affected Serum IgM normal or elevated, other Ig classes deficient
CVID	Combined genetic and environmental factors most likely	Onset at any age Immune dysregulation in addition to deficiency characteristic Autoimmune conditions and malignancies common Lymphoid hyperplasia and granuloma formation occur	T and B cells present, but numbers may be reduced Ig levels variably reduced
Isolated IgA deficiency	Probably genetic	Common – prevalence 1/500 Often asymptomatic Transfusion reactions common Increased frequency in coeliac disease, RA	
IgG subclass deficiency	Uncertain	Many asymptomatic, some develop CVID	IgG2 and IgG4 +/−IgA combined deficiencies characteristic
Specific antibody deficiency	Uncertain	Polysaccharide deficiency in infants and young children is physiological	Normal Ig/IgG subclass levels B cells present

(*Table 2.8.1 continued*)

Table 2.8.1 Continued

DISEASE	AETIOLOGY	CHARACTERISTIC CLINICAL FEATURES	CHARACTERISTIC LABORATORY FEATURES
		Repeated infections may ensue Clinical features can be as severe as that seen in full antibody deficiency syndromes Increasingly recognised	
Transient hypogamma-globulinaemia of infancy	Physiological 'immaturity' of infant immune system	Resolves by 2–3 years Increased risk in infants born prematurely	IgM is usually normal with low IgG and IgA levels
Thymoma-associated	Thymus malignancy	Middle-aged and beyond	Lymphopaenia, variable Ig deficiencies

Table 2.8.2 Secondary antibody deficiencies

B cell malignancies	Multiple myeloma; chronic lymphocytic leukaemia. Clinical immunodeficiency is related to impaired capacity to respond to polysaccharide antigens
Protein-losing states	Nephrotic syndrome, protein-losing enteropathies. Rarely of great clinical significance
Drugs	Cytotoxic agents; anti-convulsants; disease-modifying anti-rheumatic drugs. Immunodeficiency is usually due to a combination of factors related to underlying disease and therapy
Splenic	Splenectomy; hyposplenism in sickle-cell disease, coeliac disease. Overwhelming pneumococcal infection is an important complication
Extremes of age	Prematurity and old age

TREATMENT AND MONITORING

- Immunoglobulin (Ig) replacement therapy at regular intervals is the mainstay of therapy in patients with major antibody deficiencies (Section 4.8). Adequate immunoglobulin replacement *before* structural damage occurs dramatically improves patient well-being and prognosis. The role of immunoglobulin therapy in IgG subclass and specific antibody deficiencies is unclear. It is often used if antibiotic prophylaxis fails to control infection.
- Immunoglobulin supplementary therapy is useful in some patients with secondary immunodeficiencies, for example, patients with multiple myeloma and CLL with deficient specific antibody responses and a history of repeated infections. Treatment is generally not required in protein-losing states.
- Appropriate anti-microbial therapy for the treatment and prophylaxis of infections is vital.
- Gene therapies are currently not available, but may play a role in genetic antibody-deficiencies in the future.

Case 2.8.1 Immunodeficiency

A 20-year-old girl came to see her GP because of a chest infection that had failed to respond to two previous courses of antibiotics. She had a history of recurrent infections, and in the last year had had antibiotics on six occasions prior to this chest infection. These had been prescribed for an ear infection, sinusitis, bacterial pharyngitis and three previous chest infections. She gave a history of a cough, productive of 1–2 tablespoons of sputum each day, even when she did not have an infection.

The GP was concerned about the pattern of frequent infections at different sites together with failure to respond to antibiotics. Chronic sputum production in a non-smoker raised the possibility of asthma or bronchiectasis. Measurement of immunoglobulins showed undetectable IgA (immunoglobulin A) and substantially reduced IgG at 3.0 g/l (Ref. Range 6.0–13.00 g/l). She was referred to the Immunology clinic. Further assessment showed normal number of lymphocytes including B cells. High resolution CT of the lungs showed bronchiectasis affecting the right lower lobe. Sputum culture grew *Haemophilus influenzae*. A diagnosis of bronchiectasis secondary to common variable immunodeficiency was made.

The patient was treated with antibiotics and physiotherapy and replacement therapy with intravenous Ig was commenced. The patient's general health improved considerably and she no longer produced sputum daily. However, she required antibiotics twice the following year for treatment of chest infections. Unfortunately as bronchiectasis was established prior to the introduction of Ig replacement, it is likely that she will continue to have episodes of chest infection.

Cross reference

Section 4.8   Immunoglobulin Replacement Therapy

CROSS REFERENCES

Section 1.14   B Cell Activation
Section 1.15   Immunoglobulin Function
Section 1.23   Ontogeny of the Immune Response
Section 2.7   Immunodeficiency
Section 3.11   Immunodeficiency
Section 3.12   Abnormal Immunoglobulins
Section 4.8   Immunoglobulin Replacement Therapy

REFERENCES

Ballow, M. D. (2002) 'Primary immunodeficiency disorders: antibody deficiency', *J. Allerg. Clin. Immunol.*, 109: 581–91.

Consensus Document for the Diagnosis and Management of Patients with Primary Antibody Deficiencies. (1995) Published by The Marks and Spencer Publications Unit of the Royal College of Pathologists, October 1995.

Defects in T Cell-mediated Immunity

Patients with T cell-mediated immune defects are susceptible to a broader range of infections and tend to be sicker than those with pure antibody deficiency. T cell immuno-deficiency may be:

- Primary – intrinsic abnormality with diminished T cell numbers and/or function.
- Secondary – extrinsic factor causes T cell dysfunction. For example, HIV infection; immunosuppressive therapies.

Secondary defects are of varying severity and are dependent on the specific cause and the stage of involvement, for example, HIV is clinically quiescent for extended periods but eventually leads to profound T cell immunodeficiency.

T cell-mediated immune defects are rarely isolated. B cell defects usually coexist if T cell function is impaired.

CLASSIFICATION OF T CELL IMMUNODEFICIENCIES

- Severe combined immunodeficiency (SCID) – intrinsic defects cause absent or grossly deficient T cell immunity. SCID presents soon after birth and if untreated is promptly fatal. Many causes of SCID are now well characterised both clinically and at a molecular level. Genetic mutations with various patterns of T, B, and NK cell impairment are described.
- Combined immunodeficiency disorders (CID) – more moderate degrees of immuno-deficiency, occurring later and with slower progression than SCID.
- Predominantly T cell defects – rare conditions where B cell defects are limited.

SEVERE COMBINED IMMUNODEFICIENCY

Prevalence

SCID is rare, affecting an estimated 1 per 50,000 births. Less marked primary T cell deficiencies are increasingly recognised with more sensitive and wider availability of investigations. HIV infection has a huge impact globally and is discussed in more detail in Section 2.13.

Clinical presentation

Defence against intracellular pathogens is dependent on functioning T cells. Associated B cell dysfunction predisposes to pyogenic infections.

Typical infections include:

♦ Viruses – disproportionately severe, prolonged or disseminated. Pathogens include RSV (pneumonia), parainfluenzae (respiratory), CMV (disseminated), EBV (disseminated), enteroviruses (GIT), rotavirus (GIT).
♦ Bacteria – pneumonia, ear infections, skin infections, septicaemia.
♦ Fungi – persistent candidiasis, often affecting the oesophagus, *Aspergillus*.
♦ Opportunistic – *P. carinii* pneumonia, opportunistic mycobacteriae (BCG-related infections).

The following features are common:

♦ Failure to thrive – infection-related.
♦ Diarrhoea – secondary to chronic infections.
♦ Skin rash – maternal lymphocytes transferred during pregnancy or by blood transfusion can cause Graft-versus-Host disease (GvHD), which causes an erythematous skin eruption as well as internal organ dysfunction.
♦ Lymphadenopathy/hepatosplenomegaly – infections (EBV, CMV, BCG-osis); GvHD.
♦ Skeletal, cardiac, haematological and endocrine abnormalities – associated with distinct disorders (Table 2.9.1).
♦ Family history – a positive family history or a history of consanguinity may be present.

Diagnosis

SCID is a paediatric emergency. Infants with suspicious clinical features should be investigated urgently. Prompt, appropriate management is essential for survival. Infants with SCID are usually lymphopaenic (check full blood count). Absolute lymphocyte counts are normally $>2.8 \times 10^9/l$ in neonates. Lymphocyte counts $<2 \times 10^9/l$ at birth are highly suspicious of an underlying SCID disorder. Urgent referral to a specialist centre for diagnosis and therapy is essential.

Useful additional investigations are:

♦ Lymphocyte subpopulations – T, B and NK cell numbers. Subclassification into B+ and B− variants directs further investigation. More detailed phenotypic analysis, for example, CD4/CD8 T cell numbers, HLA expression, TCRβ usage are useful in specific conditions.
♦ Immunoglobulins – total isotype and IgG subclass levels, specific antibodies directed against vaccine antigens (tetanus, Hib). Antibody deficiency is usual, regardless of B cell count.
♦ *In vitro* cell function assays – lymphocyte proliferation to mitogens and specific antigens are usually impaired.
♦ ADA measurement – in T–B–SCID.
♦ HLA typing – if materno-fetal engraftment is suspected. Also required for BMT work-up.
♦ Genetic – study known genes of interest (IL-2R). Also useful in prenatal diagnosis where precise mutation is known.
♦ Microbial – expert microbiological involvement is critical.

Table 2.9.1 Classification of severe combined immunodeficiency (SCID)

CONDITION AND DEFECT	INHERITANCE	IMMUNE ABNORMALITIES	ADDITIONAL COMMENTS	FREQUENCY
T−, B+ phenotype **Mutation**				
Cytokine receptor common γ-chain (γc) Impaired cytokine signalling	X-linked	Cell-mediated immunodeficiency; B cells present but antibody deficient; NK cells absent	Typical onset and progression	50%
IL-7/IL-7R Impaired cytokine signalling	Autosomal recessive	As above but NK cells present	Typical onset and progression	10%
JAK-3 kinase Impaired cytokine signalling	Autosomal recessive	As for X-linked SCID	Typical onset and progression	5%
T−, B− phenotype **Mutation**				
ADA Lymphotoxic purine metabolite build-up	Autosomal recessive	Cell-mediated immunodeficiency; antibody deficiency; NK cells absent	Bone and neurological abnormalities. Profound lymphopaenia	20%
RAG1/2 defect DNA rearrangement defects	Autosomal recessive	As for ADA, but NK cells present		20%
Reticular dysgenesis Stem cell defect	Autosomal recessive	No haematological development	Incompatible with life	Rare
T+ phenotype **Mutation**				
Omenn syndrome ?related to *RAG* gene abnormalities	Autosomal recessive	T cells present but oligoclonal and poorly functional; B cells absent and antibody deficient; IgE elevated	Eczema, lymphadenopathy, hepatosplenomegaly, eosinophilia Occasional family history of T-B-SCID	Rare
Bare lymphocyte syndrome Class I TAP mutations	Autosomal recessive	Class I deficiency – lymphocytes present but impaired function	Varies from asymptomatic to SCID	Rare
Class II mutations in transcription factors		Class II deficiency – CD4 lymphopaenia, B cells present, variable antibody function	Variable severity	Rare
Materno-fetal engraftment	Autosomal recessive	Activated T cells (CD8+) present; poor cell and antibody-mediated immunity	GVHD; T cells are foreign – maternal or from blood Can complicate any SCID	Variable
ZAP-70; CD3 complex-impaired signal	Autosomal recessive	CD8 def (ZAP-70); variable T deficiency (CD3)	Variable defects; late onset	Rare

Management

An expert, multidisciplinary team is essential for good management.
Key aspects of treatment include:

◆ Infection management – prevention by isolation in a positive pressure area with reverse-barrier nursing and anti-microbial prophylaxis. Aggressive treatment of existing infections.
◆ Immune reconstitution – bone marrow transplantation – ideally from a HLA-identical sibling. Matched unrelated and parental donors (haploid-identical) are also used. The outlook after BMT is excellent, especially for HLA-identical grafts transplanted before serious infection-related complications develop.
◆ IVIg – required in most cases.
◆ ADA enzyme replacement therapy may improve immune function in ADA-deficient patients.

Case 2.9.1 Severe combined immunodeficiency

A 3-month-old breastfed boy was admitted to hospital for rehydration with a 2-day history of severe diarrhoea. At the time he was noted to be below the third centile for length and weight. A candidal nappy rash was present. Initial blood tests showed haemoconcentration with a raised haemoglobin, sodium and urea. Following rehydration his condition improved, and biochemical indices returned to normal. Although the diarrhoea had not completely settled, his mother was keen to return home and he was discharged with instructions to return if the diarrhoea failed to settle. One month later, he represented with a severe chest infection. The diarrhoea, although improved had never completely settled.

The possibility of immune deficiency was considered. The parents did not report any risk factors for human immunodeficiency virus (HIV), and antibody tests on mother and baby were negative. Full blood count showed marked lymphopaenia of 0.6×10^9/l. On review of the blood count taken on the previous admission this clue had been present previously, but the significance had not been considered. Lymphocyte subsets showed markedly reduced T cell count of 0.1×10^9/l, with B cells present in normal numbers. Functional testing showed a failure to proliferate in response to PHA. Immunoglobulins were not detectable. A diagnosis of T cell− B cell+ SCID (severe combined immunodeficiency) was made. Further investigation showed that the common γ-chain of the IL-2 family of cytokine receptors was absent establishing the diagnosis of X-linked SCID.

Human leucocyte antigen (HLA) typing was performed on the family members. The patient's 8-year-old brother was found to be HLA identical. Bone marrow transplantation (BMT) was performed using his HLA identical sibling. He experienced mild Graft-versus-Host Disease and a febrile episode while he was neutropenic. However, he made an excellent recovery, with full immune reconstitution.

Cross references

Section 2.27   Haemopoietic Stem Cell Transplantation
Section 3.11   Immunodeficiency

◆ SCID is the first condition successfully treated by gene therapy in humans (Table 2.9.1). Patients with X-linked SCID have had the normal gene transferred into autologous stem cells and initial results are encouraging. ADA gene therapy has been less successful. Other forms of SCID may be treatable with gene therapy.
◆ Nutritional support often with TPN is required.
◆ All blood products must be irradiated (to prevent immunocompetent donor lymphocytes causing GVHD) and CMV-negative (to prevent CMV infection).
◆ No live vaccines (BCG, MMR, oral polio) should be given, as serious infection may result.

COMBINED IMMUNODEFICIENCIES

Cell-mediated immunodeficiencies less severe than SCID are described. These conditions are not trivial. Some progress to late onset SCID. Lymphoreticular malignancies and serious non-immunological abnormalities may occur. Treatment depends on the severity of the underlying immunodeficiency (Table 2.9.2) BMT may be required. Immune support (e.g. antibody replacement therapy) may be adequate. As in SCID, untreated blood transfusions and live vaccines should be avoided.

Table 2.9.2 Combined immunodeficiencies

CONDITION AND DEFECT	INHERITANCE	IMMUNE ABNORMALITIES	COMMENTS	FREQUENCY
Purine nucleoside phosphorylase deficiency Lymphotoxic purine metabolites accumulate	Autosomal recessive	Marked T cell lymphopaenia; progressively impaired T cell function; variable antibody dysfunction	Neurological abnormalities common Onset in infancy/early childhood Usually fatal without BMT	Rare
Ataxia-telangiectasia ATM gene mutations causes impaired DNA repair	Autosomal recessive	Variable antibody and cell-mediated deficiencies; IgA deficiency with progression to generalised antibody defects; cell function variably impaired; ionising radiation sensitivity	Progressive ataxia, oculocutaneous telangiectases; lymphoreticular malignancy Onset usually in childhood Death in early adulthood if untreated; α-fetoprotein elevated. Best therapy uncertain	Frequency unknown; increased risk of CLL and breast cancer in heterozygotes
Wiskott–Aldrich syndrome WASP gene mutations leading to impaired membrane function in T cells/platelets	X-linked	Impaired polysaccharide antibodies; progression to antibody deficiency, variable cell-mediated defects	Thrombocytopaenia; severe eczema; lymphoreticular malignancies Onset in infancy/early childhood. Lymphoma in early adulthood Splenectomy for thrombocytopaenia. IVIg is usually required	Rare

Some disorders are characterised by predominant T cell defects with relative preservation of antibody-mediated immunity. Two important conditions in this category are:

DiGeorge syndrome This results from abnormal development of the pharyngeal pouches resulting in thymic hypoplasia and immunodeficiency, and abnormalities of facial, parathyroid gland and cardiac development. The genetic basis in most cases is a microdeletion on chromosome 22q11. Total DiGeorge syndrome is extremely rare and resembles SCID, however, a partial syndrome associated with chromosome 22q11 deletion is common (1/5000 population). Only 25% of those with the deletion have abnormal immunological investigations and 2–3% have clinical immunodeficiency. The syndrome is also called CATCH-22 (cardiac anomalies, abnormal face, thymic aplasia, cleft palate, hypocalcaemia with abnormalities on chromosome 22). Cell- and antibody-mediated immunity may be abnormal, and autoimmune cytopaenias are common. Management is dictated by severity of immunodeficiency. Severe cases are managed like other SCIDs. Lesser degrees of immunodeficiency are conservatively managed. Measures to avoid GvHD (irradiated blood) and iatrogenic infection (CMV negative blood, avoidance of live vaccines) may be required. Immune function may improve or deteriorate with age.

Chronic mucocutaneous candidiasis This is a condition of variable inheritance that results in defective protection against candida. Skin and mucous membranes are predominantly affected and deep-seated infection is rare. An associated endocrinopathy (parathyroid, adrenals, thyroid, ovarian) is seen in some. Gut autoimmunity is also recognised. Small numbers have a more generalised cell-mediated immunodeficiency with predisposition to other intracellular infections, akin to SCID. Anti-fungal prophylaxis and monitoring for evolving endocrine diseases are required.

CROSS REFERENCES

Section 1.12   Lymphocyte Maturation
Section 2.8   Defects in Antibody-mediated Immunity
Section 2.13   Human Immunodeficiency Virus
Section 2.27   Haemopoietic Stem Cell Transplantation
Section 3.11   Immunodeficiency

REFERENCE

Buckley, R. H. (2002) 'Primary cellular immunodeficiencies. Current reviews of allergy and clinical immunology', *J. Allerg. Clin. Immunol.*, 109: 747–57.

Neutrophil Disorders

Neutrophil disorders include abnormalities of:

*   Neutrophil number (common, usually acquired)
*   Neutrophil function (rare).

CLINICAL PRESENTATION

Typical clinical features include:

*   Skin and mucus membrane infections
*   Oral ulceration, poor dentition, infective gum disease
*   Abscesses
*   Deep-seated infections in severely affected individuals.

Common pathogens include *Staphylococci*, other catalase-positive bacteria and fungi. Infections can be recurrent or prolonged and responses to anti-microbial therapies may be impaired.

CLASSIFICATION OF NEUTROPHIL DISORDERS

Neutropaenia is defined as an absolute neutrophil count $<2 \times 10^9/l$. Mild neutropaenia is usually asymptomatic. Infection rates are increased with counts $<1 \times 10^9/l$. Neutropaenia of $<0.5 \times 10^9/l$ is associated with potentially life-threatening infection. Causes are many.
  Neutropaenic disorders are broadly categorised into:

*   *Disorders of production* (with bone marrow hypoplasia) – may be primary, where an intrinsic bone marrow disorder results in reduced neutrophil production. Congenital neutropaenic disorders are often severe and present early in life (e.g. Kostmann's syndrome), and are usually managed at expert haematology centres. In cyclical

neutropaenia neutrophil counts fall at 3-weekly regular intervals with subsequent infection, usually affecting the mouth.

The most common neutrophil-related disorder is secondary neutropaenia resulting from many therapies and disorders, including leukaemias and other myelodysplastic conditions, aplastic anaemia, cytotoxic drugs (chemotherapy regimes, and immunosuppressants), radiotherapy, other drug reactions (e.g. carbimazole), and infections.

- *Disorders of neutrophil destruction* – neutropaenia also results from excessive destruction of neutrophils despite normal or high bone marrow output. Splenomegaly of any cause can be associated with neutropaenia (e.g. Felty's syndrome in rheumatoid arthritis). Immune neutropaenia results from enhanced cell destruction due to neutrophil-specific antibodies.

NEUTROPHIL FUNCTION DISORDERS

Several rare disorders, many with known genetic defects, cause symptomatic neutrophil dysfunction. Altered function precipitated by infections, malnutrition, other illnesses (e.g. sickle-cell disease, uraemia, diabetes mellitus), or therapies (steroids, chemotherapy) also occurs but is rarely clinically important. Functional disorders are broadly classified according to the dominant dysfunction.

- Neutrophil movement (chemotaxis)
- Adhesion
- Phagocytosis (microbial uptake)
- Respiratory burst and killing.

Chronic granulomatous disease (X-linked and autosomal recessive) results from mutations in genes encoding cytochrome b/NADPH oxidase enzymes causing reduced cytotoxic oxygen radical production and impaired bacterial killing. Patients develop infections caused by catalase-positive bacteria (e.g. *Staphylococcus aureus*, *Pseudomonas*, *Serratia* and *Nocardia*) and fungi (*Aspergillus*). Skin and deep-seated abscess formation occurs. Patients develop non-caseating granulomata in different parts of the body, typically including lymph nodes, liver, spleen and gut-associated lymphoid tissues. This may represent an inappropriate response to unresolved infections. Gastrointestinal or urinary tract granulomata may cause obstructive complications. Many cases are clinically apparent from childhood but less severe phenotypes may present in adulthood. Early recognition and appropriate therapy greatly improves outcome.

Leucocyte adhesion deficiency (LAD) – adhesion molecules facilitate neutrophil movement across blood vessel walls towards sites of infection. Several genetic mutations in these adhesion molecules result in LAD, resulting in bacterial infections and abscesses. Severe forms are apparent from infancy but milder phenotypes present later. Gum disease, tooth loss, delayed separation of the umbilical cord (normally occurs within the first week of life), poor formation of pus at sites of infection, and disproportionate rises in the white cell count during infection (cells cannot pass into tissues) are characteristic.

Hyper-IgE syndrome is a disorder of uncertain aetiology. Neutrophil chemotaxis is impaired. Patients present with recurrent infections and develop staphylococcal abscesses. Atypical eczema, a characteristic coarse facial appearance (lion-like), osteopaenia with pathological fractures of the central skeleton, and abnormal dentition (failure to lose first teeth, eruption of the second teeth and dental overcrowding) are also seen. Total IgE levels are hugely elevated. An underlying defect of lymphocyte regulation rather than an intrinsic neutrophil disorder may be responsible.

Many other conditions are associated with neutrophil dysfunction. These include Chediak–Higashi syndrome, Griscelli syndrome, and specific enzyme deficiencies such as Glucose-6-Phosphate dehydrogenase, myeloperoxidase and lactoferrin deficiencies. Variable levels of clinical immunodeficiency together with non-immunological abnormalities (e.g. albinism in the case of Chediak–Higashi and Griscelli syndromes) occur.

CLINICAL INVESTIGATION

The following is an outline of investigation for patients with suspected neutrophil abnormalities. The tests are discussed in detail in Section 3.11.

- ◆ Absolute neutrophil count. If low, this is the likely cause of neutrophil abnormality.
- ◆ Blood film to assess neutrophil morphology

Patients with typical histories and normal or high numbers of morphologically normal neutrophils should be referred to an immunologist for investigation. Tests of all the components of neutrophil function are available. All require a fresh unclotted whole blood sample.

- ◆ Total IgE, Ig levels and T and B cell profiles may be useful to exclude alternative immunodeficiencies.
- ◆ Microbial analysis with special fungal cultures should be undertaken if active infection is suspected.
- ◆ Respiratory burst capacity is measured when chronic granulomatous disease (CGD) is suspected. For details see Section 3.11.
- ◆ Adhesion marker profile should be assessed in patients with suspected leucocyte adhesion deficiency (LAD).

TREATMENT

Appropriate antimicrobial therapy (for active infections and prophylaxis) is the mainstay of management. G-CSF is useful in symptomatic, severely neutropaenic patients. Prophylactic therapy with cotrimoxazole and anti-fungal therapy improves outlook for patients with CGD. IFN-γ therapy is used widely in the United States, but less so in Europe for disease suppression. Bone marrow transplantation is curative in CGD, however, risks are high in the absence of a HLA-identical donor. Patient selection is difficult as CGD may run a benign course and factors predictive of a poor outcome are unknown. BMT is also an option in some other severe neutrophil disorders (LAD). Genetic manipulation may be an option in the future.

CROSS REFERENCES

Section 1.4   Innate Immune Responses I
Section 2.7   Immunodeficiency
Section 3.11   Immunodeficiency (summarises investigations)

Complement Deficiency

Genetic deficiencies of all components of the complement cascade and many complement regulatory molecules are well recognised. Secondary deficiencies, caused by increased consumption in conditions such as active systemic lupus erthematosus (SLE) and some forms of glomerulonephritis, are more common.

Most genetic complement deficiencies are autosomal recessive in inheritance. The exceptions are properdin deficiency (X-linked) and C1 inhibitor deficiency (autosomal dominant). Inherited complement deficiency disorders are rare with C1 inhibitor deficiency being the most common. C1 inhibitor deficiency causes angioedema rather than immunodeficiency or immune complex disease (see Section 2.3). C2 deficiency is the most prevalent (1/10,000) conventional complement disorder in Caucasians. Mannan binding lectin (MBL) deficiency, caused by polymorphisms in the *MBL* gene is increasingly recognised. MBL is involved in activation of the complement cascade. The clinical significance of MBL deficiency is not fully clarified but it may be relevant when microbe-specific antibodies are defective. Partial complement deficiencies resulting from heterozygous carriage of mutated genes are usually clinically silent, although certain partial deficiencies (C2, C4 and C3) are associated with an increased frequency of specific autoimmune conditions.

CLINICAL PRESENTATION

Clinical features associated with complement deficiency include:

◆ Recurrent pyogenic infections
◆ Exquisite susceptibility to *Neisserial* infections (meningococcal infections)
◆ Immune-complex mediated disorders, especially SLE.

The precise features depend on whether the deficient component is involved in the classical (C1–C4–C2–C3), lectin (MBL–C4–C2–C3) or alternative (Factor B, Factor D, Properdin, C3, and Factors H and I) activation pathways, or in the common terminal pathway (C5–C9).

Deficiency of any component that impairs conversion of C3 to its active state increases predisposition to pyogenic infections. This occurs particularly with C3 deficiency, and with deficiencies of activating pathway components, control protein deficiencies (Factor H and Factor I), as well as in secondary C3 depletion (e.g. nephritic factor-related glomerulonephritis). Complement is particularly important in the early stages of infection and where there are low microbe-specific antibody levels.

Defective function of the classical activation pathway impairs clearance of immune complexes, increasing susceptibility to immune complex-mediated diseases, particularly SLE. Heterozygous carriers of mutated C4 and C2 genes are also at risk. Partial deficiencies of C4 are reasonably common in SLE patients, but the absolute risk of developing SLE is much greater in patients with complete C1 and C2 deficiencies.

However, on a population level, C1 and C2 deficiencies are much less prevalent than partial C4 deficiencies. Early age of onset, severe disease with critical organ involvement (renal manifestations), together with a positive family history are especially characteristic of C1 deficiencies (deficiencies of all three subunits have been described). Autoimmune serology (ANA, anti-dsDNA) may be unexpectedly negative. Unusual forms of skin involvement are also described in C2-deficient SLE.

Patients with genetic deficiencies of the terminal pathway components (C5–C8 especially, less so C9) and also Properdin are exquisitely predisposed to infections with *Neisserial* species (meningococcus and gonococcus). Patients with a history of recurring *Neisserial* infection, infection caused by unusual serotypes, and infection in adulthood warrant investigation.

INVESTIGATION

CH50 measurement – functional assessment of complement lytic capacity. Both classical and alternative pathway assays should be performed. The pattern of impairment of classical and alternative pathways indicates the part of the complement cascade involved. Measurement of specific complement components based on these findings can be performed at specialist laboratories. Further details are outlined in Section 3.10.

TREATMENT

No specific treatments are available. Meningococcal immunisation should be offered to all at risk. Antibiotic prophylaxis may also be useful. Patients should be aware of indicators of infection and the need for prompt medical care. Plasma infusions for patients with active infection have been suggested but no trials are available and some reports indicate potential adverse effects. SLE associated with genetic complement deficiencies and conditions that precipitate complement deficiency through excessive consumption are managed along usual therapeutic guidelines.

CROSS REFERENCES

Section 1.5   Innate Immune Responses II – The Complement System
Section 3.10   Complement
Section 3.11   Immunodeficiency

REFERENCE

Walport, M. (2001) 'Advances in immunology: complement', *New Engl. J. Med.*, 344: 1058–66, 1140–4.

Defective Splenic Function

The spleen is a secondary lymphoid organ, which also filters blood, removing bacteria and parasitised red blood cells (RBCs). Opsonisation increases the efficiency of particle removal. The spleen plays a particularly important role in antibody responses against polysaccharides.

CAUSES OF DEFECTIVE SPLENIC FUNCTION

The most common cause of reduced or absent splenic function are:

- Congenital absence of the spleen (asplenia)
- Surgical removal of the spleen (splenectomy), because of

  — Trauma
  — Autoimmune cytopaenias
  — Lymphoproliferative disorders.

- Functional hyposplenism

  — Coeliac disease
  — Sickle-cell anaemia.

Reimplantation of a portion of splenic tissue during splenectomy reduces the risk of hyposplenism.

DIAGNOSIS OF HYPOSPLENISM

The spleen normally removes abnormal and aged RBCs from the circulation, including RBCs released prematurely from bone marrow containing remnants of DNA (Howell–Jolly bodies) and denatured haemoglobin (Heinz bodies). Howell–Jolly and Heinz bodies are rarely seen in normal peripheral blood, but are seen in a significant percentage of RBCs in subjects with hyposplenism. Thrombocytosis and monocytosis are often present.

Radionucleotide scans measuring removal of isotope labelled particles from the bloodstream allow localisation of splenic remnants, but are rarely required to assess splenic function.

CLINICAL FEATURES OF HYPOSPLENISM

Overwhelming post-splenectomy infection (OPSI) is a major long-term risk following splenectomy, or in patients with splenic dysfunction. OPSI is a fulminant infection, often due to encapsulated bacteria, with a mortality of up to 50%. The risk of OPSI is highest in the two years post-splenectomy, but remains clinically significant lifelong. The risk is relatively reduced when splenectomy follows trauma, but is greatly increased when splenectomy is performed in patients receiving chemotherapy or radiotherapy, in children under the age of 5, and when hyposplenism is secondary to sickle-cell anaemia (SCA).

Most serious post-splenectomy infections are caused by *S. pneumoniae* (pneumococcus), *H. influenzae* type B (HiB), and *Neisseria meningitidis* (meningococcus). Salmonella infection is a particular problem in patients with hyposplenism due to SCA. Infection with *Escherichia coli*, as well as malaria, babesiosis (a tick-borne parasite) and *Capnocytophaga canimorsus* (transmitted by dog and other animal bites) are also important risks.

MANAGEMENT OF PATIENTS WITH HYPOSPLENISM

Management is aimed at reducing the risk of OPSI, and ensuring prompt and adequate therapy when infection occurs despite prophylaxis. Patients must also be educated about the other less common health risks of hyposplenism.

Patient education

The risk of OPSI must be clearly communicated, and the need to continue prophylactic antibiotics discussed. Patients should understand the risk of encouraging microbial resistance by intermittent use of antibiotics, the need to seek medical attention and start immediate therapeutic antibiotics for any febrile illness, as well as following animal bites. Travel advice should include explanation of the increased risk of malaria and babesiosis and strong advice to avoid areas where resistant malaria and/or *Plasmodium falciparum* are endemic.

Prophylactic antibiotics

Lifelong use of prophylactic antibiotics is recommended, with oral penicillin or erythromycin (if penicillin-allergic). Antibiotic prophylaxis is particularly important in children, in the first two years post-splenectomy and in those with additional defects of immune function. All patients should have a course of therapeutic antibiotics to take at the onset of a febrile, potentially infective illness. Antibiotics should be given prophylactically in the event of an animal bite.

Immunisation

The risk of infection with encapsulated bacteria is substantially reduced by vaccination, preferably two weeks before elective splenectomy. Where this is not possible, vaccination should be given prior to discharge. Hyposplenic patients not previously vaccinated should be vaccinated at the first opportunity. Vaccinations recommended include polyvalent pneumococcal vaccine (revaccinate every five years), HiB, meningitis C conjugate vaccine as well as annual influenza vaccine. Annual measurement of anti-pneumococcal antibody levels is recommended, and early revaccination may be advisable where protective antibody levels are not maintained.

Communication of risk

All healthcare providers must be aware of a patient's hyposplenism and patients should carry a splenectomy card or wear a medic-Alert bracelet.

Adequate therapy of infections

As with all immunodeficiencies prompt instigation of adequate therapy for potential infections is essential. Recommendations for febrile illness vary with prophylaxis, local patterns of penicillin resistance and penicillin allergy. However, penicillin, erythromycin or cefotaxime are commonly used. Microbiology advice should be sought immediately, however, this should not delay treatment.

REFERENCES

British Committee for Standards in Haematology Clinical Haematology Task Force. (1996) Guidelines for the prevention and treatment of infection in patients with an absent or dysfunctional spleen. *BMJ*, 312: 430–4.

Davies, J. M. (2001) 'Updated guideline', *BMJ*, Electronic letter (2 June 2001).

Human Immunodeficiency Virus

EPIDEMIOLOGY

AIDS was first described in the early 1980s and soon after attributed to infection with HIV. Globally, AIDS is a major cause of morbidity and mortality, particularly in Africa where 95% of all HIV-related deaths occur and prevalence rates are as high as 20–45%. HIV is present in body fluids – blood, semen, breast milk and saliva. Modes of virus transmission include:

Sexual

- Homosexual transmission was originally identified.
- Heterosexual transmission is increasingly important globally and is the dominant route of infection in Africa. Failure to observe safe sexual practices is a growing problem in all groups.

Parenteral

- HIV infection among haemophiliacs receiving blood-derived Factor VIII concentrates demonstrated HIV transmission by blood products. Screening and testing of all blood and organ donors has virtually eliminated HIV transmission by these routes. However, infected donors in the early phases of infection will not be identified. Blood quarantine limits this risk, but is not possible for all blood products.
- Intravenous drug users are infected by sharing of blood-contaminated needles.
- Occupational exposure to infected blood and contaminated sharps can result in infection, if correct infection control procedures are not observed.

Vertical

Transmission from mother to child during pregnancy, delivery and via breast milk is the major route of HIV infection in children.

HIV BIOLOGY

HIV, binds to and is internalized by CD4+ T cells via a surface-expressed glycoprotein molecule – gp-120. Co-binding to the chemokine receptor CCR5 is also required for uptake. Some genetic mutations in CCR5 render cells resistant to HIV infection.

The major HIV targets are:

* CD4+ T cells
* Dendritic cells
* Monocytes/Macrophages
* Follicular dendritic cells
* CNS; gut tissue.

HIV is an RNA retrovirus. It undergoes reverse transcription to DNA and subsequent integration into the cell genome. HIV is highly damaging to the immune system. This results from:

* Depletion of CD4+ T cells – the major effect
* Impaired T memory responses
* Defective cytotoxicity
* Defective antibody responses.

Surviving infected cells in lymphoid tissue, CNS and the gut act as viral reservoirs where viral replication continues at varying rates, depending on the stage of the disease. HIV is highly susceptible to mutation and this limits the effectiveness of the host response to the virus and facilitates the emergence of therapy-resistant strains (Figure 2.13.1).

Figure 2.13.1 Interaction of HIV with host immune cells.

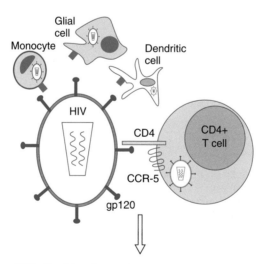

CD4+ T cell lymphopaenia

Impaired function of persisting T cells

Poor primary B cell responses with functional antibody deficiency

HIV reservoirs in secondary lymphoid tissues

CLINICAL PRESENTATIONS AND STAGING

Presentation is variable. Opportunistic, disproportionately severe or recurrent infections, and specific forms of malignancy, all related to immunodeficiency, predominate. Lymphadenopathy, gut dysfunction and distinct neurological disturbances related to HIV infection of these tissues also occurs. The features at presentation are closely related to the peripheral blood CD4+ T cell count.

A number of well-characterised stages of disease are recognised. They are:

Primary infection Frequently symptomatic approximately 2–4 weeks post-infection. Usually vague 'flu-like' symptoms. Neurological inflammation occurs rarely. CD4+ T cell numbers fall, sometimes dramatically, while HIV-specific cytotoxic T cells increase, causing a reversal of the normal CD4:CD8 ratio. HIV replication is active and detectable ('viral load'). HIV antibodies, however, are not detectable for up to 3 months post-infection. Symptom severity, HIV viral load and CD4+ T cell count at the end of this period correlate with the rate of progression to more advanced stages.

Asymptomatic disease May persist for many years. Viral replication in lymphoid tissues persists and CD4 T cell numbers gradually decline.

Mildly symptomatic disease Lymphadenopathy, weight loss, fever, diarrhoea, mucocutaneous candidiasis *but not* AIDS-defining illnesses are seen.

Acquired immunodeficiency syndrome This is defined by the development of one of a number of specified infections or malignancies, or a CD4 count below 200/mm^3.

Important AIDS-defining illnesses and the approximate CD4+ T cell number at which they pose a threat include:

- *Pneumocystis carinii* pneumonia (PCP) <200/mm^3
- Pulmonary TB – 200–500/mm^3
- Cerebral toxoplasmosis – <100/mm^3
- CNS lymphoma – 100/mm^3
- Disseminated CMV infection – <50/mm^3.

Outlook depends on the presentation. PCP-related mortality is high if specific therapy is delayed. Cerebral toxoplasmosis is highly responsive to appropriate anti-microbial therapy. CNS lymphoma has a grave prognosis.

INVESTIGATIONS

Confirmation of infection relies on demonstration of HIV antibodies in peripheral blood [enzyme linked immunosorbent assay (ELISA)/immunoblot]. Detection of HIV antigen or RNA is useful in early infection, and in neonates. HIV testing should not be undertaken without appropriate counselling and informed written consent.

Surrogate markers of infection, for example, CD4 count/CD4:CD8 ratio should never be relied upon because these parameters can be normal in HIV infection and are abnormal in many other conditions.

Sequential monitoring of CD4 T cell counts and viral load is central to the management of patients with HIV infection. Both parameters guide therapeutic decisions about:

- Specific anti-HIV therapies
- Infection prophylactic therapies
- Effectiveness of anti-HIV drugs.

Patients with HIV should also be screened and monitored for other blood-borne infections (hepatitis viruses, CMV), sexually transmitted diseases (STDs) (syphilis, other STDs), and other common immunodeficiency-related infections (cryptococcus, toxoplasmosis). Chest X-ray for TB, cervical screening in women and proctoscopy in men are also recommended.

TREATMENT

HIV infection is not curable. Avoidance of infection is essential. Education programmes suitable for all at-risk populations (almost everyone) in all settings (developed and developing countries) cannot be over-emphasised.

Outlook in HIV-positive patients has improved dramatically by the availability of anti-retroviral agents that block viral replication. The main drug categories are:

◆ Reverse transcriptase inhibitors
◆ Protease inhibitors.

Several drug combinations providing highly active anti-retroviral therapy (HAART) are widely published, and are prescribed and monitored by specialists. Benefit is proven in advanced disease and in prevention of vertical transmission. There may be benefit in seroconverters, patients with a high viral load or rapidly falling CD4 count, and post-exposure prophylaxis. HAART is associated with improved immune function (reconstitution) and rising CD4+ T cell counts in responsive patients. Adverse side-effects (rashes, GI upsets, neuropathies, metabolic upsets) occur not infrequently and can require drug discontinuation. Other patients fail to respond or become resistant.

Chemoprophylaxis – administration of antimicrobial therapies to prevent specific infections is effective against some of the microbes. Cotrimoxazole to prevent PCP (CD4 count $<200/mm^3$) is the best-known example. HAART may allow discontinuation of chemoprophylactic regimes. HAART is extremely expensive and not available in most developing countries, limiting available therapy to chemoprophylaxis. In addition, good nutritional and psychological supports are important aspects of care for HIV-infected patients.

CROSS REFERENCE

Section 3.11   Immunodeficiency

Autoimmunity

Autoimmunity results from defective self-tolerance. Autoimmune reactivity describes detectable autoantibodies or autoreactive T cells, but disease is not necessarily present. Autoimmune disease occurs when the immune system targets self tissues or organs resulting in dysfunction. Autoimmune disease may involve a single organ (organ specific autoimmune disease), or may result in multisystem disease (non-organ-specific autoimmune disease). Twin studies indicate an important genetic component in the pathogenesis of autoimmunity; however, autoimmune diseases also have significant environmental influences. The genetic diathesis in the pathogenesis of autoimmunity means that a personal or family history of one autoimmune disease increases the risk of other autoimmune disorders. Autoimmune disease is more common in premenopausal women, suggesting hormonal influences. In some conditions women may experience catamenial exacerbation of symptoms (symptoms vary with the menstrual cycle). Several types of organ specific autoimmune disease are discussed in Sections 2.15–2.21 and common non-organ specific disorders are described in Sections 2.22–2.24.

INDUCTION OF AUTOIMMUNE DISEASE

Mechanisms of induction of autoimmunity have been outlined in Section 1.28, and are summarised in Table 2.14.1. Refer to individual sections for further detail.

Kawasaki syndrome is a vasculitis, usually seen in children, characterised by inflammation of medium-sized vessels with a predilection for coronary arteries. Patients develop prolonged fever, conjunctivitis, mucositis, cervical lymphadenopathy, rash and desquamation of the hands and feet. The disease often follows *Staphylococcal* or *Streptococcal* infections, leading to the hypothesis that immune activation by bacterial superantigens plays a pathogenic role. Aneurysm formation particularly in coronary vessels is a serious complication. Early treatment with high dose IVIg and aspirin reduces the risk of aneurysm formation.

Table 2.14.1 Mechanisms of autoimmunity

MECHANISM	EXAMPLE	COMMENTS
Molecular mimicry	Rheumatic fever	Section 2.25
Release of sequestered antigen	Sympathetic ophthalmia	Section 1.27
Cryptic epitopes	SLE	Section 2.23
Altered self	Drug-induced SLE	Section 2.23
	Drug-induced haemolytic anaemia	Section 2.16
Polyclonal activation by superantigen	Kawasaki syndrome	Section 2.24
Antigen presentation by infected organs	? viral infection of islets in insulin-dependent diabetes mellitus	Section 2.15
Genetic defect in immune-regulatory molecule	AIRE mutation (Type I autoimmune polyendocrinopathy)	Section 2.15

Figure 2.14.1 The presence of autoantibodies does not invariably imply a pathogenic role.

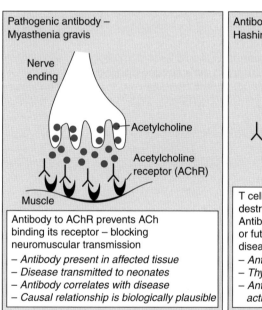

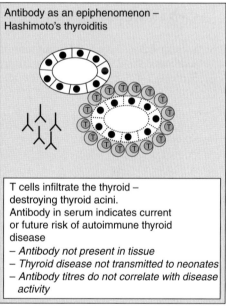

AUTOANTIBODIES

Autoimmune disease may result from Types II, III or IV hypersensitivity, or combinations of these mechanisms. Autoantibodies are produced in many autoimmune diseases, but their presence does not imply a pathogenic role (Figure 2.14.1). Establishing that an antibody is pathogenic requires demonstration of:

♦   The presence of antibody in the diseased organ
♦   Disease transfer across the placenta or to animals following antibody infusion

- Correlation of antibody level with disease activity
- Biological plausibility.

Autoantibodies play a pathogenic role in conditions including autoimmune haemolytic anaemia, anti-GBM disease, myasthenia gravis and some autoimmune blistering skin diseases. Autoantibodies may contribute to tissue injury in several other conditions. However, even as epiphenomena, autoantibodies frequently provide valuable diagnostic tests.

Most autoimmune diseases result in inflammation, and in non-organ specific autoimmune disease, an acute phase response is detectable (increased ESR or CRP, and polyclonal hypergammaglobulinaemia). Immune complex deposition diseases (Type III hypersensitivity disorders) are characterised by immune complex deposition and complement activation, resulting in complement consumption. Serial measurement of complement levels are of value. Complement components are also acute phase reactants and the effects of inflammation (raising levels) may mask the effects of consumption (reduced levels). Hence results must be interpreted with caution. Measurement of organ dysfunction is essential in diagnosis, assessment of extent of non-organ specific autoimmune disease, as well as monitoring disease activity and response to therapy.

CROSS REFERENCES

Section 1.28	Autoimmunity
Sections 2.15–2.24	Various common autoimmune disorders
Sections 3.4–3.8	Autoantibodies useful in diagnosis of autoimmune disorders

Autoimmune Endocrinopathies

Organ specific autoimmune disease can affect any endocrine gland, however, the thyroid is most commonly affected. Patients with autoimmune endocrine disease also have an increased prevalence of other organ specific and non-organ specific autoimmune disorders, reflecting an underlying predisposition to autoimmunity. There are well-described polyglandular syndromes where several autoimmune endocrinopathies occur, with or without non-endocrine features. Some of these are heritable and a genetic defect in an immunoregulatory molecule (Autoimmune regulator, AIRE) is known to be the basis of autoimmune polyendocrinopathy syndrome Type I. Treatment of autoimmune endocrinopathies is by replacement of hormone deficiency resulting from gland destruction. Immunosuppression is not routinely used.

AUTOIMMUNE THYROID DISEASE

Autoimmune thyroid disease can cause:

* Goitre (enlargement of the thyroid gland)
* Hypothyroidism (thyroxine deficiency)
* Hyperthyroidism (excessive production of thyroxine).

Thyroid autoreactivity also occurs in patients who have thyroiditis, and thyroid cancer.

Hashimoto's thyroiditis

This is a lymphocytic thyroiditis of unknown cause, initially causing hyperthyroidism (often subclinical), followed by hypothyroidism when thyroid destruction has occurred. Older women are frequently affected, and goitre is common. Associated autoimmune disease is common.

Gland destruction is due to cellular mechanisms, however, 90% of patients have high-titre antibodies to thyroid peroxidase (TPO), providing a useful diagnostic test.

Antibodies to thyroglobulin are only found in the absence of anti-thyroid peroxidase in about 1% of patients.

Graves' disease

Graves' disease usually presents with hyperthyroidism and goitre. Females are predominantly affected. The majority of patients have anti-TPO antibodies, which are useful indicators of the autoimmune process, but are not pathogenic. Graves' disease has a clear genetic predisposition, with concordance in identical twins of 30%.

Stimulating antibodies to the TSH receptor and growth promoting antibodies, which bind the insulin-like growth factor receptor, play a pathogenic role. Transplacental transfer of stimulating antibodies may cause neonatal hyperthyroidism.

Graves' disease may be associated with exophthalmos, due to inflammation in retro-orbital fat and connective tissue. Different autoantibodies to unidentified antigens in connective tissue are implicated. Thyroid acropachy may also be seen.

Diagnosis is based on clinical findings, thyroid function tests and imaging, and anti-thyroid antibodies. Remission can be induced using anti-thyroid drugs. If relapse occurs, definitive treatment with surgery or radiolabelled iodine is undertaken. Immuno-suppression is not used for the thyroid disease, but may be necessary in severe eye disease, if this becomes sight-threatening.

Thyroiditis and other thyroid disease

Thyroiditis may be due to infection of the thyroid or unidentified causes. The resulting granulomatous inflammation causes a painful goitre and abnormal thyroid function. Patients often have weakly positive anti-thyroid antibodies.

Thyroiditis can occur in pregnancy, usually causing hyperthyroidism, followed by hypothyroidism before finally resolving. Thyroiditis may be associated with post-natal depression. Anti-thyroid antibodies found during pregnancy are predictive of hypo-thyroidism during or after the pregnancy.

Thyroid antibodies are found in non-immune thyroid disease, including thyroid cancer, probably produced secondary to thyroid damage. The presence of anti-thyroid antibodies in patients with thyroid nodules is not an indication of autoimmune disease.

INSULIN-DEPENDENT DIABETES MELLITUS

Insulin-dependent diabetes mellitus (IDDM) or Type I DM results from autoimmune destruction of the islets of Langerhans, leading to insulin deficiency. Genetic predisposition is significant with 50% concordance in identical twins. Unusually, males and females are at equal risk. Several HLA-types contribute to genetic susceptibility, while possession of DR2 appears to be protective. Environmental factors implicated in genetically susceptible individuals include viral infections.

Destruction of the islets is primarily mediated by cytotoxic T cells, however, autoanti-bodies to islets, glutamic acid decarboxylase (GAD) and insulin are detectable before, and 1–2 years following onset of disease. Interestingly there is sequence homology between GAD-67 (the pancreatic isozyme) and coxsackie viruses, one of the infections epidemio-logically linked to IDDM.

IDDM is diagnosed by demonstrating elevated glucose. Autoantibodies are not useful at diagnosis or in establishing prognosis. However, in patients with other autoimmune dis-ease, anti-islet antibodies indicate current or future risk of developing IDDM. IDDM is associated with coeliac disease, and anti-endomysial antibodies should be measured, even in the absence of gastrointestinal symptoms.

Aggressive immunosuppression at the onset of disease or in antibody-positive siblings can delay the need for insulin therapy. However, the toxicity and risks of therapy greatly exceed the benefits. In the future, tolerogenic therapies for people at high risk of IDDM may become a reality.

ADDISON'S DISEASE

In the developed world, the commonest cause of adrenal destruction is autoimmune adrenalitis, however, on a worldwide basis tuberculosis remains the most common cause. Other infections, malignancy, sarcoidosis and haemorrhage also cause hypoadrenalism.

Destruction of the adrenal is due to cellular responses, however, autoantibodies are produced in about 80% of patients and are useful in confirming the diagnosis. Occasionally anti-adrenal antibodies can be detected in patients with hypoadrenalism for other causes, including up to 5% of patients with malignancy. There is a clinical association with ovarian failure and anti-ovarian antibodies should also be requested.

OVARIAN AUTOIMMUNITY

Premature ovarian failure occurs in 1% of women. This is associated with autoimmune polyglandular syndrome in 20% of cases. Antibodies to ovarian tissue and often adrenal gland are detectable. Autoimmune ovarian failure can occur in the absence of other autoimmune endocrine disease, however, there is a future risk of other autoimmune endocrinopathies.

Table 2.15.1 Features of autoimmune polyglandular syndromes

TYPE	DIAGNOSTIC FEATURES	COMMONLY ASSOCIATED AUTOIMMUNE DISORDERS	INHERITANCE AND MOLECULAR BASIS	COMMENTS
Type I PGA or APECED	Addison's disease, hypoparathyroidism, chronic mucocutaneous candidiasis	Chronic active hepatitis; GI involvement with malabsorption; pernicious anaemia; alopaecia; primary hypogonadism	Most autosomal recessive. Some autosomal dominant. Mutation in *AIRE* gene	Onset usually in childhood; male predominance
Type II PGA; Schmidt syndrome	Addisons disease and autoimmune thyroid disease and/or IDDM	Gonadal failure; other features of PGA I rare	Autosomal dominant, variable penetrance or multifactorial	Typically middle aged women. Do not develop hypoparathyroidism or candidiasis
Type III PGA	Autoimmune thyroid disease and one or more autoimmune disorders		Unknown	Do not develop Addison's disease

POLYGLANDULAR AUTOIMMUNE SYNDROME (PGA)

Multiple autoimmune endocrinopathies occur, sometimes associated with non-endocrine autoimmune disease. Three distinct patterns are described, and are summarised in Table 2.15.1.

CROSS REFERENCES	
Section 1.28	Autoimmunity
Section 2.14	Autoimmunity
Section 3.7	Autoantibodies Associated with Endocrine Diseases and Pernicious Anaemia

REFERENCES

Anderson, M. A. (2002) 'Autoimmune endocrine disease', *Curr. Opin. Immunol.*, 14: 760–4.

Autoimmune polyendocrinopathy syndrome, Type I, Entry # 240300 and Schmidt syndrome, Entry # 269200.

Online Mendelian Inheritance in Man (OMIM) www.ncbi.nlm.nih.gov/Omim/searchomim.html

Immune-mediated Haematological Conditions

Autoimmunity can cause autoimmune cytopaenias, aplastic anaemia and even thrombophilia. Autoimmune haematological disorders can occur in isolation or as components of a systemic autoimmune disorder.

IMMUNE-MEDIATED THROMBOCYTOPAENIA

Immune-mediated thrombocytopaenia (ITP) may be alloimmune or autoimmune. Alloimmune thrombocytopaenia is rare and affects babies of women sensitised to platelet antigens by transfusion or previous pregnancy. Maternal antibody to platelet antigens not expressed by the mother crosses the placenta and damages fetal platelets. ITP is much more common, resulting from autoantibodies against platelets.

ITP may be:

* An isolated abnormality
* In association with autoimmune haemolytic anaemia (Evans syndrome)
* Part of systemic autoimmune disorders such as SLE
* Due to immune dysregulation complicating immunodeficiency (e.g. CVID)
* Associated with lymphoid malignancy (e.g. CLL)
* Associated with infections (e.g. HIV).

ITP is characterised by a low platelet count, and decreased platelet survival as antibody-coated platelets are removed by the reticuloendothelial system. Megakaryocyte numbers in the bone marrow are increased in a compensatory effort. Patients can present at any age with unexplained bleeding and petechiae.

Diagnosis of ITP is based on the platelet count, bone marrow findings and sometimes the presence of anti-platelet antibodies. Exclusion of infection, immunodeficiency, malignancy and systemic disease is essential. Effective treatments include steroids, anabolic steroids, immunosuppression, high dose IVIg (short-term effect only), cytotoxic agents (to reduce antibody production) and splenectomy (to reduce removal of platelets from circulation).

ANTIBODY-MEDIATED HAEMOLYTIC ANAEMIA

Antibody-mediated haemolytic anaemia includes:

+ Alloimmune haemolytic anaemia
+ Drug-induced haemolytic anaemia
+ Autoimmune haemolytic anaemia.

Red blood cells (RBCs) are vulnerable to complement-mediated lysis as, unlike nucleated cells, they are unable to repair their cell membrane following insertion of the membrane attack complex. Antibody-coated RBCs may also be removed by the reticuloendothelial system. Antibodies to RBCs may be detected by the direct and indirect Coomb's tests.

Alloimmune haemolysis

This complicates ABO incompatible transfusion and preformed isohaemagglutinins lead to potentially fatal massive haemolysis. Rhesus disease of the newborn occurs when maternal anti-D from a sensitised Rhesus-negative mother crosses the placenta and damages Rhesus-positive RBCs in the foetus. Rhesus-negative mothers develop anti-Rhesus antibodies in response to transfusions or pregnancies. Sensitisation following pregnancy is prevented by giving Rhesus-negative mothers anti-D, destroying Rhesus-positive cells before an immune response is generated.

Drug-induced haemolysis

This occurs by three different mechanisms:

+ Drug binds to the RBC acting as a hapten. Anti-drug antibodies bind the drug and incidentally destroy the RBC. Haemolysis usually stops once the drug is withdrawn.
+ RBCs may be destroyed as innocent bystanders. Protein bound drug in the vicinity of the RBC is bound by antibody and complement activation leads to destruction of the nearby RBC.
+ Some drugs such as methyldopa can trigger a true autoimmune haemolytic anaemia, which persists for months despite drug withdrawal.

Autoimmune haemolytic anaemia

Autoimmune haemolytic anaemia (AIHA) is divided into warm and cold types, depending on whether the pathogenic antibody is functional at 4°C or 37°C (Table 2.16.1).

Warm AIHA often runs a relapsing-remitting course, and may be associated with splenomegaly. Treatment includes removal or treatment of any underlying cause, steroids, cytotoxics, high dose IVIg and possibly splenectomy.

Cold AIHA usually presents with haemolysis aggravated by cold, often associated with Raynaud's phenomenon. Infection associated cases may be transient. Treatment includes treatment of the underlying cause, keeping the patient warm and occasionally alkylating agents.

IMMUNE-MEDIATED NEUTROPAENIA

Alloimmune neutropaenia can result from transplacental transfer of maternal antibody. Autoimmune neutropaenia may occur in isolation or more commonly as part of a systemic

Table 2.16.1 Classification of autoimmune haemolytic anaemia

WARM AIHA	COLD AIHA
Idiopathic	Idiopathic
Secondary	Secondary
SLE and other CTDs	Infections (mycoplasma, EBV)
B cell malignancy	Lymphoproliferative disease
Common variable	Paroxysmal cold haemaglobinuria
immunodeficiency	(Donath–Landsteiner antibody) – may
Drugs (e.g. methyldopa)	be associated with syphilis

Figure 2.16.1 Antibody-mediated haemopoietic cell destruction.

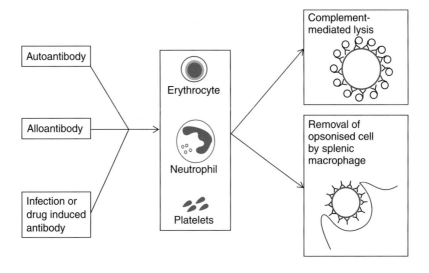

autoimmune disorder (e.g. SLE) or secondary to infection, drugs, lymphoproliferative disorders or immunodeficiency. Bone marrow examination shows increased numbers of myeloid precursors and anti-neutrophil antibody (either free or neutrophil bound) may be demonstrated by flow cytometry.

High dose IVIg may be of value but is less effective than in ITP. Splenectomy may be necessary. Antibiotic prophylaxis and G-CSF may be used to decrease the risk associated with profound neutropaenia (Figure 2.16.1).

APLASTIC ANAEMIA

Aplastic anaemia (AA) causes reductions in all three cell lines and the bone marrow appears empty. AA occurs in response to toxins including drugs, infections or may be idiopathic. Many idiopathic cases are due to a cellular immune response against haematological precursors. This may respond to ATG and cyclosporin. Bone marrow transplantation may be curative.

ANTIPHOSPHOLIPID SYNDROME

Antiphospholipid syndrome (APS) is an immune-mediated cause of thrombophilia. Antibodies against negatively charged phospholipids involved in the coagulation cascade induce a prothrombotic state. Antibody binding to the phospholipid cardiolipin is dependent on the presence of a co-factor called β_2-glycoprotein 1. β_2-glycoprotein 1 is an anticoagulant, and its inhibition may contribute to the procoagulant state.

APS may occur in isolation (primary APS) or associated with connective tissue disease, usually SLE (secondary APS). Establishing a diagnosis of APS requires clinical and laboratory criteria.

Laboratory criteria include:

* Moderate or strong IgG or IgM anti-cardiolipin antibody in a β_2-glycoprotein 1 dependent assay.
* Lupus anticoagulant.

The laboratory abnormality must be demonstrated on two occasions, at least 8 weeks apart. Many patients are positive for both lupus anticoagulant and anti-cardiolipin antibodies, 10% are positive in one test only.

Clinical criteria for the diagnosis include:

* Vascular thrombosis, venous or arterial, in the absence of another cause.
* Pregnancy associated morbidity, including early delivery of a baby before 32 weeks because of severe pre-eclampsia or intrauterine growth retardation; pregnancy loss due to miscarriage or intrauterine death in the second or third trimester; three first trimester miscarriages.

Other clinical features of APS include thrombocytopaenia, livedo reticularis, transverse myelopathy and migraine. However, these features are not specific enough to be diagnostic criteria.

Treatment consists of high dose aspirin or life long anticoagulation in patients who have experienced thrombotic complications. Management of pregnancy is particularly challenging, requiring self-administration of heparin (warfarin is teratogenic) together with very close monitoring of the pregnancy. Immunosuppressive therapy is not routinely indicated for APS, but may be used in specific circumstances under the guidance of a specialist.

CROSS REFERENCES

Autoimmune Liver Diseases

Chronic hepatitis is defined as persistent lymphoid inflammation of portal tracts, liver lobules, or bile ducts (intrahepatic and/or extrahepatic) lasting more than 6 months. Progression to cirrhosis and liver failure occurs in many cases. Predisposition to hepatocellular carcinoma is a feature in some patients. Many factors are implicated in causation. These include:

◆ Infections (Hepatitis B and C viruses)
◆ Toxins (most notably alcohol; some drugs)
◆ Metabolic/genetic (haemachromatosis; Wilson's disease; alpha-1 antitrypsin deficiency).

Autoimmunity is implicated in a number of important clinical entities. Specific patterns of autoantibody reactivity, association with other autoimmune conditions and, in the case of chronic autoimmune hepatitis (CAH), good responses to steroid therapy are characteristic.

AUTOIMMUNE (CHRONIC ACTIVE) HEPATITIS

Clinical features

This is predominantly a disorder of young and middle-aged women. Symptoms of acute but persisting hepatitis (jaundice, malaise, profound tiredness) are common. Clinical recovery followed by later relapse occurs, but about half of patients continue to manifest clinical features of ongoing inflammation. Some patients present for the first time with features of hepatic compromise indicating cirrhosis (bleeding varices, ascites, encephalopathy).

Characteristically, extrahepatic features are present. Arthralgia, autoimmune endocrine disease, immune-mediated haematological disorders, inflammatory bowel disease and vitiligo are all described.

Laboratory diagnosis

Elevated transaminases and hypergammaglobulinaemia (IgG mainly) are typical findings. Hepatitis virus screening is negative as are tests for other aetiological factors as outlined above. Lymphoid inflammation of varying extent and severity with features of established cirrhosis is seen on biopsy material. Distinct patterns of autoantibody positivity are highly supportive of the diagnosis. A number of sub-types are now recognised based on the precise patterns of autoantibodies detected.

Type 1 – Autoimmune 'lupoid' hepatitis

This sub-type represents the classical form of autoimmune hepatitis and is also called lupoid hepatitis because of the prevalence of extrahepatic features common in SLE (e.g. arthralgia). Lupoid also refers to the usual finding of high titres of ANA. High titre smooth muscle antibodies and ds-DNA antibodies are also detected. Most cases occur in women and presentation in the thirties is usual.

Type 2 – LKM hepatitis

Antibodies to liver/kidney microsomes (LKM) are seen in some patients with autoimmune CAH where the typical ANA/smooth muscle autoantibody pattern is absent. This antibody interacts specifically with cytochrome P450. This pattern tends to occur in cases presenting in childhood. Girls are predominantly affected. Extrahepatic manifestations are prominent and progression is rapid.

Type 3 – CAH

Soluble liver antibodies (anti-SLA) distinguish this type of CAH. Less commonly, ANA and anti-smooth muscle antibodies are detected. Adult women are again predominantly affected. Characteristically, extrahepatic manifestations are not common.

Type 4 – CAH

This refers to cases of CAH where anti-mitochondrial antibody reactivity coexists. The latter antibody is found in high titres in most cases of primary biliary cirrhosis – a condition discussed later in this section. Outlook in these patients is less clear than in classical autoimmune hepatitis but is probably poorer.

Treatment

Control of inflammation and support of liver function are the mainstays of therapy.

- Steroids are effective, although variation in responsiveness of the different sub-types may occur. More detailed studies are required to identify best therapy options for each subtype.
- Azathioprine is commonly used as a steroid sparing agent with good effect. Other immunosuppressants like Cyclosporin A are less commonly used.
- Liver failure regime and even liver transplantation may be required in patients with progressive decompensation.

Case 2.17.1 Autoimmune hepatitis

A 30-year-old woman presented with a 6-month history of fatigue and joint pains. For the preceding 4 weeks she had upper abdominal pain and nausea, as well as pruritis. On examination her liver was enlarged and tender. Her GP suspected that she may have liver disease, and liver function tests suggested hepatitis with serum transaminases over 10 times the upper limit of normal. Alkaline phosphatase was only mildly elevated.

Further investigations showed a strongly positive anti-smooth muscle antibody, together with a positive ANA and marked polyclonal hypergammaglobulinaemia (IgG 28 g/l). Viral studies were negative. A liver biopsy showed periportal inflammation with lymphocytes and plasma cells present, together with necrosis of hepatocytes. A diagnosis of autoimmune hepatitis Type I was made.

Treatment with corticosteroids and azathioprine was commenced. Within one month she felt much better and liver function tests had improved considerably. Liver chemistry and immunoglobulins (Igs) were normal after 3 months. Steroid therapy was gradually tapered over the following months and azathioprine was continued to reduce the risk of relapse.

Cross references

Section 4.2   Corticosteroids
Section 4.3   Immunosuppression (I)

PRIMARY BILIARY CIRRHOSIS

Clinical features

Primary biliary cirrhosis (PBC) is a condition of middle-aged and older women. The pathological lesion is one of progressive destructive fibrosing inflammation in the intrahepatic bile ducts leading to cholestasis and eventual cirrhosis. Tiredness and intractable itch are marked features. Progression is associated with features of hyperlipidaemia, fat-soluble vitamin deficiencies (e.g. osteoporosis due to vitamin D deficiency) and eventual cirrhosis and decompensation. PBC is associated with other autoimmune conditions, most notably Sjögren's syndrome, CREST variant of scleroderma and autoimmune thyroid disease.

Laboratory findings

An elevated alkaline phosphatase level is the dominant biochemical disturbance at presentation and is a persisting feature. Variable elevations in transaminases and other evidence of hepatic decompensation occur with progression. Hypergammaglobulinaemia, mainly IgM, is common. Most patients have detectable mitochondrial antibodies (AMA) by IIF and this is a highly useful diagnostic tool. There are many subtypes of AMA but the M2 subtype is typical in PBC. The target antigen is the E2 component of pyruvate dehydrogenase. The role of the antibody in pathogenesis is unclear. Antibody titres do not vary with progression.

Treatment

- Symptomatic relief of itch (cholestyramine), control of cholesterol (statin therapy, diet) and osteoporosis prevention (calcium and vitamin D supplements, exercise) are all important therapeutic interventions.
- Steroids are contraindicated because of the potential to worsen osteoporosis.
- Many immunosuppressive agents have been used but results are disappointing.
- Ursodeoxycholic acid, a bile acid, is widely used. Biochemical improvement is seen and rate of progression is slowed.
- Liver transplantation is the treatment of choice in advanced cases.

SCLEROSING CHOLANGITIS

Stricturing patchy inflammation of the intra- and extra-hepatic bile ducts with episodic cholangitis characterises this disorder. Progression to cirrhosis is typical. Cholangiocarcinoma occurs with increased frequency. There is a strong association with ulcerative colitis.

Biochemical findings are similar to those found in PBC. Mitochondrial antibodies are not found. An atypical ANCA is detected in some patients.

Immunosuppression is unhelpful. Ursodeoxycholic acid may improve outlook and is usually prescribed. Transplantation is indicated in patients with advanced hepatic dysfunction. This is contraindicated if cholangiocarcinoma has developed so detailed investigation to rule out this complication is needed in the pre-transplant work-up.

CROSS REFERENCES
Section 1.28   Autoimmunity
Section 2.14   Autoimmunity
Section 3.6   Autoantibodies Associated with Liver and Gastrointestinal Diseases

Immune-mediated Gastrointestinal Disorders

The gut is constantly exposed to food antigens and both commensal and pathogenic bacteria. In health, the distinct mucosal immune system tolerates innocuous antigens while also maintaining effective immunity against pathogens. Immunodeficiency, allergy, lymphoid malignancy and transplantation all affect the gut as outlined below.

IMMUNODEFICIENCY

- Infections – giardiasis, cryptosporidosis, salmonellosis, chronic enteroviral infections.
- Malabsorption/coeliac-like disorder.
- Inflammatory conditions – lymphoid hyperplasia; granulomatous enterocolitis.
- Malignancies – lymphoma and Kaposi Sarcoma; increased frequency of other gut tumours.

ALLERGIC DISORDERS

Ingested antigens affect allergic conditions in GIT and other systems (see Section 2.4).

LYMPHOID MALIGNANCY

- MALToma; immunodeficiency-related lymphomas; coeliac disease-associated T cell lymphoma.

TRANSPLANTATION

- Graft-versus-Host disease in allogeneic haematological transplantation.
- Immunosuppression-related gut infections.

SPECIFIC IMMUNE-MEDIATED GASTROINTESTINAL DISEASE

Atrophic gastritis and pernicious anaemia

Atrophic gastritis results in lymphocytic infiltration, mucosal atrophy, impaired acid production and deficiency of intrinsic factor. Autoreactive T cells damage the proton pump in gastric parietal cells (GPC). Anti-GPC antibodies, present in 90% of patients, are epiphenomena. Atrophic autoimmune gastritis is usually asymptomatic.

Atrophic gastritis may progress to pernicious anaemia (PA), if vitamin B_{12} absorption is compromised due to depletion of GPCs or the additional effect of anti-intrinsic factor (IF) antibodies, which block the action of IF. PA results in a megaloblastic anaemia and neurological complications (peripheral neuropathy, subacute combined degeneration and dementia), which can be reversed by regular parenteral vitamin B_{12} if treatment is initiated early.

PA is associated with other organ-specific autoimmune disease, particularly thyroid disease, as well as an increased risk of gastric cancer.

Coeliac disease

Coeliac disease results from a hypersensitivity reaction to gliadin (present in wheat, barley and rye glutens) occurring in the small intestine of genetically susceptible individuals. Predisposing factors include Celtic origin, positive family history, IgA deficiency, expression of a particular HLA haplotype (HLA-B8, DR3, DQ2), insulin-dependent diabetes mellitus and Down's syndrome. Prevalence in western European countries may be as high as one per hundred of the population.

Pathological changes are most marked in the proximal GIT and include lymphocytic inflammation and villous atrophy. Anti-endomysial and anti-tissue transglutaminase antibodies (>95%) and anti-gliadin antibodies (>50%) are typically present in serum.

The cause appears to be an abnormal immune response to gluten – gluten exposure is essential and gliadin-specific T cells appear in the small intestine within hours of gluten exposure.

Clinical presentation is variable:

- Failure to thrive; fatigue; weight loss
- Anaemia
- Osteoporosis, osteomalacia
- Infertility
- Recurrent aphthous ulceration
- Malabsorption
- Associated dermatitis herpetiformis
- Small bowel lymphoma (rarely)
- Hyposplenism
- Asymptomatic.

While originally described as a paediatric disease, coeliac disease is often diagnosed in adults, even in the elderly. The availability of serological tests, together with a higher awareness has improved detection.

Diagnosis requires a high index of suspicion. Serological tests for IgA anti-endomysial, anti-tissue transglutaminase, and anti-gliadin antibodies are useful. If IgA deficiency is present, serology is less helpful. Small bowel biopsy showing typical features remains the gold standard.

Treatment requires lifelong dietary exclusion of gluten. Failure to comply increases symptoms, as well as anaemia, osteoporosis and the risk of developing small bowel lymphoma. Supplements (iron, folate, vitamin D and calcium) may be required.

Inflammatory bowel diseases

Crohn's disease and Ulcerative Colitis (UC) are chronic, relapsing and remitting, inflammatory bowel diseases (IBD). There are distinct epidemiological, clinical and pathological features, however, in some patients it is difficult to differentiate Crohn's disease from UC.

IBDs are most prevalent in Western countries (combined incidence 15–20/100,000 population). Crohn's disease incidence continues to grow.

There are racial and genetic (high twin concordance; 10% have positive family history) risk factors. However, environmental triggers including diet and smoking appear to play a role.

Pathogenesis remains unclear, however, dysregulated inflammatory responses to antigens, possibly normal bowel flora, in genetically predisposed individuals is probably important. Unidentified persistent infection remains possible, but unlikely. Pro-inflammatory TH1-type cytokines like TNF-α mediate the inflammation of Crohn's disease.

Pathological features are distinct. Crohn's disease affects any part of the GIT from mouth to anus, often with a patchy distribution (skip-lesions); UC is limited to the colon and rectum, most severe distally with continuous proximal spreading. Stricture and fistula formation are highly suggestive of Crohn's disease. Crohn's inflammation is transmural with non-caseating granulomata and fibrosis. UC is limited to the mucosal layer and crypt abscesses are typical. Intermediate histological features occur sometimes making precise classification difficult.

Clinical presentation depends on the location and severity of inflammation. Common presenting features include diarrhoea, rectal bleeding, abdominal pain, peri-anal disease, fistulae, malnutrition and systemic upset due to inflammation. Extra-intestinal manifestations (sero-negative arthritis, uveitis, erythema nodosum, pyoderma gangrenosum, sclerosing cholangitis, aphthous ulceration) occur in both conditions. Long-standing UC can be complicated by colon cancer.

Diagnosis is based on clinical presentation together with endoscopic, radiological and histological findings. Haematological, biochemical and inflammatory markers help to monitor disease severity. P-ANCA (non-MPO) activity is detected in the serum of some IBD patients and may indicate those at increased risk of developing primary sclerosing cholangitis.

Treatment includes:

- Anti-inflammatory drugs – aminosalicylic acid derivatives and corticosteroids (topical and systemic).
- Immunomodulation – Azathioprine, 6-Mercaptopurine, Cyclosporin A and Methotrexate. Anti-TNF therapies (e.g. infliximab) have revolutionised management of severe Crohn's disease.
- Nutritional support, elemental diets for severe small bowel Crohn's disease.
- Probiotic microbes may play a role in prevention and treatment of IBD in the future.
- Antibiotics and surgery may be required.

CROSS REFERENCES

REFERENCES

Farrell, R. J. and Kelly, C. P. (2002) 'Celiac sprue', *N. Engl. J. Med.*, 346: 180–8.
Podolsky, D. K. (2002) 'Inflammatory bowel diseases', *N. Engl. J. Med.*, 347: 417–29.

Immune-mediated Neurological Disease

The brain is relatively isolated from the immune system by the blood brain barrier (BBB), which consists of endothelium with tight junctions, a basal lamina and perivascular end-feet of astrocytic processes. Functionally the BBB prevents large molecules and most cells from crossing cerebral vessels. BBB permeability increases at sites of inflammation, allowing entry of cells and plasma proteins.

The brain is poorly supplied by lymphatics, however, CNS antigens, and some glial cells with antigen presenting capabilities can exit the CNS, migrate to cervical lymph nodes, and elicit an immune response.

The brain, spinal cord and nerves are targets of several immune-mediated diseases. Some solely involve the CNS, however, neurological disease may occur in non-organ specific autoimmune disease such as SLE.

MYASTHENIA GRAVIS

In myasthenia gravis (MG), antibodies to the acetylcholine receptor (AChR) inhibit neuromuscular transmission, causing weakness and fatigability of muscles. Disease severity varies from weakness of orbital muscles, causing drooping of the eyelid and double vision, to profound weakness involving respiratory muscles that may be life threatening. Thymoma or thymic hyperplasia is often associated.

Table 2.19.1 Common immune-mediated neurological diseases

TYPE OF HYPERSENSITIVITY	EXAMPLES
Type I (IgE mediated)	Not relevant
Type II (antibody-mediated)	Myasthenia gravis
Type III (immune complex)	Systemic lupus erythematosus
Type IV (delayed hypersensitivity)	Multiple sclerosis

Anti-AChR antibodies are pathogenic and transplacental passage of anti-AChR causes transient disease in neonates. Antibodies bind the AChR, blocking receptor function. Anti-AChR also activates complement, resulting in internalisation of AChR and damage to the motor endplate.

Treatment of MG is usually with anticholinesterase drugs, which increase the amount of acetylcholine present at the motor endplate, improving impulse conduction, often with immunosuppression to reduce autoantibody production. Antibody removal by plasmapheresis is also useful.

SYSTEMIC LUPUS ERYTHEMATOSUS (SLE)

SLE is an immune complex deposition disease, discussed in detail in Section 2.23. Involvement of cerebral blood vessels can cause highly variable neurological symptoms including seizures, neuropsychiatric disorders and focal neurological signs.

MULTIPLE SCLEROSIS

Multiple sclerosis (MS) is an autoimmune disease in which episodes of inflammation occur in the CNS disseminated in time and place. MS may run a relapsing-remitting or progressive course. The effects of inflammation may be visualised as plaques on MRI scanning. Inflammation damages the myelin sheath around nerves, and demyelination slows nerve conduction causing symptoms. Inflammation and demyelination also lead to secondary axonal loss, leading to long-term disability. Suspected diagnosis is usually based on history and MRI appearances. Oligoclonal bands of immunoglobulin in the CSF support the diagnosis.

Attacks of MS may be shortened by treatment with high dose steroids, which reduce inflammation. IFN-β reduces the number and severity of attacks in a number of patients, through an unknown mechanism. IFN-β causes fever and flu-like symptoms, which many MS patients are unable to tolerate.

CROSS REACTIVITY AND IMMUNE-MEDIATED NEUROLOGICAL DISEASE

Several autoimmune disorders are thought to result from cross-reactivity between self-antigen and pathogens or tumours.

Guillain–Barré syndrome (GBS)

GBS is an inflammatory demyelinating polyneuropathy, thought to be due to cross-reactivity of gangliosides in nerves and bacteria, particularly *Campylobacter jejuni*. Anti-GM1 antibodies, frequently found in GBS, cross-react with lipopolysaccharides present in this microbe. GBS presents with ascending weakness, which may progress rapidly to involve respiratory and bulbar muscles. Sensory symptoms are mild, but autonomic involvement may be life-threatening. Most patients recover, often over months or years.

The progression of GBS may be halted by early treatment with plasmapheresis or high-dose immunoglobulin. Plasmapheresis is dangerous if autonomic instability is present and therefore immunoglobulin is more commonly used.

Chronic inflammatory demyelinating polyneuropathy

Chronic inflammatory demyelinating polyneuropathy (CIDP) is a chronic form of GBS. Diagnosis is based on history, neurophysiological demonstration of demyelination and exclusion of other causes of neuropathy. Autoantibodies to gangliosides are often present, however, a clear history of infection preceding onset is rare. Weakness is prominent but sensory symptoms can also be disabling. Treatment is usually with high-dose IVIg but may also include steroids, immunosuppressive agents, and plasmapheresis.

Cross-reactivity with tumours – paraneoplastic syndromes

Paraneoplastic syndromes are distant non-metastatic effects of tumours. Cerebellar degeneration causing ataxia is a frequent manifestation of these rare conditions, although varied presentations are described. Paraneoplastic neurological syndromes result from antibodies raised against neoantigens on tumour cells cross-reacting with brain tissue. The tumour is often very small – held in check by an aggressive immune response. However, this immune response causes severe neurological disease. Patients usually present with neurological disease and the tumour may only become apparent later or even at autopsy. Paraneoplastic syndromes are associated with tumours of lung, breast and ovary most commonly.

CROSS REFERENCES

Section 2.14   Autoimmunity
Section 4.9   High Dose Immunoglobulin Therapy
Section 4.12   Plasmapheresis and Plasma Exchange

Immune-mediated Skin Disease

Intact skin forms a natural barrier to infection. Skin contains specialised antigen presenting cells (APCs) (Langerhan's cells), which take up antigen and migrate to regional lymph nodes. While essential in fighting infection, this efficient capacity to present antigen to the immune system facilitates the development of hypersensitivity and autoimmune disease. Skin may be involved in many multisystem autoimmune diseases, and skin biopsy often with direct immunofluorescence provides an easy means to establish the diagnosis (Figure 2.20.1).

Skin involvement is common in some types of immunodeficiency – T cell defects result in viral and fungal eruptions, while neutrophil dysfunction may present with boils and abscesses. Many immunodeficiencies are associated with immune dysregulation, which may result in eczematous rashes.

IMMUNE-MEDIATED BLISTERING SKIN CONDITIONS

Pemphigus

Pemphigus vulgaris and pemphigus foliaceus are serious diseases characterised by intraepidermal blister formation. Autoantibodies react with components of the desmosome (adhesion complexes which maintain the integrity of the epidermis). Antibody binding results in complement activation, weakening the desmosome. Keratinocytes separate resulting in blister formation. Biopsy findings are of intraepidermal blister formation, while direct immunofluorescence shows linear staining with IgG and often C3 in a chicken wire pattern, surrounding keratinocytes. Indirect immunofluorescence (often using monkey oesophagus as a substrate) detects circulating antibody, and the antibody titre is useful for monitoring disease. Treatment is with high dose steroids and additional immunosuppression with an agent such as azathioprine.

Bullous pemphigoid

Bullous pemphigoid (BP) is a blistering disease, predominantly affecting elderly patients. Itchy tense blisters develop on the trunk and limbs, and mucous membranes are affected in

Table 2.20.1 Hypersensitivity and the skin

TYPE OF HYPERSENSITIVITY	EXAMPLES	COMMENT
Type I (IgE mediated)	Urticaria	Section 2.2
	Eczema	Section 2.1
Type II (cytotoxic antibody)	Pemphigus	
	Pemphigoid	
Type III (immune complex)	Lupus erythematosus	Section 2.23
	Dermatitis herpetiformis	
	Immune complex vasculitis	Section 2.24
Type IV (delayed hypersensitivity)	Contact dermatitis	

about 30%. Skin biopsy shows subepidermal blisters, and direct immunofluorescence (DIF) shows linear deposition of IgG, often with C3 along the dermoepidermal junction (DEJ). This autoantibody is thought to be pathogenic and is directed against components of the hemidesmosome, which anchors keratinocytes to the basement membrane. Antibody binding and resultant complement activation leads to an infiltration of neutrophils. Neutrophils discharge proteases, weakening the hemidesmosome, allowing subsequent blister formation. Antibodies are detected in serum in about 70% of patients, however, autoantibody titre does not reflect disease activity. Mild disease may respond to topical steroids, however, oral steroids often with additional immunosuppression are usually required.

Cicatricial pemphigoid

This is a mucosal variant of BP, which affects conjunctivae, oral mucosa and vaginal mucosa. Subepithelial fibrosis can occur. Systemic treatment is usually required.

Herpes gestationis

Herpes gestationis (HG) is a BP variant, occurring only in pregnancy and the puerperium. Linear C3 is found on DIF. The baby may be affected due to transplacental passage of antibody.

SKIN MANIFESTATIONS OF LUPUS ERYTHEMATOSUS

These may occur in isolation or associated with systemic disease. Skin manifestations include:

◆ Photosensitivity
◆ Butterfly rash associated with systemic disease
◆ Discoid lesions
◆ Subacute cutaneous lupus (skin lesions, photosensitivity and often anti-Ro and anti-La antibodies).

Skin biopsy helps to confirm the nature of skin-limited disease, and over 50% of patients with chronic lesions are found to have granular deposition of immunoglobulins (varying isotypes) usually with complement along the dermoepidermal junction.

DERMATITIS HERPETIFORMIS

Dermatitis herpetiformis (DH) is an intensely itchy, blistering disease, involving extensor surfaces, often associated with coeliac disease or subclinical gluten sensitivity. Skin biopsy demonstrates accumulations of neutrophils in the papillary tips. Direct immunofluorescence shows deposits of IgA and occasionally C3 and/or fibrin in the papillary tips. Anti-endomysial antibodies are present in up to 70% of patients. DH may respond to gluten withdrawal or treatment with dapsone.

IMMUNE COMPLEX VASCULITIS

This condition usually presents with palpable purpura but occasionally with urticarial lesions or angioedema. Immune complexes deposited in dermal blood vessels activate complement and attract neutrophils. Histological examination of a fresh lesion shows vasculitis (inflammation of the vessel wall), leucocytoclasis (breakdown of neutrophils) and fibrinoid necrosis of the vessel wall. DIF shows granular deposits of immunoglobulins and complement in vessel walls. Causes include Type III hypersensitivity to drugs, infection including bacterial endocarditis, connective tissue diseases and cryoglobulinaemia.

Figure 2.20.1 Immune-mediated skin disorders: direct immunofluorescence.

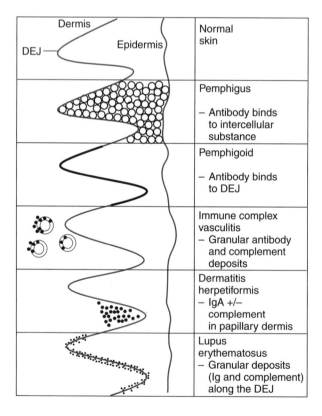

Note: See Figure 3.17.1 for DIF plates.

CONTACT DERMATITIS

This condition is due to delayed hypersensitivity to allergens adsorbed to keratinocytes. These allergens frequently act as haptens, forming neoantigens, which are taken up by Langerhan's cells, and transported to regional lymph nodes where they activate T cells. The expanded clones of allergen-reactive T cells migrate to skin and activate macrophages as well as releasing proinflammatory cytokines. The diagnosis may be made on the clinical appearance of the rash and its distribution, as well as a careful history of exposure to possible sensitisers. Patch testing is then used to confirm the putative causative agents, and avoidance measures determined.

CROSS REFERENCES

Section 1.29 Hypersensitivity
Section 2.1 Clinical Manifestations of Atopy
Section 2.3 Urticaria and Angioedema
Section 3.8 Other Organ-specific Autoimmunity

Immune-mediated Renal Disease

Immune-mediated renal disease may be isolated or result from kidney involvement in systemic disease. Clinically, kidney disease presents with:

- Renal impairment – kidneys fail to clear waste material normally. Renal impairment (or failure) may be acute or chronic, and result from pre-renal, renal or post-renal causes.
- Haematuria which may be frank (visible to the patient) or microscopic (only detectable on urinalysis).
- Nephritic syndrome – haematuria, hypertension and oliguria (reduced urinary output).
- Proteinuria.
- Nephrotic syndrome – proteinuria (>3g/24 hours), hypoalbuminaemia and oedema.

No type of presentation is specific for immunological disease. All types of hypersensitivity can cause renal disease (Table 2.21.1). Renal biopsy is often required to establish the diagnosis, and in suspected immunological disease a portion of the biopsy should be frozen for direct immunofluorescence examination.

Allergic interstitial nephritis may result from an infection or drug exposure (NSAIDs and antibiotics commonly). Connective tissue diseases can also cause interstitial nephritis. An underlying cause is not always identified. Fever, rash and eosinophilia may be present. Haematuria, pyuria and white cell casts in the urine may precede renal impairment. Eosinophils may also be present in the urinary sediment. Histological examination of renal tissue shows a mononuclear infiltrate with eosinophilia associated with tubular injury. Antibody deposition may be seen along the tubular basement membrane. The essential aspect of treatment is discontinuation of the offending drug, and corticosteroids may be helpful.

Goodpasture's disease is a classic antibody-mediated disease. Antibodies to glomerular basement membrane (GBM) bind to glomeruli, activate complement and cause severe glomerular inflammation, resulting in severe crescentic glomerulonephritis. Clinically rapidly progressive renal failure with haematuria ensues. Antibodies to GBM can bind to pulmonary basement membrane, causing pulmonary haemorrhage. When suspected, anti-GBM are measured as an emergency. Treatment includes plasmapheresis to remove antibodies rapidly, corticosteroids and potent immunosuppression with cyclophosphamide.

Table 2.21.1 Mechanisms of immune-mediated renal diseases

MECHANISM	EXAMPLES
Type I hypersensitivity (? + other)	Allergic interstitial nephritis
Type II hypersensitivity	Goopasture's disease
Type III hypersensitivity	IgA nephropathy
	Membranous nephropathy
	Membranoproliferative GN
	Post-infectious glomerulonephritis
	Lupus nephritis
Type IV hypersensitivity	Acute cellular transplant rejection
Other	ANCA-associated focal segmental necrotising glomerulonephritis

Case 2.21.1 Pulmonary renal syndrome

A 28-year-old male smoker complained of breathlessness and cough productive of blood-stained sputum. He had been unwell for 3 weeks, and his GP arranged for urgent admission to hospital. While in the admissions unit he had a large haemoptysis of approximately 500 mls of blood. Chest X-rays showed alveolar shadowing in both lower lobes. Urinalysis revealed microscopic haematuria, and serum creatinine was raised at 130 μmols/l. Urgent measurement of anti-GBM (glomerular basement membrane) antibodies and ANCA (anti-neutrophil cytoplasmic antibody) demonstrated the presence of anti-GBM.

He was started on plasmapheresis together with cyclophosphamide and steroids. He continued to produce blood stained sputum for a further three days. By day 4, haematuria was reduced to a trace and serum creatinine had fallen to 80 μmols/l. Anti-GBM antibodies were no longer detectable. Plasmapheresis was stopped and the steroid dose was tapered. Cyclophosphamide was continued for several months and then azathioprine was given for a further year. He remained anti-GBM antibody negative, and had no recurrence of haemoptysis or haematuria.

Cross references

Section 4.4   Immunosuppression (II)
Section 4.12   Plasmapheresis and Plasma Exchange

IgA NEPHROPATHY

This is the commonest glomerular disease identified in native kidney biopsies. IgA-containing immune complexes (ICs) are deposited in the mesangium extending into capillary loops in severe disease (Figure 2.21.1). IgA deposits are usually associated with mild mesangial changes, however, occasionally crescents and severe glomerular inflammation are seen. Clinically, patients present with microscopic or frank haematuria. Proteinuria indicates severe

Figure 2.21.1 Patterns of immune complex deposition I.

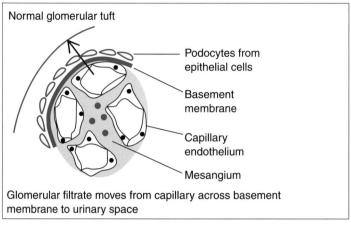

Normal glomerular tuft

Podocytes from epithelial cells

Basement membrane

Capillary endothelium

Mesangium

Glomerular filtrate moves from capillary across basement membrane to urinary space

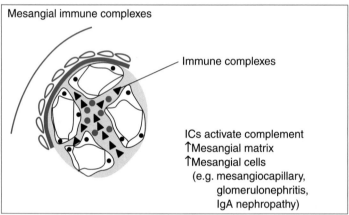

Mesangial immune complexes

Immune complexes

ICs activate complement
↑Mesangial matrix
↑Mesangial cells
(e.g. mesangiocapillary,
glomerulonephritis,
IgA nephropathy)

disease. Renal impairment can occur with progression to renal failure usually over many years. Severe disease can be treated with steroids and cytotoxic therapy, however, toxicity is significant. In mild disease management it is limited to blood pressure control with no specific therapy. Renal involvement in Henoch–Schönlein purpura is histologically indistinguishable from IgA nephropathy. IgA nephropathy can recur following transplantation.

MEMBRANOUS GLOMERULONEPHRITIS

Deposition of immune complexes on the epithelial side of the GBM is seen. Rapid urine flow washes away complement and chemoattractants, so an inflammatory response to ICs does not occur. Patients present with nephrotic syndrome, and renal impairment may progress slowly. Underlying causes include tumours, infections, drugs and SLE, however, most cases are idiopathic. Spontaneous remission may occur, particularly where a remediable cause is corrected. Some patients are treated with intensive steroids and chlorambucil, which is beneficial but highly toxic.

MEMBRANOPROLIFERATIVE GLOMERULONEPHRITIS

Three major types of *membranoproliferative glomerulonephritis* (MPGN) are described. MPGN Type I results from deposition of ICs predominantly on the endothelial side of the GBM while MPGN Type III is characterised by both subendothelial and subepithelial ICs. Complement activation results in marked inflammation. MPGN Type II is due to complement activation and deposition by an autoantibody, nephritic factor. MPGN is often idiopathic, but may be associated with chronic infection, complement deficiency, cryoglobulinaemia and some tumours. The clinical presentation may be nephritic syndrome, haematuria, incidental proteinuria or nephrotic syndrome. Low complement levels are typical. Most patients progress to renal failure, although at highly differing rates (Figure 2.21.2). Treatments include steroids and anti-platelet agents. MPGN frequently recurs in transplanted kidneys.

POST-INFECTIOUS GLOMERULONEPHRITIS

This may follow several bacterial, viral and parasitic infections, with post-streptococcal glomerulonephritis the best characterised example. Presentations vary from transient haematuria and proteinuria to nephritic syndrome and occasionally renal failure. ICs are deposited in the mesangium and subepithelial areas. C3 and IgG may be identified on DIF. Hypocomplementaemia is typical, and serological evidence of infection may be identified. When spontaneous recovery occurs, biopsy is unnecessary.

RENAL INVOLVEMENT IN SLE

This manifests as one of a variety of types of glomerulonephritis and is part of a systemic IC deposition disease. Lupus nephritis commonly shows a diffuse proliferative pattern like MPGN or a membranous pattern of injury.

ANCA-ASSOCIATED FOCAL NECROTISING GLOMERULONEPHRITIS

This condition may be renal-limited, or a manifestation of systemic disease. The mechanism of tissue injury remains to be fully elucidated, however, ANCA may play a pathogenetic role. Patients frequently develop rapidly progressive renal failure, however, the clinical course may be insidious. Haematuria is usually present in active disease. Renal biopsy shows a focal necrotising glomerulonephritis with crescents indicating severe glomerular injury. Immune deposits are not seen in renal tissue. When suspected, ANCA should be requested on an urgent basis as renal failure progresses rapidly. Early treatment with steroids, cyclophosphamide and occasionally plasmapheresis may reverse renal failure, even in patients who are dialysis-dependent.

Figure 2.21.2 Patterns of immune complex deposition II.

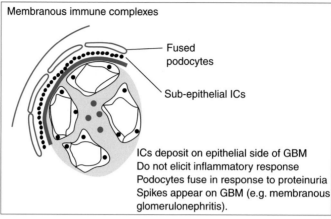

Membranous immune complexes

Fused podocytes

Sub-epithelial ICs

ICs deposit on epithelial side of GBM
Do not elicit inflammatory response
Podocytes fuse in response to proteinuria
Spikes appear on GBM (e.g. membranous glomerulonephritis).

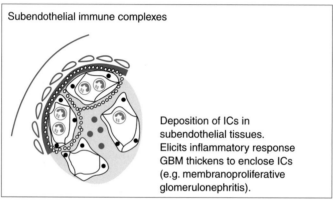

Subendothelial immune complexes

Deposition of ICs in subendothelial tissues.
Elicits inflammatory response
GBM thickens to enclose ICs
(e.g. membranoproliferative glomerulonephritis).

MINIMAL CHANGE DISEASE

This is the most common cause of nephrotic syndrome in children. Renal biopsy appears normal on light microscopy and direct immunofluorescence, however, fusion of podocytes is seen on electron microscopy. The disease is thought to be T cell mediated, and treatment with steroids is usually successful. If steroids fail, or relapse occurs after tapering steroids, cyclophosphamide or cyclosporin are used.

CROSS REFERENCES

Section 1.29   Hypersensitivity
Section 3.5   Autoantibodies Associated with Vasculitic Syndromes and Renal Diseases
Section 3.10   Complement
Section 3.17   Direct Immunofluorescence

Rheumatoid Disease and Spondylarthropathies

Rheumatoid disease (RA) is a multisystem disease, typically characterised by inflammatory arthritis. However, many organs may be affected, with or without joint involvement (Figure 2.22.1).

RA affects approximately 1% of Caucasian populations, with a higher prevalence in some Native American populations, and lower rates in oriental and rural African populations. Peak age of onset is uncertain and female : male ratio is 3 : 1. There is a well-recognised genetic predisposition, explained in part by expression of particular alleles of *DR4* and closely related *DR1* alleles. The disease-associated *HLA* alleles show close similarities in the antigen-binding groove, suggesting that all are capable of presenting identical or similar disease related peptide(s).

Typically RA is characterised by stiff inflamed joints, in a symmetrical pattern. Several joints, particularly the small joints of the hands are involved. Approximately 20% of patients have rheumatoid nodules in subcutaneous tissues, found over bony prominences. Up to 90% of subjects are rheumatoid factor (RF) positive, however, weakly positive RF is not specific for RA. Detection of antibodies against citrullinated peptides are promising as a tool in early diagnosis. X-rays of hands or other affected joints may show bony erosions.

RA can cause vasculitis (inflammation in blood vessels), and this complication may affect small blood vessels (usually associated with active arthritis), or medium-sized vessels (occurring even when joint disease is quiescent). A small proportion of patients with RA develop neutropaenia and splenomegaly, a triad known as Felty's syndrome. Pulmonary manifestations include pulmonary nodules (which are usually asymptomatic), pleural effusions, interstitial lung disease and bronchiolitis obliterans (a devastating scarring process in the small airways carrying a very poor prognosis). Ocular complications include dry eyes (usually indicating associated Sjögren's syndrome), episcleritis and scleritis (inflammation on the surface and in the sclera). Occasionally scleritis may be severe, resulting in scleromalacia and perforation of the orbit. As in other chronic inflammatory conditions, patients may develop amyloidosis, a non-inflammatory deposition of extracellular material resulting in organ dysfunction associated with a poor prognosis.

The pattern of progression of RA is variable. Arthritis may present abruptly or insidiously and may involve one or several joints at the outset. Occasionally patients may have

Figure 2.22.1 Clinical features of rheumatoid disease and spondylarthropathies.

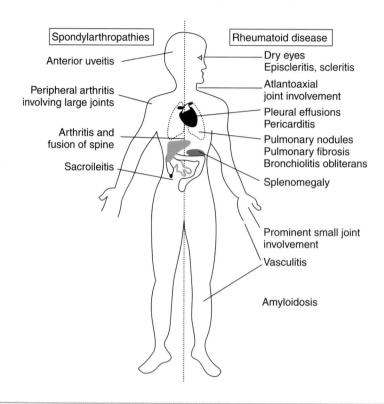

only extraarticular disease with no evidence of joint disease. The majority of patients follow a relapsing and remitting course, however, a small subgroup follows a relentless progressive course. Up to 20% of patients have a monocyclic disease followed by recovery.

Analgesic and anti-inflammatory drugs are used for symptom control. Immunosuppressing agents used either singly or in combination are a central component in disease control. Early intervention with such drugs is increasingly used. Cytokine blockade (anti-TNF-α, IL-1) is revolutionising treatment of RA.

The pathology of affected joints shows a chronic widespread synovitis with lymphocytic infiltration and evidence of macrophage activation.

The inflamed synovium gives rise to pannus, at the synovial interface with cartilage and bone. Pannus is unique to RA and is locally invasive, destroying cartilage and bone and giving rise to marginal erosions. Joint destruction is thought to be driven by T cell activation of macrophages. It remains controversial how much Type III hypersensitivity (resulting from immune complex formation by RF and normal Ig) contributes to joint damage (Figure 2.22.2). Rheumatoid vasculitis is thought to be primarily an immune complex mediated (Type III) process.

SPONDYLARTHROPATHIES

The spondylarthropathies are a group of seronegative (RF negative) inflammatory arthritides. Ankylosing spondylitis is the typical example, primarily affecting the spine and

Figure 2.22.2 Joint pathology in rheumatoid disease.

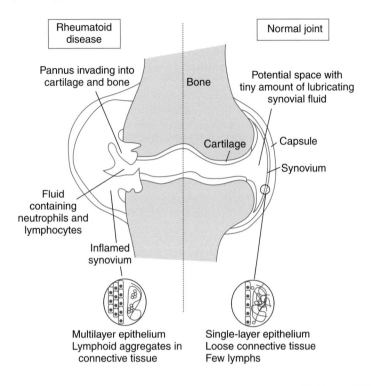

sacroiliac joints. Inflammation in the spine gradually progresses and results in fusion and deformity of the spine. Peripheral joints may also be involved. There is a striking association with expression of HLA-B27. Many patients have antibodies to *Klebsiella* species, suggesting previous infection, however, organisms are not isolated from the joint. The observation that anti-*Klebsiella* antibodies can bind HLA-B27 has raised interest in molecular mimicry as the possible mechanism for autoimmunity in this condition. However, cross reactivity with HLA-B27 cannot explain why the disease localises in the spine, sacroiliac joints and occasionally the eyes. Elucidating the mechanisms underlying this disorder will probably give considerable insights into autoimmunity.

Closely related spondylarthropathies include reactive arthritis, arthritis associated with inflammatory bowel disease, and a form of psoriatic arthritis. The spondylarthropathies may be associated with inflammation in the anterior chamber of the eye (anterior uveitis or iritis).

Reactive arthritis follows a gastrointestinal or genitourinary infection with organisms such as *Chlamydia, Campylobacter, Shigella* or *Yersinia*. As with ankylosing spondylitis, there is a striking association with HLA-B27. The association with infection and a particular HLA type again suggests some form of immune cross-reactivity, however this has not been conclusively demonstrated. In many patients, reactive arthritis resolves after several months, however, in others the disease follows a relapsing or chronic course. This suggests loss of self-tolerance, resulting in ongoing inflammation, even after elimination of the pathogen.

Case 2.22.1 Inflammatory polyarthritis

A 30-year-old woman developed pain, stiffness and swelling in the small joints of her hands. A few weeks later her wrists and feet became affected. Her GP prescribed nonsteroidal anti-inflammatory drugs (NSAIDs). Six weeks later she returned to her GP as her joints became more swollen. Blood tests showed a normochromic, normocytic anaemia, and raised erythrocyte sedimentation rate (ESR) and C-reactive protein (CRP) consistent with an inflammatory process. Rheumatoid factor was strongly positive, and anti-nuclear factor was also positive. Anti-double stranded deoxyribonucleic acid (DNA) and antibodies to extractable nuclear antigens were negative. Her GP prescribed stronger anti-inflammatory and referred her to a rheumatologist.

She was seen in the Rheumatology clinic, 6 months after her symptoms had begun. X-ray of her hands showed two erosions. A diagnosis of rheumatoid arthritis was made based on clinical findings, positive rheumatoid factor and erosions.

The presence of erosions and a strongly positive rheumatoid factor are poor prognostic factors, and her symptoms were not controlled on NSAIDs. She was commenced on methotrexate, an anti-rheumatic drug that reduces erosion formation. After six months on methotrexate, her symptoms continued to cause considerable discomfort and disability and an anti-TNF monoclonal antibody was commenced. After three infusions there was a dramatic improvement in pain and stiffness, and she was able to resume all normal activities. Acute phase markers returned to normal. She continues to get maintenance infusions of anti-TNF less frequently. Methotrexate was continued for its anti-rheumatic effect and to reduce the risk of developing anti-chimeric antibodies.

Cross reference

Section 4.7   Other Antibody Therapies

CROSS REFERENCES

Section 1.28   Autoimmunity
Section 3.4   Autoantibody Profiles in Connective Tissue Diseases and Rheumatoid Disease

Connective Tissue Diseases

The connective tissue diseases (CTDs) are chronic autoimmune conditions characterised by inflammation in blood vessels and connective tissues. CTDs are also known as collagen vascular disorders reflecting the prominence of vascular pathology and abnormal collagen deposition. The prototypic disease is SLE. Related disorders include polymyositis, systemic sclerosis, mixed connective tissue disease, Sjögren's syndrome and rheumatoid disease.

SYSTEMIC LUPUS ERYTHEMATOSUS (SLE)

SLE is an immune complex (IC) mediated disease, which can affect any organ. Clinical presentations are protean, and patients may present to virtually any medical speciality. Skin-limited variants include discoid lupus erythematosus and subacute cutaneous lupus. A minority of patients with apparently skin-limited disease ultimately progress to systemic disease.

SLE affects up to 1 : 1000 of the population, being more common in women than men (9 female : 1 male). Incidence peaks in the second/third decades as well as in later life. Concordance in monozygotic twins is 60% demonstrating a significant genetic influence.

SLE is an IC deposition disease, where inflammation and ultimately organ dysfunction are due to deposition of ICs in the vasculature of affected organs. Patients produce an array of autoantibodies, including ANA, anti-dsDNA antibodies, ENA antibodies, and antibodies to blood cells. Type II hypersensitivity is involved in the immune-mediated cytopaenias, which are common.

Clinical manifestations of SLE vary substantially between patients. Mildly affected patients may only have skin and joint disease, however, severe renal or cerebral disease can occur. SLE causes considerable morbidity and despite treatment continues to cause mortality.

Common clinical features of SLE (Figure 2.23.1) include:

- Erythematous facial rash (butterfly rash) most prominent on the cheeks and bridge of the nose.
- Chronic discoid plaque-like lesions.
- Photosensitivity.

Figure 2.23.1 Common clinical features of SLE.

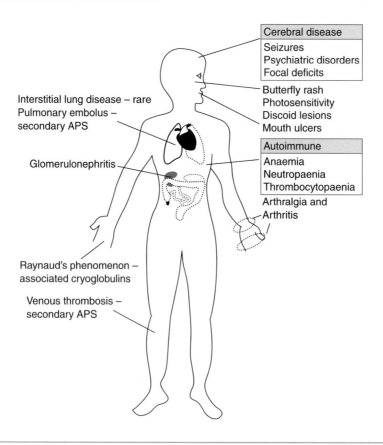

Cerebral disease
Seizures
Psychiatric disorders
Focal deficits

Butterfly rash
Photosensitivity
Discoid lesions
Mouth ulcers

Autoimmune
Anaemia
Neutropaenia
Thrombocytopaenia
Arthralgia and
Arthritis

Interstitial lung disease – rare
Pulmonary embolus –
secondary APS

Glomerulonephritis

Raynaud's phenomenon –
associated cryoglobulins

Venous thrombosis –
secondary APS

- ◆ Arthralgia and arthritis.
- ◆ Haematological abnormalities – particularly haemolytic anaemia, immune thrombocytopaenia, autoimmune neutropaenia.
- ◆ Renal abnormalities – proteinuria, haematuria, nephrotic syndrome and acute renal failure.
- ◆ Cerebral disease – seizures, focal neurological disorders or neuropsychiatric disorders for which no other cause is identified.
- ◆ Mouth ulcers and occasionally ulceration of nasal mucosa.

The majority of patients are ANA and anti-dsDNA positive (if sensitive methods are used). Antibodies to the Sm (Smith) antigen are present in 30% of patients and are specific for SLE. Anti-Ro and occasionally anti-La are also found in a minority of patients with SLE.

Approximately 30% of patients have antibodies to phospholipids, with detectable anti-cardiolipin antibodies or lupus anticoagulant. Only some of these patients develop clinical features of the anti-phospholipid syndrome (pregnancy associated morbidity and/or vascular thrombosis).

Disease activity in SLE is significantly affected by hormonal status. Women may experience flares during pregnancy or in the puerperium. Some women describe catamenial fluctuations in symptoms. Transplacental passage of antibodies, particularly anti-Ro antibodies, may result in neonatal lupus. Neonatal lupus causes skin lesions similar to discoid lupus in approximately half the infants. Congenital heart block is also a risk because Ro antibodies cross-react with tissue in the cardiac conducting bundle. Occasionally liver disease and thrombocytopaenia may also occur. Pregnancy may be complicated by miscarriage or preeclampsia in patients with associated anti-phospholipid syndrome (see Section 2.16).

Drug-induced lupus may complicate the use of several drugs including salazopyrine, hydralazine, penicillamine, several anticonvulsants and etanerocept. Breaking self-tolerance due to presentation of altered self (drug interacts with self-antigen), is thought to be the mechanism involved. Drug-induced lupus is usually mild, generally resolving when the offending drug is stopped.

Treatment of SLE depends on the severity of the disease. Skin lesions usually respond to topical steroids and hydroxychloroquine, and joint disease is treated with anti-inflammatory drugs and hydroxychloroquine. Serious systemic involvement requires steroid therapy usually with other immunosuppressive drugs that inhibit antibody formation. Anti-phospholipid syndrome associated with SLE is treated in the same way as primary anti-phospholipid syndrome, with aspirin or anti-coagulation.

POLYMYOSITIS

Polymyositis is an inflammatory muscle disease caused by damaging T cell responses to muscle antigens. Proximal muscles are prominently involved, becoming painful, tender and weak. Creatine kinase and aldolase (muscle enzymes) are markedly elevated together with an acute phase response. Approximately 30% of patients have anti-Jo-1 antibodies, which are associated with a syndrome comprising polymyositis, Raynaud's phenomenon, interstitial lung disease and thickening of the fingers ("mechanics' hands").

Dermatomyositis is a related condition where muscle inflammation is associated with skin lesions. The pathogenesis appears to be related to immune complex deposition in the vasculature of muscles resulting in muscle injury. Dermatomyositis and more rarely polymyositis may be associated with underlying malignancies. Anti-Jo-1 associated polymyositis has not been associated with tumours to date.

SCLERODERMA AND CREST

Scleroderma (also called systemic sclerosis) is characterised by abnormal deposition of collagen in blood vessels and connective tissues. Skin involvement is prominent and skin thickening impairs mobility and function. Sclerodactyly (thickening of the skin on the fingers) and tightening of the mouth are common. Collagen deposition in the gastrointestinal tract, lungs and kidneys impair function. The diagnosis is predominantly clinical, however, anti-Scl-70 antibodies are present in 30% of patients. Anti-Scl-70 is specific and is associated with a poor prognosis.

CREST syndrome (Calcinosis, Raynaud's phenomenon, oesophageal dysmotility, sclerodactyly and telangiectasia) is a mild variant of scleroderma usually without visceral involvement. Raynaud's phenomenon may be troublesome and associated with digital ischaemia. Recently an association with pulmonary hypertension has been recognised, suggesting that this may not be as benign as previously thought. Centromere pattern ANA is characteristically found in this variant of systemic sclerosis.

MIXED CONNECTIVE TISSUE DISEASE

Features of different CTDs frequently overlap, and patients are often difficult to classify. Mixed connective tissue disease (MCTD) is a tightly defined overlap syndrome, combining features of SLE, polymyositis and scleroderma, and the presence of anti-RNP antibodies. Serious visceral involvement is rare, and the response to steroid therapy is usually good.

SJÖGREN'S SYNDROME

Sjögren's syndrome (SS) is characterised by infiltration of glands and organs by autoreactive T cells. Lacrimal and salivary glands are typically destroyed, resulting in dry eyes and dry mouth (sicca syndrome). Patients may also develop arthritis, systemic symptoms, lung disease and vasculitis. Anti-Ro antibodies are present in up to 70% of patients and anti-La antibodies are less commonly found. Anti-salivary gland duct antibodies may also assist diagnosis. Patients with SS are at significant risk of developing lymphoma. While manifestations of the disease respond to steroids and immunosuppression, the latter increases the risk of lymphoma considerably.

CROSS REFERENCES

Section 1.28   Autoimmunity
Section 2.16   Immune-mediated Haematological Conditions
Section 3.4   Autoantibody Profiles in Connective Tissue Diseases and Rheumatoid Disease

Vasculitis

Vasculitis means inflammation in the walls of blood vessels, disrupting the internal elastic lamina (Figure 2.24.1). The symptoms and signs of vasculitic disorders are due to generalised inflammation, and the consequences of vascular inflammation, causing dysfunction of organs supplied by vasculitic vessels. Clinical manifestations vary depending on the size of vessel involved and the type of inflammation. Vasculitis may result from Type III or Type IV hypersensitivity, however, in many clinical vasculitic syndromes the precise mechanism of vascular inflammation remains elusive.

PRIMARY VERSUS SECONDARY VASCULITIS

Vasculitis may be primary (with no recognised underlying cause) or secondary to many causes including:

- Drugs
- Infections
- Abnormal proteins (e.g. cryoglobulins)
- Other connective tissue diseases.

Primary and some forms of secondary vasculitis are treated with immunosuppression. Secondary vasculitis, particularly due to underlying infection or drugs must be excluded prior to initiating immunosuppression. This section will focus on the primary vasculitides – some secondary vasculitides are discussed elsewhere in this book.

CLINICAL MANIFESTATIONS AND INVESTIGATIONS

Clinical features are due to widespread inflammation or direct consequences of vascular inflammation (Figure 2.24.2). Inflammation causes fatigue, weight loss, fever and raised inflammatory markers such as CRP and ESR.

Figure 2.24.1 Pathological changes in an artery in vasculitis.

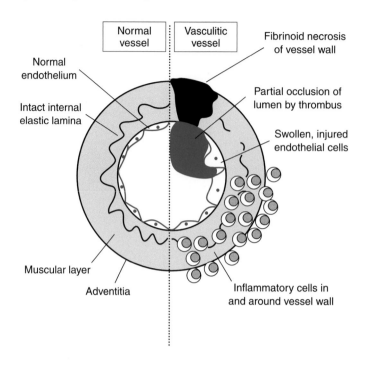

Vascular inflammation in large or medium vessels may result in vascular occlusion and dysfunction of organ(s) distal to the inflammation. In large vessel vasculitides, absent pulses or tenderness over involved vessels may occasionally be detected on physical examination. Vascular inflammation may weaken the vessel wall resulting in aneurysm formation. Inflammation in small vessels increases vessel permeability. In the lung this results in pulmonary haemorrhage; in the kidney severe glomerulonephritis resulting in haematuria, and in skin raised (palpable) purpura and/or bruising is typically seen. Skin, kidneys, lungs and joints are commonly affected, however, organ involvement varies between individual patients.

Several classifications of the primary vasculitides have been proposed. A clinically useful scheme based on vessel size and the presence or absence of granulomata is shown in Table 2.24.1.

For many patients a diagnosis of vasculitis leads to long-term immunosuppression, associated with considerable morbidity and even mortality. The gold standard diagnostic test remains histological demonstration of vasculitis. When this is not possible, angiographic evidence of aneurysm formation and beading of inflamed vessels, or occasionally positive serology may be the only possible diagnostic information.

Until the late 1980s biopsy and angiography were the only methods available to diagnose primary vasculitis. Recognition of anti-neutrophil cytoplasmic antibodies (ANCA, Section 3.5) was a major advance, providing a blood test which was positive in a large percentage of patients with small vessel vasculitis and which varied with disease activity. However, as false positive ANCA occur, a positive ANCA is usually confirmed by biopsies of affected organ(s). ANCA have some pro-inflammatory effects and this may constitute a

Figure 2.24.2 Clinical features of systemic vasculitis depend on the size and location of involved vessels.

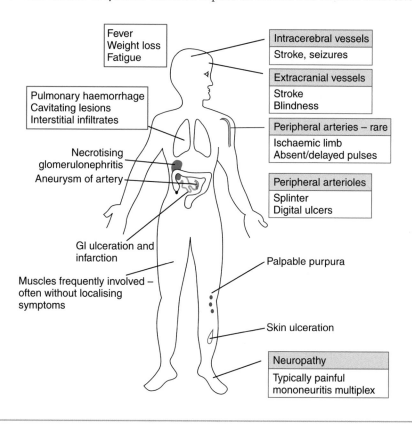

Table 2.24.1 Classification of primary vasculitic conditions

SIZE OF DOMINANT VESSEL AFFECTED	GRANULOMATOUS	NON-GRANULOMATOUS
Large	Temporal arteritis Takayasu arteritis	—
Medium	Churg–Strauss syndrome	Classical polyarteritis nodosa Kawasaki disease
Small	Wegener's granulomatosis	Microscopic polyangiitis Henoch–Schönlein purpura

novel mechanism of hypersensitivity producing tissue damage in ANCA-associated vasculitis – however this remains controversial.

The clinical features of the vasculitic syndromes are highly variable between patients, and considerable overlap between the defined syndromes is seen. Typical features of these conditions are shown in Table 2.24.2, however, virtually any organ can be affected by most types of vasculitis.

Table 2.24.2 The vasculitic syndromes

DISEASE	PATHOLOGY	COMMON CLINICAL FEATURES	TREATMENT
Wegener's granulomatosis	Small vessel vasculitis Granulomata Necrosis Kidney – pauciimmune cresentic GN 95% ANCA positive – usually PR3 ANCA	1. Acute renal failure 2. Pulmonary haemorrhage 3. Upper respiratory tract involvement 4. Non-specific systemic illness	Steroids Cyclophosphamide Relapsing and remitting course
Microscopic polyangiitis	Small vessel vasculitis No granulomata Kidney – as WG 95% ANCA positive – usually MPO–ANCA	1. Acute renal failure 2. Pulmonary haemorrhage 3. Rarely involves upper respiratory tract	Steroids Cyclophosphamide Relapsing and remitting course Often, more insidious than Wegener's granulomatosis
Henoch–Schönlein purpura	May follow infection Small vessel vasculitis IgA deposits in blood vessels and kidneys	1. Skin rash 2. Haematuria 3. Abdominal pain and GI bleeding	Usually resolves in children. Adults may need steroids +/– other treatment
Churg–Strauss syndrome	Medium vessel vasculitis Granulomata Eosinophilia in tissue and blood 30% ANCA positive	1. Asthma 2. Vasculitic illness – frequently involves lungs, kidneys and peripheral nervous system	Steroids and cyclophosphamide
Polyarteritis nodosa	Medium vessel vasculitis Aneurysm formation No granulomata Angiography useful in diagnosis Some associated with Hep B Most ANCA negative	1. PUO and systemic illness 2. Renal failure 3. Skin lesions 4. Abdominal pain 5. Neuropathy	Steroids and cyclophosphamide
Temporal arteritis (often associated with polymyalgia rheumatica)	Large vessel vasculitis Predilection for extracranial vessels Giant cells and granulomata present Elevated ESR ANCA negative	1. Common in elderly 2. Headache/Scalp tenderness 3. Pain in proximal muscles 4. Untreated can progress to cause blindness and stroke	Rapid response to steroids If fail to respond to steroids, reconsider the diagnosis
Takayasu's syndrome	Cellular infiltration of large vessel walls often with occlusion	1. 'Pulseless disease' 2. Widespread bruits 3. Rare in Caucasians – most cases in oriental women	Steroids ? Cytotoxics Bypass surgery

Case 2.24.1 Systemic vasculitis

A 60-year-old woman presented with pain and numbness affecting her hands and feet which had developed gradually over the previous 3 weeks. In the last few days she had noticed increasing weakness in her hands, making normal daily activities difficult. She had been generally unwell in the preceding 6 months and had required medication for asthma for the last 10 years. Neurological examination suggested a mononeuritis multiplex. Bloods revealed anaemia and eosinophilia, an acute phase response and normal glucose.

The neurologist suspected possible vasculitis because of the painful neuropathy and evidence of inflammation. Anti-neutrophil cytoplasm antibody (ANCA) was positive and follow-up testing demonstrated a strong proteinase 3 (PR3)-ANCA. Electrophysiological testing confirmed a mononeuritis multiplex. A nerve biopsy showed demyelination and some axonal loss but did not establish a cause. However, a muscle biopsy performed simultaneously showed vasculitis, with abundant eosinophils in the inflammatory infiltrate and granulomata. The clinical picture of a vasculitic illness, history of asthma and eosinophilia, together with the biopsy findings established a diagnosis of Churg–Strauss syndrome, a vasculitis that predominantly affects medium-sized vessels.

She was treated with cyclophosphamide and steroids and made an excellent recovery over the next two months. Following resolution of her symptoms and normalisation of the eosinophil count and acute phase markers, steroids were tapered and cyclophosphamide was changed to azathioprine, a weaker but less toxic immunosuppressive drug.

Cross references

Section 3.5   Autoantibodies Associated with Vasculitic Syndromes and Renal Diseases
Section 4.2   Corticosteroids
Section 4.3   Immunosuppression (I)

CROSS REFERENCES

Section 1.29   Hypersensitivity
Section 3.5   Autoantibodies Associated with Vasculitic Syndromes and Renal Diseases

Hypersensitivity Induced by Pathogens

The immune system evolved to protect us from pathogens. However, overzealous immune responses to pathogens result in tissue injury, contributing to the morbidity and even mortality associated with some infections. All types of hypersensitivity reaction can be induced by infection. Pathogen-induced hypersensitivity may be clinically apparent during infection or may follow recovery from the inciting infection.

TYPE I HYPERSENSITIVITY

Type I reactions protect against multicellular parasites, and when successful eliminate the parasites. However, when parasites are not eliminated, ongoing immune responses can cause tissue injury. Schistosomiasis is a water-borne infection occurring when schistosoma enter the body through breaches in skin. Adult worms migrate to the liver and lay eggs. Worms elicit IgE mediated responses, and the chronic response produces eosinophil-dominated inflammation. Eosinophils degranulate depositing toxic granule contents on the worm, usually killing the parasite. If unsuccessful, ongoing inflammation provokes scarring ultimately leading to cirrhosis and bladder disease.

TYPE II HYPERSENSITIVITY

Antibodies that bind tissue components and activate complement are implicated in rheumatic fever, a multisystem inflammatory disorder caused by strains of Group A β-haemolytic streptococci. Rheumatic fever is uncommon in the developed world due to improved living standards and the availability of penicillin but remains important, from a global perspective. Several outbreaks have occurred in the United States in the last decade.

Rheumatic fever occurs in genetically susceptible individuals, 1–4 weeks after a streptococcal pharyngitis. Antibodies that bind some Streptococcal M proteins and cross-react with cardiac myosin have been found in some patients. Carditis, arthritis, chorea (involuntary rapid movements), rash, subcutaneous nodules and fever are clinical features.

Diagnosis is primarily clinical, requiring the presence of two major criteria (carditis, polyarthritis, chorea, subcutaneous nodules, erythema marginatum) or one major and two minor criteria (fever, arthralgia, prolonged PR interval on ECG, increased ESR or CRP) in a patient with evidence of recent streptococcal infection (culture or serological).

Treatment includes antibiotics to eliminate residual infection, high-dose salicylates for fevers and arthritis, and steroids for cardiac and possibly neurological involvement. Supportive therapy for cardiac failure may be required. Recurrence of rheumatic fever is a risk, and secondary prophylaxis, with long-term antibiotic therapy to prevent streptococcal colonisation or infection is indicated. About 60% of patients who have had carditis develop valvular damage – rheumatic heart disease. These patients are at future risk of endocarditis.

Other examples of infection induced Type II hypersensitivity include infection induced haemolytic anaemia, which can complicate Mycoplasma infection.

TYPE III HYPERSENSITIVITY

Infection is associated with formation of immune complexes (ICs), however, physiological methods of IC disposal usually prevent IC disease. Infection-induced IC disease typically follows indolent chronic bacterial infections, which provoke a strong antibody response. Examples include vasculitis complicating subacute bacterial endocarditis (SBE), post-streptococcal glomerulonephritis, shunt nephritis and cryoglobulinaemia complicating hepatitis C infection.

High-titre antibody combines with antigen from bacteria resulting in IC formation. When physiological disposal mechanisms are overwhelmed, ICs get trapped in blood vessels, commonly in the skin and kidneys. Complement activation and influx of inflammatory cells result in organ dysfunction.

SBE is a chronic infection of heart valves, usually precipitated by episodes of bacteraemia in people with pre-existing valvular damage. Clinical manifestations are due to further valve damage (murmur and haemodynamic effects), effects of inflammation (APR, hypergammaglobulinaemia, fever and weight loss) and IC deposition. Manifestations attributable to ICs include splinter haemorrhages, nail-fold infarcts, Roth spots, skin rash and haematuria (due to mild glomerulonephritis). Diagnosis depends on identification of the organism in blood cultures or demonstration of vegetations (infected masses) on the heart valves at echocardiography.

Post-streptococcal glomerulonephritis can follow 2–4 weeks after streptococcal pharyngitis or skin infection. ICs deposited in the kidney activate complement, and on kidney biopsy, C3 is usually the prominent immunoreactant. C3 levels are reduced and there is serological evidence of streptococcal infection (positive ASOT or anti-DNAase B).

Infection of a ventriculoperitoneal shunt (used to drain hydrocephalus) may be indolent, resulting in chronic immune stimulation and IC deposition usually causing skin rash (leucocytoclastic vasculitis) and nephritis. Treatment involves removal of the shunt and prolonged antibiotic therapy.

TYPE IV HYPERSENSITIVITY

Type IV hypersensitivity is characterised by macrophage activation by TH1 lymphocytes. When chronic, this can result in granuloma formation. This type of response protects against organisms that are phagocytosed by macrophages but capable of prolonged intra-cellular survival. This includes mycobacteria and some fungi.

The clinical manifestations of leprosy vary greatly depending on the host's immune response to the organism. Leprosy is caused by *Mycobacterium leprae*, which resist killing by macrophages, unless macrophages are activated by TH1 cells. Patients who produce a predominantly TH2 response develop an ineffective antibody-mediated response with poor cellular immunity. Mycobacteria proliferate and spread through the body, and biopsies of lesions show numerous mycobacteria with little inflammatory response. The patient remains highly infectious. At the other end of the spectrum, patients who produce a strong TH1-dominated response develop effective cell-mediated immunity, and lesions show granuloma formation and few mycobacteria – tuberculoid leprosy. These patients are minimally infective to others, however, the granulomatous inflammation causes destruction of skin and peripheral nerves. Severe neuropathy results in progressive tissue damage particularly to the fingers and toes. Many patients have intermediate responses between these extremes. However, tuberculoid leprosy is an example of tissue destruction arising from a vigorous response to infection (Figure 2.25.1).

Figure 2.25.1 Pathological features of tuberculoid and lepromatous leprosy.

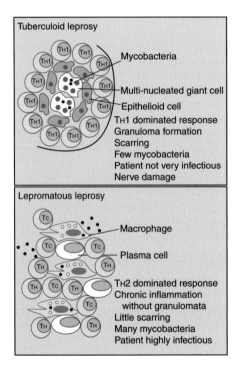

CROSS REFERENCES

Section 1.29 Hypersensitivity
Section 2.14 Autoimmunity
Section 2.24 Vasculitis

REFERENCE

Davies, D. H., Halablab, M. A., Clarke, J., Cox, F. E. G. and Young, T. W. K. (1999) *Infection and Immunity*. Taylor & Francis, London, UK.

Transplantation

In clinical practice, transplantation (or grafting) of bone marrow (or haemopoietic stem cells) as well as solid organs and tissues has become routine treatment.

Transplantation may be:

- Autologous – the individual's own tissue, usually bone marrow or haemopoietic stem cells are returned to the body.
- Syngeneic – tissue is transplanted from a genetically identical individual (identical twin).
- Allogeneic – tissue is transplanted from a non-identical individual, from the same species.
- Xenogeneic – tissue is transplanted from one species to another.

Rejection is not a risk in autologous and syngeneic transplantation but is a major problem in allogeneic transplantation. Xenotransplantation carries a high risk of rejection, which together with concerns about infection have prevented clinical trials.

WHAT IS TRANSPLANTED?

Clinical transplantation may be divided into haemopoietic stem-cell (HSC) transplantation, solid organ transplantation and tissue transplantation.

HSCs are progenitor cells that develop into the cellular elements of blood and the immune system. Until recently, bone marrow was the only viable source of HSCs, however, these cells are now harvested from peripheral blood after mobilisation by growth factors, and from umbilical cord blood.

Solid organ transplantation is used to treat irreversible failure of kidneys, liver, heart, lung and pancreas. Small bowel transplantation remains experimental.

Tissue transplantation refers to transplantation of non-vascularised tissues. The lack of blood-supply protects from rejection. However, when tissues expressing HLA-antigens are transplanted, sensitisation may result. Tissues routinely transplanted include cornea, bone and human and porcine heart valves. Islet cell transplantation has been successfully performed, and techniques are being refined.

IMMUNOLOGICAL ASPECTS

HSC transplantation replaces the bone marrow and immune system of the recipient. The recipient's body is foreign to the new donor immune system, which may mount an attack on this 'foreign' tissue. This is termed graft-versus-host disease (GvHD).

In solid organ transplantation, the donor organ is foreign to the recipient's immune system. Rejection occurs when the recipient's immune system attacks the transplanted organ.

Non-vascularised tissue is generally not rejected, and systemic immunosuppression is not required. However, a corneal graft that becomes vascularised may be rejected.

CROSS REFERENCES
Section 2.27   Haemopoietic Stem Cell Transplantation Section 2.28   Solid Organ Transplantation

Haemopoietic Stem Cell Transplantation

INDICATIONS

Pluripotential haemopoietic stem cell (HSC) transplantation refers to a range of procedures that restore haemopoietic function. Bone marrow, peripheral blood and umbilical cord blood are sources of HSCs. Indications for HSC grafting are many and include:

- Haematological malignances

  — lymphoid – acute lymphoblastic leukaemia (ALL), if it falls within a poor prognostic category or for relapsing disease
  — Hodgkin's and non-Hodgkin's lymphomas (relapsed; high grade) multiple myeloma (young, poor prognosis)
  — myeloid – acute myeloid leukaemia (AML) – (1st/2nd remission); chronic myeloid leukaemia.

- Primary haematological diseases

  — aplastic anaemia
  — thalasaemias
  — sickle-cell disease
  — myelodysplasia.

- Primary Immunodeficiencies

  — SCIDs
  — progressive combined immunodeficiencies
  — severe neutrophil-related immunodeficiencies (CGD and LAD).

- Inborn errors of metabolism

  — Gaucher's disease
  — mucopolysaccharidoses (Hurler's)
  — osteopetrosis
  — leucodystrophies.

- Solid organ malignancies – rescue from marrow-ablating chemotherapy (breast; lung; testis; ovary; Ewing's sarcoma; neuroblastoma)
- Autoimmune disorders – experimental in severe, therapy-resistant conditions (scleroderma etc.).

TYPES OF TRANSPLANT

Haemopoietic transplants are either autologous or allogeneic. Autologous HSC transplantation is relatively straightforward, however, allogeneic HSC transplantation is more challenging, and may be complicated by:

- Non-engraftment (recipient rejects donors cells, which never 'take')
- Graft-versus-Host Disease.

Autologous transplantation

The use of auto-grafts is increasing because of the lack of rejection and GvHD complications as well as quicker marrow recovery. This type of transplant is suitable in:

- Haematological malignances – stem cells obtained during remission are used to restore marrow function following intensive, marrow-ablating chemotherapy.
- Non-haematological malignancy – restoration of marrow function following ablative therapy.
- Autoimmune disease – currently limited to clinical trials.

Transplantation of residual tumour cells is a risk. Increasingly sensitive detection and eradication of minimal residual disease from stem cell preparations has increased success rates.

Allogeneic transplantation

Allografts are used when there is an intrinsic fault in HSCs.

- Congenital abnormalities – immunodeficiency, haemoglobinopathies and metabolic disorders (e.g. mucopolysaccharidoses). HSC transplantation is not used if the risks of the transplant procedure outweigh the benefit of correcting the underlying disease (e.g. X-linked agammaglobulinaemia).
- Some haematological malignancies – for example, CML, myelodysplasia, aplastic anaemia. Immune non-identity may have some positive effects. Graft recognition and elimination of leukaemic cells (graft versus leukaemia effect), reduces relapse rate.

While allogeneic transplants may offer cure (SCID) or improved outlook in very serious conditions (CML, aplastic anaemia), there are significant risks as outlined:

- Rejection – failure of engraftment is more common than in autologous transplantation.
- GvHD may be acute, occurring immediately post-transplant phase or chronic. Preventive measures include limitation of marrow mismatch, pre-treatment of stem cell transplant (T cell depletion) and immunosuppression of the host (Figure 2.27.1).

Figure 2.27.1 Bone marrow transplantation.

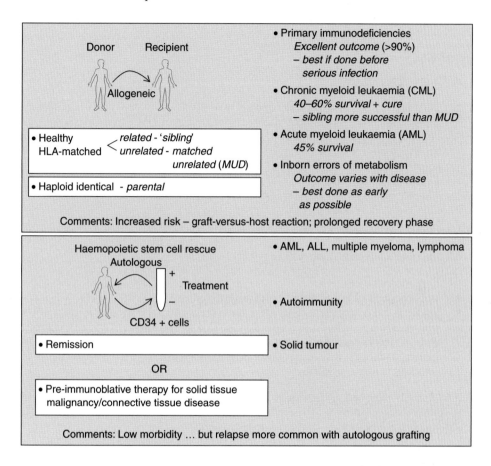

Adverse effects

The following complications occur after both autologous and allogeneic HSC transplantation, but are more common and severe with allografts:

♦ Severe marrow dysfunction, is more prolonged in allogeneic transplants, requiring intensive transfusion support and infection prevention measures (isolation, reverse-barrier nursing, antibiotic prophylaxis). Severe mucositis and alopoecia are almost inevitable. Bacterial, fungal, and certain viral infections occur frequently. CMV-negative donors are preferable and anti-viral prophylaxis is required if the donor was CMV-positive.

♦ Immunodeficiency is profound immediately post-transplant and some compromise is common for up to two years. In SCID, T cell restoration usually occurs, however, if B cells do not reconstitute long-term antibody support is required. Immune reconstitution is delayed and deficient in patients with GvHD.

♦ Veno-occlusive disease – occurs with pre-existing liver disease, intensive conditioning, or if undergoing second transplant.

- Secondary malignancies – skin; EBV-related lymphomas.
- Endocrine – infertility.
- Psychological – symptoms are common.

Sources of HSCs

HSCs are obtained from:

- Bone marrow – aspirated under general anaesthetic, from puncture of the iliac crests.
- Peripheral blood – a viable and convenient source of HSC, particularly with improved cell harvesting and separation techniques. Treating the donor with haemopoietic growth factors increases numbers of HSCs. The outcome post-grafting with PBSCs is often better than with bone marrow transplantation.
- Cord blood – is a rich source of immature stem cells of limited immunogenicity. The number of cells that can be retrieved limits this application.

Donors

All potential allogeneic donors must:

- Give informed consent.
- Undergo screening for blood-borne infections.
- Undergo HLA typing – The ideal but rarely available donor is an HLA-matched sibling. HLA-matched unrelated donors (MUD transplants), usually identified from bone-marrow registries, are a less-favoured option. Haploid-identical matching (parental donors will share one HLA haplotype) has been successful in SCID, as rejection is not a problem.

Incompletely matched grafts can be assessed prior to transplantation for the likelihood of problems using a number of specialised immunological tests (mixed lymphocyte reaction, and precursor lymphocyte frequency measurement).

In autologous transplantation, HSC must be harvested during clinical remission.
Outlook for graft recipients is optimised by:

- Appropriate pre-transplant conditioning (enough to eradicate diseased cells and to make enough physical space for the new bone marrow to develop)
- Aggressive infection prophylaxis and treatment
- Good supportive care.

GvHD prophylaxis is given if there is a significant risk. The underlying condition also influences outcome. SCID patients generally do very well even with haploidentical donors. SCID patients are usually managed at specialist immunodeficiency transplant centres.

CROSS REFERENCES
Section 2.26   Transplantation
Section 2.28   Solid Organ Transplantation
Section 2.30   Leukaemia and Lymphoma

Solid Organ Transplantation

The most commonly transplanted solid organ is the kidney, however liver, heart, lung and pancreas transplantation are routine treatments for irreversible failure of these organs. Islet cell transplantation techniques are being refined, and small bowel transplantation remains experimental treatment.

INDICATIONS

General indications for solid organ transplantation are:

* Irreversible organ failure
* Underlying condition with acceptable risk of recurrence
* Recipient free from infection and malignancy
* Recipient fit for major surgery.

TRANSPLANT ASSESSMENT

Patients are thoroughly assessed before going on the waiting list to ensure:

* Medical and surgical fitness for transplantation
* Psychologically suitable for surgery and post-transplantation therapy
* Understanding of the process and willingness to give informed consent.

Laboratory assessment includes viral studies, blood grouping, HLA typing and identification of anti-HLA antibodies which could damage grafts. Anti-HLA antibodies develop when individuals are exposed to foreign HLA antigens. HLA sensitising events include pregnancy, blood transfusions and previous transplants.

PREPARATION FOR TRANSPLANTATION

The waiting time depends on the number of patients awaiting transplantation, clinical priority for the patient and the donor rate in the organ sharing area. Living-related (or unrelated) kidney transplantation may be considered, and is associated with superior outcomes for the recipient. Organ allocation policies vary between organs – size is a major determinant in thoracic transplantation, while HLA matching receives more attention in renal transplantation. A graft bearing HLA-antigens to which a patient has antibodies is not acceptable. Such anti-HLA antibodies will be identified at initial or ongoing assessments, well in advance of a donor becoming available.

When a patient is considered for an organ, cross-matching is performed as a final check that the patient does not have anti-donor-HLA antibodies, which would cause hyperacute rejection. If cross-match results are acceptable, surgery may proceed. Every effort is made to minimise the ischaemic time of the organ. In the case of heart transplants acceptable ischaemia is limited to 4 hours, whereas kidneys can withstand over 24 hours in appropriate conditions. Longer ischaemia is associated with inferior outcomes.

COMPLICATIONS

Patients experience different complications at different times post transplantation. The prevalence of each complication depends on the organ transplanted and in some cases, the patient's primary disease. Problems include:

- Surgical – bleeding, anastomotic leaks, wound infection
- Thrombosis of arteries and veins
- Rejection
- Infection
- Malignancy – post-transplant lymphoproliferative disorder (PTLD); skin cancers; other tumours
- Drug toxicity – steroid-induced osteoporosis; hirsutism and gingival hypertropy with cyclosporin
- Recurrence of primary disease in transplanted organ
- Rejection is a common occurrence following transplantation as the immune system attacks the graft (non-self).

REJECTION: WHAT MOLECULES DOES THE IMMUNE SYSTEM SEE?

The immune system responds to molecules that differ between the donor and recipient. These may be divided into:

- Major antigens – HLA (MHC) antigens, which are recognised by the immune system without processing, and elicit strong cellular and antibody responses. Routine typing and cross-matching usually identifies these antigens.
- Minor antigens – numerous molecules, not identified by tissue typing techniques. Minor antigens require processing, and are presented to the recipient's immune system complexed with recipient HLA molecules (indirect presentation). They elicit T cell responses, weaker than those elicited by HLA molecules.

Classification of rejection

Classification of rejection is based on the mechanism of tissue damage – different types being common at different times post transplantation (Table 2.28.1).

Mechanisms of graft damage

ANTIBODY-MEDIATED REJECTION

Binding of antibody results in complement activation and deposition of the membrane attack complex (MAC). Graft endothelium becomes damaged, and the coagulation cascade is activated. Biopsy shows thrombi, neutrophil infiltration and severe tissue injury. DIF demonstrates deposition of antibody and complement. Anti-donor antibody is frequently detectable in the serum. Antibody mediated rejection occurs in about 1% of renal transplant recipients.

T CELL-MEDIATED REJECTION

Acute cellular rejection   T cells infiltrate the graft interstitium and renal tubules. Cytotoxic T cells directly injure the allograft, and cytokines produced by helper and cytotoxic T cells attract more inflammatory cells and up-regulate HLA antigen expression thus amplifying the process (Figure 2.28.1). Cellular rejection is seen in about 20% of renal allograft recipients.

Chronic rejection   The mechanisms of chronic rejection are poorly understood. It appears that early damage to the graft (due to rejection, reperfusion injury, cytomegalovirus) initiates an inflammatory process leading to scarring and tissue remodelling. Virtually all long-surviving solid organ grafts show evidence of chronic rejection.

Episodes of rejection are a common complication, even with modern immunosuppression, in recipients of all solid organs.

The risk can be reduced by:

- Optimal HLA matching (however, not possible for patients with rare HLA types)
- Improved cross matching (reducing antibody-mediated rejection)
- More potent immunosuppression (but also increases the risk of infection and malignancy).

Table 2.28.1 Types of rejection

TYPE OF REJECTION	TIME POST Tx	MECHANISM OF TISSUE DAMAGE
Hyperacute	<24 hours	Preformed antibody, complement, coagulation
Acute cellular	Common < 6 months	Cytotoxic T cells
Acute humoral	Common < 6 weeks	Antibody produced post-transplant
Chronic	Months–years	Uncertain. Scarring in response to injury

Figure 2.28.1 Mechanisms of graft rejection.

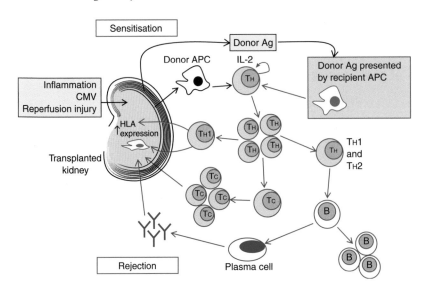

Table 2.28.2 Graft survival figures

ORGAN	KIDNEY	HEART	LUNG	LIVER
1 year graft survival	>87%	83%	70%	77%
Median survival	11 years	9 years	5 years	8 years

SURVIVAL

Graft survival is longest for kidneys, followed by heart, liver and lung (see Table 2.28.2). Survival is affected by:

◆ Donor factors (age, sex, cause of death)
◆ Perioperative events (cold ischaemia time, surgical aspects)
◆ Recipient factors (age, sex, comorbidity, sensitisation, HLA match, adherence to therapy).

THERAPY

Immunosuppression includes 3–4 agents, typically steroids, cyclosporin/tacrolimus and azathioprine/mycophenylate with additional antibody therapy added in high-risk patients. Acute cellular rejection is treated with high dose steroids, and occasionally T cell-depleting antibodies. Antibody-mediated rejection is treated with plasmapheresis to rapidly remove antibodies, and augmented immunosuppression. Currently there are no treatments for chronic rejection.

Case 2.28.1 Renal transplantation

A 25-year-old woman complained of ankle swelling, facial swelling in the mornings and weight gain of 4 kg. She had been generally unwell for the preceding two months, and also had joint pains and stiffness. On examination, blood pressure was elevated (170/100 mm/Hg), there was synovitis affecting small joints in her hands, pitting oedema to the midcalf and urinalysis showed large amounts of protein and blood in her urine. The GP suspected glomerulonephritis, possibly related to systemic lupus erthematosus (SLE) and arranged for urgent admission.

Anti-nuclear antibody and anti-double stranded DNA were strongly positive. C3 and C4 were undetectable, ESR was >100 mm/hour, albumin was low (20 g/l) and urinary protein was 5 g/24 hours. Renal biopsy showed a membranoproliferative pattern of injury with glomerular deposits of C3, C4, IgA, IgG and IgM. Creatinine had risen to 500 µmol/l. A diagnosis of SLE with active, severe nephritis was made.

She was immediately treated with high dose intravenous methylprednisolone and monthly pulses of cyclophosphamide, and her disease became less active over the ensuing months. She required dialysis for a short period, but renal function improved and she became dialysis independent with a creatinine of 200 µmol/l. Unfortunately 5 years later, despite good control of the SLE her creatinine began to climb. Repeat biopsy showed extensive scarring without significant active inflammation. Once more she became dialysis dependent, and was listed for a cadaveric renal transplant.

After waiting for 2 years she received a renal transplant. The kidney functioned immediately and she was maintained on tacrolimus, azathioprine and corticosteroids. She remains well 5 years post transplant with normal renal function. As with many SLE patients her disease has remained quiescent since her transplant, as post-transplant immunosuppression is usually more than adequate to control SLE.

Cross references

Section 2.23   Connective Tissue Diseases
Sections 4.2–4.4   Corticosteroids and immunosuppression

CROSS REFERENCES

Section 1.5   Innate Immune Responses II – The Complement System
Section 1.9   Human Leucocyte Antigen (HLA) Molecules
Section 1.15   Immunoglobulin Function
Section 3.15   Transplantation
Section 3.17   Direct Immunofluorescence
Sections 4.2–4.6   Immunosuppression

REFERENCE

Cecka, J. M. and Terasaki, P. I. (published annually, 2004) 'Clinical transplants', UCLA Immunogenetics Center, Los Angeles.

Lymphoid Malignancies

OVERVIEW

These are a diverse group of conditions, arising from malignant transformation of a single (monoclonal) lymphocyte population. B cell malignancies are more common (80%+), with most others being of T cell lineage. NK cell malignancies are very rare. Malignant transformation results in arrest of development and uncontrolled proliferation or persistence of a monoclonal lymphoid population. This can occur at any stage of maturation or activation. The microscopic appearance, pattern of CD− and antigen receptor molecule expression, distribution within the lymphoid system, and behaviour of malignant lymphocytes is highly variable, depending on the developmental or activation stage from which they originate (Figure 2.29.1). Malignant lymphocytes closely mirror the features of normal lymphocytes at similar stages of differentiation.

Lymphoid malignancies are sub-divided into:

- Leukaemia – malignant proliferation originates and accumulates in the bone marrow, usually with peripheral blood involvement.
- Lymphoma – focussed in tissues of the secondary immune system – lymph nodes, liver, spleen, MALT. Bone marrow and peripheral blood involvement may occur.

The incidence of lymphoid malignancies of all types approximates 25/100,000 population per year. Patients of all ages are affected. Distinct age profiles are seen in some conditions. ALL occurs in children predominantly. It accounts for a third of all malignancies in this age group. In contrast, chronic leukaemias (e.g. CLL) and plasma cell malignancies are rare before the age of 40 years and increase in prevalence with increasing age. Incidence of Hodgkin's lymphoma peaks in young adulthood with a further peak in later life. The incidence of non-Hodgkin's lymphoma (NHL) has increased dramatically in recent decades.

Figure 2.29.1 Lymphoid population and their malignant counterparts. The relationship of lymphoid malignancies to normal lymphoid counterparts is shown.

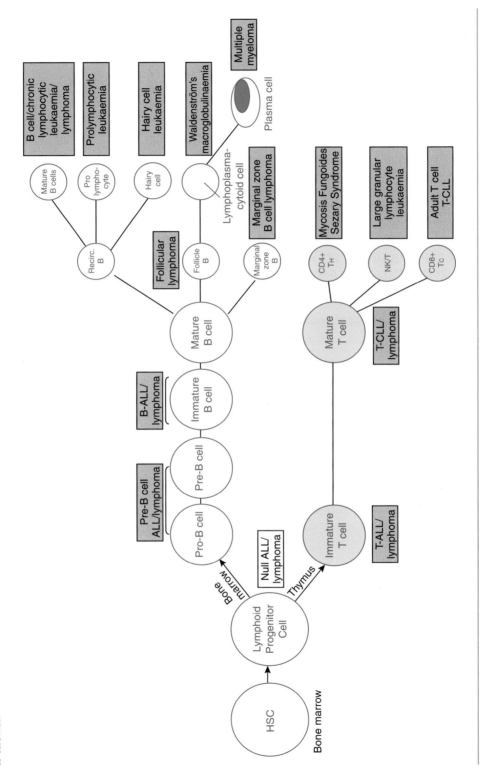

CLINICAL CHARACTERISTICS

Clinical presentations distinct to particular conditions will be discussed in Section 2.30. Generally, clinical manifestations of lymphoid malignancies are due to:

- Accumulation of malignant cells – enlargement of lymphoreticular organs, especially in lymphomas. Thymic involvement in some T cell leukaemias. Extranodal masses occur anywhere, especially in the gut, brain and skin.
- Suppression of non-malignant blood cell lines – anaemia, thrombocytopaenia and neutropaenia.
- Immune dysregulation – antibody immunodeficiency in plasma cell malignancies; cell-mediated abnormalities in Hodgkin's disease; production of autoantibodies causing several complications, for example, haemolytic anaemia and immune thrombocytopaenia in CLL, acquired C1 inhibitor deficiency in NHL.

FACTORS ASSOCIATED WITH THE DEVELOPMENT OF LYMPHOID MALIGNANCIES

The pathogenesis of some specific lymphoid malignancies has been elucidated. However, aetiology is usually complex and probably multifactorial. Causative factors include:

Genetic

There is an increased incidence in:

- Identical twin of patient with leukaemia.
- Down's syndrome.
- Fanconi anaemia.
- Specific genetic translocations, often involving oncogenes/antigen receptors – t8:14 (c-myc/IgH) in Burkitt's lymphoma; t14:18 (IgH/bcl-2) in follicular lymphoma; Philadelphia chromosome/t9:22 (bcr/c-abl fusion) in CML and in bad prognosis ALL.
- Other cytogenetic variations, for example, hyperploidy (too many chromosomes) or deletions are also seen.

Microbial

- EBV is a causative factor in Burkitt's lymphoma. EBV is also implicated in diffuse large B cell lymphoma associated with immunodeficiency (e.g. post-transplant), in CNS lymphoma affecting HIV positive patients and in Hodgkin's lymphoma.
- Lymphomas occur with increased frequency in patients with advanced HIV infection. EBV-related CNS lymphoma and Human herpesvirus-8 (HHV-8)-related extranodal lymphomas are well-recognised.
- HTLV-1 is a human retrovirus implicated in an aggressive adult-onset T cell leukaemia endemic in the Caribbean and Japan.
- *Helicobacter pylori* is associated with MALToma involving the gastric mucosa.

Immunodeficiency

- Virus-driven NHLs are seen in secondary immunodeficiency states like HIV infection and in the setting of post-transplant immunosuppression.

◆ Lymphoma occurs with increased frequency in patients with primary immunodeficiencies, possibly due to susceptibility to lymphoma-triggering infections. This risk is especially pronounced in X-linked lymphoproliferative disease, Wiskott–Aldrich syndrome, CVID, Chediak–Higashi syndrome and in disorders of DNA repair.

Others

◆ Radiation exposure (e.g. Hiroshima, Chernobyl, extensive radiological exposure); chemicals (benzene); cytotoxic drugs; chronic immune stimulation/dysregulation, for example, in connective tissue diseases and coeliac disease, are all possible factors.

CROSS REFERENCES

Section 2.30   Leukaemia and Lymphoma
Section 2.31   Plasma Cell Diseases
Section 3.16   Immunophenotyping Leukaemias and Lymphomas

Leukaemia and Lymphoma

CLASSIFICATION

Neoplastic blood cell proliferations are classified into three groups:

* Lymphoid – B, T, or NK cell origins
* Myeloid – granulocyte, monocyte, red blood cell, platelet origins
* Histiocytic – dendritic cell origin.

Haematological malignancies are classified as leukaemias or lymphomas. Lymphomas are further sub-divided into:

* Hodgkin's lymphoma – HD – a condition with distinct histological and clinical features
* Non-Hodgkin's lymphoma (NHL) comprise all other forms.

Acute leukaemias originate from immature/precursor cells. Chronic leukaemias arise from mature populations. Lymphoid and myeloid leukaemias are described. Acute leukaemias develop and manifest quickly and survival without therapy is short. Chronic leukaemias are slow growing, survival may be prolonged, and many are clinically silent. Transformation to more active disease occurs with varying frequency in different chronic leukaemias. Classification of lymphoid neoplasms is complex and many different systems are described. The Revised European American Lymphoma (REAL) classification is the most widely used. Both leukaemias and lymphomas of lymphocytic origin are included.

Myeloid counterparts of lymphomas are not described. Enlargement of lymphoreticular organs may occur, either due to deposition of myeloid malignant cells or as a result of blood cell production occurring outside the bone marrow (extramedullary haematopoiesis). Histiocytic conditions are rare. They typically involve extramedullary tissues.

ACUTE LYMPHOBLASTIC LEUKAEMIA (ALL)

ALL arises from malignant transformation of bone marrow immature lymphoblasts. Four types are categorised using immunophenotyping techniques:

- Pre-B/'common' – 85%
- T – 10%
- B – <5%
- 'null' – <5%.

Subdivision according to cell size and variability (FAB classification) is also used and has prognostic implications.
  ALL is the single commonest childhood malignancy. Adults are less frequently affected. Onset is usually sudden and florid.
  Clinical features include:

- Bone marrow failure
- Bone pain/tenderness
- CNS – meningism, nerve palsies
- Lymphadenopathy/hepatosplenomegaly
- Testicular enlargement
- Thymic enlargement with SVC obstruction (T-ALL, older boys).

ALL is highly sensitive to chemotherapy; >90% achieve complete remission and 70% are cured. Presentation in the first year of life or in adolescence and adulthood, or Philadelphia chromosome positivity are poor prognostic indicators. BMT during first remission in these groups may offer a better outlook.

CHRONIC LYMPHOCYTIC LEUKAEMIA (CLL) AND VARIANTS

CLL is the most common adult leukaemia and represents malignant transformation in a mature B cell population. It predominantly affects the elderly. Presentations include:

- Coincidental
- Lymphadenopathy/hepatosplenomegaly
- Constitutional upset
- Marrow failure
- Autoimmune haemolytic anaemia/thrombocytopaenia
- Hypogammaglobulinaemia with recurrent bacterial infections.

Therapeutic approach varies with stage.

- Monitor only – asymptomatic
- Chlorambucil – more advanced
- Purine nucleoside analogues (fludarabine/2-CDA) or MAbs (alemtuzumab/rituximab) – aggressive/relapsing.

Approximately 30% undergo transformation into more aggressive states including prolymphocytic leukaemia or diffuse large cell lymphoma (Richter's syndrome) following which survival is decreased.
  Other mature leukaemias similar to CLL are:

- Prolymphocytic leukaemia – more aggressive. Major lymphocytosis, anaemia, thrombocytopaenia, massive splenomegaly and constitutional symptoms are typical.

Case 2.30.1 Chronic lymphocytic leukaemia

A 55-year-old woman complained of bruising and nose bleeds. She had been unusually fatigued for the last 6 months. Her GP checked a full blood count, which showed a lymphocytosis of 6×10^9/l and thrombocytopaenia, with a platelet count of 35×10^9/l. She was referred to the haematology clinic, where these initial findings were confirmed. Immunophenotyping of peripheral blood showed an excess of CD5+ CD19+ B cells, the typical phenotype of chronic lymphocytic leukaemia (CLL). Bone marrow examination revealed an excess of B cells, as well as increased numbers of megakaryocytes (platelet precursors), which suggested that the low platelet count was due to excessive destruction in the periphery. She had no lymphadenopathy, and liver and spleen size were normal clinically, however, mild splenomegaly was detected radiologically. Anti-platelet antibodies were positive. A diagnosis of CLL complicated by immune thrombocytopaenia was made.

Initial treatment with steroids improved her platelet count to between 90 and 100×10^9/l. As the lymphocyte count was stable, no treatment was required for the CLL, which frequently runs an indolent course. One year later, the patient was admitted with a severe pneumonia. In the preceding 6 months she had required monthly antibiotics for bacterial infections. Immunoglobulin (Ig) measurement showed a low IgG at 4 g/l (Ref 6–13 g/l), undetectable IgA and normal IgM. Test vaccination with Pneumovax II showed low prevaccination level, with no response to vaccination. Hypogammaglobulinaemia secondary to CLL is common, and contributes to the morbidity and mortality of the condition. The patient was commenced on intravenous Ig replacement therapy. Over the next two years she only required antibiotics twice per year, and her lymphocyte count remains stable.

Cross references

Characteristic cell morphology is diagnostic. Combination chemotherapy or the newer CLL therapies may be of benefit.

- Hairy cell leukaemia – usually indolent condition with characteristic 'hairy' appearance of malignant cells. Usually affects older males. Massive splenomegaly and pancytopaenia are typical. Symptomatic disease is exquisitely sensitive to purine analogues and IFN-γ treatment.
- Splenic lymphoma with villous lymphocytes (SLVL) – is indolent. Splenomegaly and constitutional upset are common. Distinct morphology and immunophenotype and minimal marrow involvement characterise SLVL. Treatment is similar to CLL. Splenectomy may be required.

HODGKINS'S DISEASE

This is a common malignancy in young adults particularly affecting male Caucasians from high socio-economic groupings. EBV is probably involved in pathogenesis. The

Reed–Sternberg cell, with distinctive histological and immunophenotypic features (binucleate large cell with prominent nucleoli), is essential for diagnosis. Different sub-classes are defined according to the relationship of Reed–Sternberg cells to other white cell populations and to patterns of fibrosis within the affected tissues. The histological pattern influences prognosis.

Presenting features of HD are:

- Painless lymphadenopathy – superficial, supra-diaphragmatic. Internal nodes may cause compressive effects. Direct spread along chains of nodes is typical.
- Constitutional upset – 'B symptoms'. Fever, night sweats, weight loss, alcohol-related lymph node pain highly suggestive.

Stage of disease partly predicts outcome. This is established on the basis of the extent of lymph node involvement and presence or absence of 'B' symptoms. Radiotherapy may adequately treat localised disease. More extensive disease requires chemotherapy. Outlook is good even in the latter group. Myeloid leukaemias, other malignancies and lung damage are complications of therapy.

NON-HODGKIN'S LYMPHOMAS (NHLs)

NHLs vary from low-grade, indolent lymphoid expansions through to aggressive disease, which may be fatal. NHLs are dramatically increasing in frequency throughout the Western world. Response to therapy is not as successful as with HD.

Distinct entities are described according to:

- Developmental stage from which the malignant clone originates (e.g. lymphoblastic, follicular, small mature lymphocytic, diffuse large B cell, plasma cell)
- Type of lymphocyte (B, T, NK)
- Cytogenetic and other molecular mutation patterns
- Clinical features, for example, aggressive (high-grade), indolent (low-grade), location (nodal, extranodal), associated features (hyperviscosity, splenomegaly, skin involvement, immune dysfunction).

Clinically, grade (rate of proliferation) is the most important prognostic factor. Approximately 1/3 of cases are high-grade, diffuse large B cell, a further 1/3 are follicular B cell and the remainder are varied in origin. NHLs are typically more widespread than HD at presentation.

As with CLL, many low-grade lymphomas may not require immediate therapy. Indications for therapy include systemic symptoms, symptomatic lymphadenopathy and bone marrow failure. Survival may be prolonged even in the absence of therapy, but cure is rare. In contrast, patients with high-grade NHLs require immediate chemotherapy. Initial response rates are high, but relapse is common and outlook poor if this occurs. BMT may be indicated in some cases. Radiotherapy is beneficial in distinct disorders, for example, CNS lymphoma. Antibiotic therapy is potentially curative in *Helicobacter* – related MALToma.

CROSS REFERENCES	
Section 1.12	Lymphocyte Maturation
Section 2.27	Haemopoietic Stem Cell Transplantation
Section 3.16	Immunophenotyping Leukaemias and Lymphomas

Plasma Cell Diseases

Plasma cell diseases (dyscrasias) comprise several conditions of varying clinical presentation and severity characterised by monoclonal plasma cell proliferation. The intensity and dissemination of plasma cell expansion, amount and type of the monoclonal immunoglobulin secreted, and associated systemic features (e.g. renal failure, hypercalcaemia, hyperviscosity) are important in classification. Conditions associated with paraprotein production are also called gammopathies.

MULTIPLE MYELOMA

Multiple myeloma (MM) is the commonest malignant disorder of plasma cells and accounts for 1% of all malignancies in Caucasians, usually occurring after 50 years. The cause of MM is unknown, but autocrine secretion of IL-6 may play a role. Disseminated monoclonal expansion of paraprotein-secreting plasma cells in the bone marrow is the hallmark of the disease. The paraprotein is IgG in 60% of cases, IgA in 20%, and light chains alone in 15–20%. Rare cases are IgD- or IgE-secreting, occasionally non-secreting, or biclonal (two different paraproteins). True IgM MM is rare.

Diagnosis

At least two of the following criteria must be present to make a diagnosis of MM:

*   Increased percentage of abnormal looking bone marrow plasma cells (>20% of nucleated cells or 12% if monoclonality confirmed)
*   Paraprotein in blood and/or urine. Suppression of non-myeloma immunoglobulins is common
*   Bone destruction with osteoporosis or lytic lesions.

Clinical presentation

The major clinical features of MM are:

- Bone disease – found in 70% of cases at presentation. Bone breakdown activated by IL-6, IL-1 and TNF-α (osteoclast activating factors) is exaggerated. Osteoporosis and punched-out lytic lesions affecting the skull and axial skeleton are commonly seen on X-ray. Back pain is common. Myeloma screening is indicated in unexplained back pain over 40 years. Spinal cord compression is a dangerous complication. Pain at other sites and pathological fractures occur. Extensive bone breakdown leads to hypercalcaemia. Classically, the alkaline phosphatase level is normal even when significant bone involvement is present.
- Renal impairment is present in 25% at presentation, developing in 50% at some stage. The mechanisms are multiple. Hypercalcaemia and dehydration are important potentially reversible causes. Increased light-chain excretion can cause renal tubular obstruction leading to atrophy and necrosis with renal failure. Forced diuresis and treatment of the underlying myeloma can rarely improve renal function. Renal amyloidosis, and renal vein thrombosis are other causes of renal impairment.
- Haematological – anaemia is common and dominates presentation in 20% of cases. Causes include marrow failure, and renal impairment. Full-blown marrow failure more often complicates intensive therapies. Hypergammaglobulinaemia (paraprotein) and anaemia may greatly elevate the ESR (>100 mm/hour). Large paraprotein concentrations, especially IgA and IgG3 may cause hyperviscosity. Coagulopathy occurs in a small number of cases.
- Immunological – Suppression of non-paraprotein immunoglobulins (immunoparesis) and functional antibody deficiency, predisposing to pyogenic infections is common. 10% of patients present with bacterial infection (most often pneumococcal). Infection is also a common cause of death.

Prognosis and monitoring

MM is a serious condition. Death occurs within a year in most untreated cases and with treatment the 5-year mortality rate is 75%.

Poor prognostic features include:

- Anaemia (<8.5 g/dl)*
- Hypercalcaemia (>3.0 mmol/l)*
- Widespread bone disease*
- High levels of paraprotein (IgG > 70 g/l; IgA > 50 g/l; BJP > 12 g/24 hours)*
- Renal impairment
- High % of plasma cells, circulating cells; abnormal plasma cell morphology
- High β_2-microglobulin
- High IL-6 (CRP surrogate marker).

Prognosis is related to the tumour mass, calculated from the asterisked parameters (Durie–Salmon staging system – '0' – indolent $\rightarrow$ III – advanced). Alternatively, β_2-microglobulin (corrected for serum creatinine) and CRP can be used, with poorest outlook when both parameters are elevated. Monitoring of MM includes serial measurement of the above parameters. Occasionally patients meeting diagnostic criteria for MM (excess plasma cells and paraprotein) have a small tumour burden, normal haematological, biochemical and bone indices with stable paraprotein levels. Such cases are called smouldering or indolent myeloma and do not require immediate treatment. Monitoring for progression is important.

Management

MM is rarely curable. Therapy aims to reduce tumour burden to a plateau level with stable haematological and biochemical parameters and bone lesions. Relapse and progression is inevitable in most cases.

The principle points of management are:

- Good Supportive Management – analgesia for bone pain; radiotherapy for localised bone pain; re-hydration, loop diuretics and bisphosphonates for correction of hypercalcaemia; rehydration and renal replacement therapy in renal impairment; antibiotic treatment of infection; antibiotic prophylaxis or Ig replacement therapy in functional antibody deficiency; blood transfusion for anaemia; plasma exchange for hyperviscosity.
- Standard Therapy – cyclical melphalan and prednisolone administered monthly until plateau is achieved.
- Newer approaches – more intensive chemotherapy (e.g. VAD) induce plateau phase more rapidly, but are more toxic. Rapid response is of benefit in bone marrow failure and renal disease, however, benefit in other situations is less clear cut.
- Marrow ablation and HSC transplantation is still being evaluated and is an option for young patients. IFN-α can prolong the plateau phase but does not improve overall survival. Bisphosphonates reduce progression of bone disease.

OTHER PLASMA CELL DISEASES

Plasmacytoma is a single, localised deposit of monoclonal plasma cells, usually in bone, causing localised pain. Paraproteins are detected in about 50% of cases. Local radiotherapy is effective in controlling symptoms. Monitoring is important as 50% advance to MM.

Waldenström's macroglobulinaemia occurs mainly in patients over 50 years and is relatively benign. The paraprotein is of IgM isotype and may cause hyperviscosity. Proliferative, invasive and dysfunctional characteristics of malignant plasma cells are rare. The malignant cell is of lymphoplasmacytoid morphology. Mild anaemia and ESR > 100 mm/hour are common. Moderate lymphoid enlargement is also seen. Renal involvement and amyloidosis is rare. Bone involvement does not occur. Hyperviscosity symptoms usually appear at serum viscosity levels >4 (IgM usually >40 g/l) but individual sensitivity to rises in viscosity varies.

Symptoms of hyperviscosity include:

- Headaches, confusion; light-headedness – impaired cerebral circulation
- Acute deterioration in eyesight – blood vessel tortuosity, dilations, retinal haemorrhages
- Nose bleeds and easy bruising.

Immediate reduction in the serum viscosity by plasmapheresis is indicated in symptomatic patients, especially if visual acuity is impaired. Plasmapheresis is continued until symptoms resolve and serum viscosity improves following which maintenance plasmapheresis is provided at intervals. Chemotherapy similar to that used in CLL is indicated if viscosity or systemic features are difficult to control. Occasional cases are aggressive with major lymphoid enlargement and marrow failure requiring more intensive therapy. Outlook is poor in such cases.

Other rare plasma cell disorders include:

Heavy-chain diseases – rare conditions in which monoclonal plasma cells produce incomplete heavy chain. IgA heavy-chain disease is most common, with IgA-producing plasma cell proliferation in gut mucosa and presenting features of diarrhoea, malabsorption, and weight loss. Transition to an aggressive lymphoma may occur. Other heavy-chain diseases are extremely rare and present like NHL.

Primary amyloidosis – monoclonal light chains deposit as amyloidosis usually complicating MM. Renal, neurological and cardiac dysfunctions are common. Occasionally MM is not present.

Paraprotein-associated neurological syndromes – these include paraprotein-associated neuropathy with a peripheral demyelinating neuropathy caused by paraprotein, usually of IgM isotype, specific for myelin-associated glycolipids. Low-grade B cell neoplasms are sometimes identified. Plasmapheresis and chemotherapy for underlying lymphoproliferation may be useful. POEMS is a syndrome characterised by polyneuropathy, organomegaly,

---

Case 2.31.1 Monoclonal gammopathy of unknown significance

A 60-year-old man presented with tingling and numbness in his fingers and toes, in a glove and stocking distribution. Investigations for causes of neuropathy showed that he had non-insulin dependent diabetes, and this was felt to be the cause of his symptoms. However, an additional incidental finding was of an IgM Kappa monoclonal band on serum electrophoresis.

Further investigation showed that the paraprotein was present in small quantities (4 g/l) and there was no immune paresis detectable. Urine electrophoresis showed only a trace of albuminuria, and no paraprotein or Bence–Jones proteins. Serum calcium was normal, as was alkaline phosphatase and skeletal survey was normal. Bone marrow aspirate and trephine biopsy were within normal limits – specifically there was no increase in plasma cells. There was no clinical or radiological evidence of lymphadenopathy. Following exclusion of multiple myeloma and detectable lymphoproliferative disease, a diagnosis of monoclonal gammopathy of unknown significance was made.

The patient remained well and was followed up regularly in the haematology clinic, with regular monitoring of the amount of paraprotein and β_2-microglobulin. Eight years after presentation the amount of paraprotein detected at a routine visit had doubled. Full workup did not reveal evidence of myeloma. However, the paraprotein level continued to rise, and one year later Bence–Jones proteins became detectable in the urine. Repeat bone marrow showed an excess of plasma cells. In view of progression of monoclonal gammopathy of uncertain significance to myeloma, the patient was commenced on chemotherapy.

Cross reference

Section 3.12   Abnormal Immunoglobulins

endocrine disturbances and skin changes with a monoclonal band. Lymph nodes show monoclonal plasma cell hyperplasia. Symptomatic therapies are indicated.

MONOCLONAL GAMMOPATHY OF UNCERTAIN SIGNIFICANCE

Detection of paraprotein in serum becomes increasingly prevalent with age. In some healthy, asymptomatic patients, paraproteins are identified coincidentally and no underlying causes are found despite careful investigation. This is monoclonal gammopathy of uncertain significance (MGUS) – a diagnosis of exclusion. This is a common problem occurring in 1% of 50 year-olds, 3% of 70 year-olds and 10% of 80 year-olds.

Typical features in MGUS are:

- Lower paraprotein level than in malignant conditions (usually <10 g/l)
- Bence–Jones protein rare (<5%)
- Marrow plasma cell percentage is <10%
- Immunoparesis is rare
- Other laboratory and radiological investigations are normal (myeloma screen)
- No evidence of other paraprotein-related disorder.

The previous term used for this condition – Benign Monoclonal Gammopathy – is not accurate. On long-term follow-up, about 20% of these patients evolve into true MM. On-going clinical and laboratory monitoring is essential. This should be done on a 3–6 month basis indefinitely in all cases.

CROSS REFERENCES

Section 1.13   Immunoglobulin Structure
Section 2.29   Lymphoid Malignancies
Section 3.12   Abnormal Immunoglobulins

Self Assessment

Section 1

State whether the following statements are true or false

2.1a. Genetic factors are more important than environmental factors in explaining the recent rise in atopic disease.
2.1b. *In utero* the immune system is biased towards producing TH2 type responses.
2.1c. In the absence of a history of atopy in one or other parent, a child is unlikely to develop atopy.
2.1d. Overuse of sympathomimetic decongestants can cause a type of chronic rhinitis.
2.1e. SPTs are commonly positive in children with atopic dermatitis and are reliable predictors of clinical response to allergen avoidance.

2.2a. Aspirin-sensitive asthma is commonly associated with nasal polyps.
2.2b. Long-term treatment of asthma is aimed at relaxing bronchial smooth muscle.
2.2c. Cough in the absence of wheeze is a well-recognised presentation of asthma.
2.2d. Histamine is the prominent mediator of the late phase of the allergic response.
2.2e. In the asthmatic airway the number of ciliated cells is increased.

2.3a. C1 Inhibitor deficiency may present with crampy abdominal pain, caused by mucosal oedema.
2.3b. Aspirin sensitivity causes urticaria and angioedema through an IgE-mediated mechanism.
2.3c. Chronic urticaria is rarely due to food allergy, and routine allergy assessment of patients is generally unhelpful.
2.3d. Thyroid disease can present with chronic urticaria.
2.3e. Individual lesions in acute allergic urticaria last for more than 24 hours and resolve with bruising.

2.5a. Anaphylaxis can be differentiated from anaphylactoid reactions on clinical grounds.
2.5b. Elevation of mast cell tryptase proves that mast cell degranulation has occurred, and differentiates anaphylactic reaction to an anaesthetic drug from other anaesthetic accidents.
2.5c. Infection, alcohol and exercise can all exacerbate allergic reactions.
2.5d. Beta-blockers can safely be used in patients with severe allergies.
2.5e. Asthma must be well controlled in patients at risk of an anaphylactic reaction.

2.8a. Severe antibody deficiencies present in the first few weeks after birth.
2.8b. Recurrent bacterial infection is the most common presentation of hypogammaglobulinaemia.
2.8c. All types of hypogammaglobulinaemia may be associated with granulomatous inflammation in lungs and lymphoid tissues.
2.8d. Antibody deficiencies that require replacement therapy present in childhood.
2.8e. Full assessment of humoral immunity should be performed in patients with bronchiectasis.

2.9a. Patients with SCID rarely require intravenous immunoglobulin.
2.9b. Transfusion associated GvHD is a life-threatening complication of SCID, which can be prevented by using irradiated blood products.
2.9c. Vaccination should proceed according to schedule unless a definitive diagnosis of SCID is established.
2.9d. Antibiotic prophylaxis against *Pneumocystis carinii* pneumonia is indicated in SCID.
2.9e. Lymphopaenia is usually present in SCID.

2.10a. Severe gum disease may indicate defects of neutrophil function.

2.10b. The most common neutrophil disorder is primary neutropaenia.

2.10c. Delayed separation of the umbilical cord due to a defective inflammatory response may be the first sign of leucocyte adhesion defects.

2.10d. Neutrophil function testing is unnecessary if there are normal numbers of morphologically normal neutrophils.

2.10e. Prophylactic antibiotics are useful in patients with defective neutrophil function.

2.11a. C1 Inhibitor deficiency is associated with pyogenic infections and immune complex disease.

2.11b. C3 deficiency is the most severe type of complement deficiency.

2.11c. C2 deficiency is the most common complete complement component deficiency in Causacians.

2.11d. Complement deficiency is unlikely if C3 and C4 levels are normal.

2.11e. Patients with deficiencies of terminal attack complex components are particularly susceptible to meningococcal infections.

2.12a. Hyposplenism due to sickle-cell anaemia is associated with a high incidence of salmonella infection.

2.12b. If vaccination cannot be performed pre-splenectomy it should be deferred for at least 6 weeks.

2.12c. Overwhelming post-splenectomy infection rarely occurs in patients under 5 years of age.

2.12d. Howell–Jolly bodies are composed of denatured DNA and are detected on a routine full blood count.

2.12e. Vaccination against pneumococci is effective lifelong post splenectomy.

2.13a. HIV infection can be reliably diagnosed using antibody-based tests within 1 month of infection.

2.13b. Chemoprophylaxis against PCP should be initiated as soon as HIV infection is diagnosed.

2.13c. Anti-retroviral therapy during pregnancy greatly reduces the risk of vertical transmission from a HIV infected mother to their child.

2.13d. HIV rarely mutates – therefore patients who respond to HAART tend to remain responsive.

2.13e. Heterosexual transmission of HIV is rare.

2.15a. In Hashimoto's thyroiditis the presence of autoantibodies indicate that the disease is mediated by humoral immune mechanisms.

2.15b. Immunosuppression may be required for severe eye involvement in Grave's disease.

2.15c. Strongly positive anti-thyroid antibodies in a patient with a thyroid nodule reliably excludes thyroid cancer.

2.15d. IDDM is associated with coeliac disease, and all patients should be screened for anti-endomysial antibody.

2.15e. Addison's disease is frequently the presenting feature of an autoimmune polyglandular syndrome.

2.16a. Diagnosis of ITP requires demonstration of antiplatelet antibodies.

2.16b. Haemolytic disease of the newborn can be fatal and once maternal sensitisation has occurred future pregnancies are extremely difficult to manage.

2.16c. Drug-induced haemolytic anaemia usually remits when the drug is stopped, but recurs if drug is given in the future.

2.16d. Diagnosis of the antiphospholipid syndrome requires demonstration of a laboratory abnormality on at least 2 occasions 8 weeks apart.

2.16e. Aplastic anaemia is a potentially fatal disorder, in which T cell responses to precursors of all three lineages can produce an empty marrow.

2.24a. Active systemic vasculitis is accompanied by an APR that may be quite marked.

2.24b. Biopsy evidence of vasculitis proves that the patient has an autoimmune disorder.

2.24c. ANCA is useful in Wegener's granulomatosis and microscopic polyarteritis, as the majority of patients with active systemic disease are positive. Other types of vasculitis are usually ANCA negative.

2.24d. Henoch–Schönlein purpura usually resolves in children, but is more serious in adults.

2.24e. Rapid introduction of steroids is essential to prevent blindness in patients with temporal arteritis.

2.27a. Autologous HSC transplantation can be used for all of the indications for allogeneic transplantation.

2.27b. In the leukaemias, allogeneic transplantation is preferred.

2.27c. Even in successful HSC transplantation, reconstitution of humoral immunity may not be complete.
2.27d. HSC can only be harvested from bone marrow.
2.27e. GvHD is usually easy to treat, and rarely occurs in a well-matched graft.

2.28a. Hyperacute rejection occurs when an organ is transplanted into a patient with preformed antibodies against the graft, and leads to immediate loss of the graft.
2.28b. In renal transplantation, chronic allograft nephropathy (rejection) is rare.
2.28c. In solid organ transplantation, lung transplantation is associated with the best graft survival.
2.28d. Survival of a renal allograft is primarily determined by recipient factors.
2.28e. Tissue typing routinely types for both major (HLA) and minor (non-HLA) polymorphic molecules.

2.31a. MM can be confidently excluded by a normal serum protein electrophoresis.
2.31b. Renal impairment is rare in MM.
2.31c. Waldenström's macroglobulinaemia is associated with high concentration IgM paraproteins, which frequently cause hyperviscosity.
2.31d. Paraprotein associated neuropathies are usually demyelinating and may respond to plasmapheresis or high-dose intravenous immunoglobulin.
2.31e. MGUS is a benign condition, and patients can be reassured and discharged from follow-up.

Section 2

Match the gene defect from the list on the right with the resulting immunodeficiency on the left.

1.	DiGeorge Syndrome	a.	ADA mutation
2.	X-linked SCID	b.	btk mutation
3.	Hyper-IgM syndrome	c.	Chromosome 22q11 deletion
4.	X-linked agammaglobulinaemia	d.	CD40L mutation
5.	T–B–NK–SCID	e.	Cytokine receptor common gamma-chain mutation.

Match the immunodeficiency from the list on the left with the typical infection/organism on the right.

6.	Chronic Granulomatous Disease	a.	*Pneumocystis carinii*
7.	C5 deficiency	b.	*Enterovirus infection*
8.	X-linked agammaglobulinaemia	c.	*Staphylococcal abscess*
9.	Common variable immunodeficiency	d.	*Meningococcal meningitis*
10.	Severe combined immunodeficiency	e.	*Pneumococcal septicaemia.*

Match the condition from the list on the left with the correct mechanism from the list on the right.

11.	Coeliac disease	a.	IgE-mediated allergy
12.	Migraine	b.	IgE cross-reactivity between pollens and fruit
13.	Anaphylaxis	c.	Food aversion
14.	Oral allergy syndrome	d.	Sensitivity to amines in food
15.	Avoids large numbers of unrelated foods	e.	Non-IgE-mediated immune response to gluten.

Match the condition from the list on the left with the correct mechanism from the list on the right.

16.	Penicillin-induced haemolytic anaemia	a.	Type III hypersensitivity
17.	Skin rash following use of antibiotic cream	b.	Type I hypersensitivity – early phase
18.	Anaphylaxis following IV penicillin administration	c.	Type IV hypersensitivity
19.	Serum sickness following ATG administration	d.	Type I hypersensitivity – late phase
20.	Eosinophilic airway inflammation in asthma.	e.	Type II hypersensitivity.

Match the condition from the list on the left with the correct causative factor from the list on the right

21.	Chronic myeloid leukaemia	a.	EBV
22.	Burkitt's lymphoma	b.	t8:14 (*c-myc/IgH* fusion)
23.	MALToma	c.	HTLV-1 infection
24.	T cell leukaemia	d.	*Helicobacter pylori*
25.	Post-transplant lymphoproliferative disorder	e.	Philadelphia chromosome (*bcr/c-abl* fusion).

Match the condition from the list on the left with the correct causative factor from the list on the right. Each item on the right may be used more than once or not at all.

26.	Rheumatic fever	a.	Cryptic epitopes
27.	Sympathetic ophthalmia	b.	Superantigens
28.	Kawasaki syndrome	c.	Sequestered antigens
29.	Idiopathic SLE	d.	Molecular mimicry
30.	Type I autoimmune polyglandular syndrome	e.	Altered-self
		f.	Genetic defect in immune regulatory gene.

Match the condition from the list on the left with the most appropriate treatment from the list on the right. Each item on the right may be used more than once or not at all.

31.	Coeliac disease	a.	Interferon-β
32.	Guillain–Barré syndrome	b.	Anticholinesterases
33.	Multiple sclerosis	c.	Dietary manipulation
34.	Myasthenia gravis	d.	Anti-TNF-α
35.	Crohn's disease	e.	Interferon-α
		f.	High-dose IVIg.

Match the condition from the list on the left with the correct causative factor from the list on the right.

36.	Pemphigus vulgaris	a.	Antibody binding to blood vessel
37.	Dermatitis herpetiformis	b.	Antibody binding to hemidesmosome
38.	Leucocytoclastic vasculitis	c.	Cellular immune response
39.	Bullous pemphigoid	d.	IgA deposition in dermal papillae
40.	Contact dermatitis	e.	Antibody binding to desmosome
		f.	Immune complex deposition in dermal blood vessels.

Match the condition from the list on the left with the most typical presentation from the list on the right.

41.	ANCA associated GN	a.	Haematuria
42.	IgA nephropathy	b.	Nephrotic syndrome – normal complement
43.	MPGN	c.	Rapidly progressive renal failure
44.	Post-streptococcal GN	d.	Nephritic syndrome
45.	Membranous GN	e.	Hypocomplementaemia with variable renal abnormalities.

Match the condition from the list on the right with the most typical clinical manifestation from the list on the left.

46.	Rheumatoid arthritis	a.	Calcinosis
47.	CREST	b.	Photosensitive rash
48.	SLE	c.	Dry eyes and dry mouth
49.	Sjögren's syndrome	d.	Anterior uveitis
50.	Ankylosing spondylitis	e.	Erosive arthritis.

Section 1 – Answers

2.1a.   False. Environmental factors are more important, given that dramatic increase in prevalence has occurred within a generation.
2.1b.   True.
2.1c.   False. With neither parent atopic, a child has a 10% risk of atopy.
2.1d.   True.
2.1e.   False. SPTs are poor predictors of response to allergen avoidance.

2.2a.   True.
2.2b.   False. Main aim is to treat mucosal inflammation.
2.2c.   True.
2.2d.   False. Histamine is involved in the early phase. Hence antihistamines play no role in management of asthma.
2.2e.   False. Ciliated cells are replaced by mucus-producing cells.

2.3a.   True.
2.3b.   False. Mechanism is not IgE mediated.
2.3c.   True.
2.3d.   True.
2.3e.   False. These features are suggestive of urticarial vasculitis.

2.5a.   False. These types of reaction are clinically indistinguishable.
2.5b.   True.
2.5c.   True.
2.5d.   False. Will inhibit the action of adrenaline if resuscitation is required.
2.5e.   True. Poorly controlled asthma prior to a severe allergic reaction is associated with increased mortality.

2.8a.   False. Usually after 6 months, following depletion of maternal antibody.
2.8b.   True.
2.8c.   False. Granulomatous inflammation is a complication of CVID.
2.8d.   False. CVID and secondary antibody deficiencies commonly present in adult life.
2.8e.   True.

2.9a.   False – they usually do.
2.9b.   True.
2.9c.   False – lifethreatening error! All live vaccines must be withheld until immunodeficiency is excluded.
2.9d.   True.
2.9e.   True.

2.10a. True.
2.10b. False. Secondary neutropaenia.
2.10c. True.
2.10d. False. The opposite. If neutrophil counts are low, or neutrophils look abnormal formal neutrophil function testing rarely adds to patient management.
2.10e. True.

2.11a. False – associated with angioedema.
2.11b. True.
2.11c. True (not so in some other racial groups).
2.11d. False. Need to check classical and alternative haemolytic assays.
2.11e. True.

2.12a. True.
2.12b. False – vaccinate as soon as possible, and definitely before discharge.
2.12c. False – High-risk group
2.12d. False. Must request a blood film. Howell–Jolly bodies are not detected by routine automated haematology analysers.
2.12e. False. Revaccination is recommended at five years, and sooner if anti-pneumococcal antibodies are not maintained.

2.13a. False. Seroconversion may take up to 3 months, and may never occur in neonates. PCR is useful in these situations.
2.13b. False. Only required when CD4 T cell count falls significantly.
2.13c. True.
2.13d. False – frequently mutates, and patients may become resistant to HAART.
2.13e. False – now a major problem. Observation of safe sex practices could greatly reduce transmission by this route.

2.15a. False. Autoantibodies are epiphenomena.
2.15b. True.
2.15c. False. About 30% of patients with thyroid cancer have anti-thyroid antibodies.
2.15d. True.
2.15e. True.

2.16a. False. Diagnosis can be inferred from platelet counts and marrow examination.
2.16b. True. Hence appropriate use of anti-D to prevent sensitisation is essential (see Section 4.7).
2.16c. True.
2.16d. True.
2.16e. True.

2.24a. True.
2.24b. False. Vasculitis can also be secondary to infection and drugs. While such cases are rare, it is essential to distinguish secondary vasculitis before instituting immunosuppression.
2.24c. True.
2.24d. True.
2.24e. True.

2.27a. False. Cannot be used in diseases where stem cells are abnormal.
2.27b. True. Despite higher risk of GvHD, graft-versus-leukaemia effect and avoidance of regrafting malignant cells, there are significant advantages.
2.27c. True.
2.27d. False. HSC can be mobilised with growth factors and harvested from peripheral blood, as well as from umbilical cord blood.
2.27e. False. GvHD is a common cause of morbidity and mortality.

2.28a. True.
2.28b. False. Will ultimately occur in virtually all transplants unless graft is lost from some other cause first.
2.28c. False. Lung transplantation remains a major challenge, and is associated with relatively poor outcomes.
2.28d. False. Donor factors and perioperative events also exert a major influence.
2.28e. False. Routine typing is only available for major (HLA) antigens.

2.31a. False. SPEP normal in about 15%. Must also exclude BJPs. True non-secretory myeloma accounts for 1% of cases.
2.31b. False. Occurs in 50% of cases.
2.31c. True.
2.31d. True.
2.31e. False. Approximately 20% will progress to myeloma. Regular follow-up is essential.

Section 2 – Answers

1c;	2e;	3d;	4b;	5a;	6c;	7d;	8b;	9e;	10a;
11e;	12d;	13a;	14b;	15c;	16e;	17c;	18b;	19a;	20d;
21e;	22b;	23d;	24c;	25a;	26d;	27c;	28b;	29a;	30f;
31c;	32f;	33a;	34b;	35d;	36e;	37d;	38f;	39b;	40c;
41c;	42a;	43e;	44d;	45b;	46e;	47a;	48b;	49c;	50d.

PART 3

IMMUNOTECHNIQUES AND DIAGNOSTIC TESTS USED IN CLINICAL IMMUNOLOGY

INTRODUCTION

The aim of this part is to describe the diagnostic tests that are performed in a clinical immunology laboratory. The principles underlying immunological techniques are explained and illustrated. There is a concise description of each specific test that includes clinical indications, principles of the test, interpretation and potential pitfalls. This part is cross-referenced with Clinical Immunology (Part 2) and provides the practical information that is necessary for the effective use of a clinical immunology laboratory.

REFERENCES

Gooi, H. C. and Chapel, H. (eds) (1990) *Clinical Immunology: A Practical Approach*, Oxford University Press, Oxford.

Rose, N. R., deMacario, E. C., Folds, J. D. *et al.* (eds) (1997) *Manual of Clinical Laboratory Immunology*, ASM Press, Washington D.C., USA.

Zola, H., Roberts-Thomson, P. and McEvoy, R. (1995) *Diagnostic Immunopathology: Laboratory Practice and Clinical Application*, Cambridge University Press, Cambridge.

Laboratory Tests in Clinical Immunology

CLINICAL INDICATIONS

Before requesting a test, it is important to decide what clinically useful information will be obtained from the result, that is, the clinical indication for testing.

The value of laboratory tests in the care of patients varies greatly and they may be grouped as follows:

* Essential for diagnosis and monitoring
* Useful for subtyping disorders with different complications and outcomes
* Limited to research applications (with potential for future use in the diagnostic laboratory).

No matter how good a test is, it will not be helpful if ordered in inappropriate circumstances.

HOW GOOD IS A TEST?

The ideal test distinguishes all patients with a particular condition (true positives) from all patients with conditions other than the one of interest, and from healthy individuals (true negatives). In real life, this rarely occurs. Correct interpretation of test results is dependent on many parameters including patient characteristics, laboratory techniques, operator characteristics, predictive values of particular tests and quality performance. Some factors that influence test performance are outlined here along with terms widely used to describe laboratory test systems. This is by no means a complete account, but rather highlights important concepts in laboratory test evaluation.

PARAMETERS THAT INFLUENCE TEST PERFORMANCE

Predictive value of tests

There are four possible relationships between test result and disease status (Table 3.1.1).

Erroneous conclusions (i.e. false positive and false negative results) are possible with almost all test systems. Several terms are used to indicate test performance in this regard:

Specificity Diagnostic specificity is the ability of a test to indicate a negative result in the absence of disease. It is the percentage of patients who do not have the disease and whose test result is negative.

$$\text{Specificity} = \frac{\text{Number of true negatives} \times 100}{\text{Number of true negatives} + \text{Number of false positives}}$$

A positive result in a test that is very specific for a disease or clinical state may be used to confirm clinical diagnosis.

The term specificity is also used to describe the ability of an assay to measure one component without interference from others (i.e. absence of cross-reactivity).

Sensitivity Diagnostic sensitivity is the ability of a test to indicate a positive result in the presence of disease. It is the percentage of patients with the disease whose test result is positive.

$$\text{Sensitivity} = \frac{\text{Number of true positives} \times 100}{\text{Number of true positives} + \text{Number of false negatives}}$$

A negative result in a test that is very sensitive may be used to exclude disease.

The term sensitivity is also used to describe the ability of a test to detect small quantities of the protein or antibody being measured.

Positive and negative predictive values The positive predictive value (PPV) of a test is the proportion of patients with positive tests who have disease. It measures how well the test establishes a diagnosis. PPV is critically dependent on the prevalence of the disease in the population tested. The prevalence of disease is the total number of cases of a particular disease existing in a population at a certain time.

$$\text{PPV \%} = \frac{\text{Number of true positives} \times 100}{\text{Number of true positives} + \text{Number of false positives}}$$

The negative predictive value (NPV) of a test is the proportion of patients with negative results who do not have disease. It measures how well the test rules out disease. It is also dependent on the prevalence of the disease tested.

$$\text{NPV \%} = \frac{\text{Number of true negatives} \times 100}{\text{Number of true negatives} + \text{Number of false negatives}}$$

Table 3.1.1 Relationships between disease status and test outcome

	DISEASE PRESENT D+	DISEASE ABSENT D−
Test positive T+	True positive TP	False positive FP
Test negative T−	False negative FN	True negative TN

Accuracy and precision

◆　Accuracy is the ability of an assay to obtain results that are very close to the true value.
◆　Precision refers to an assay's ability to obtain reproducible results when it is repeated on different occasions.

Inaccuracy and imprecision arise from two types of error. Systematic error refers to an ongoing bias in test performance that hinders results, for example, persisting problems with test technique such as worn machinery, deteriorated control or test specimens. Random errors occur when variability in techniques, for example, measuring, timing or counting, impair quality; specimen error is usually due to inadequate specimen labelling.

Reference ranges

Without a well-constructed reference range, accuracy and precision are meaningless. Testing of a large population of healthy individuals, and in some cases patients with diseases other than that of interest, is required to define the level of the analyte in this unaffected population. The larger this group, the more reliable the reference range will be (at least 100). The sample should be representative of the general population with regard to age, sex and ethnicity. The reference range is usually defined as the range of values that fall within two standard deviations (SD) of each side of the mean result. If results are normally distributed, this will include 95% of the normal population. The percentage of patients with disease who have an abnormal result depends on the test sensitivity.

When a reference range is being selected, it is important to decide whether sensitivity or specificity is more important. A reference range with high sensitivity (nearly all patients with a disease will have a positive result) is desirable in a screening test like anti-nuclear antibody (ANA) (for SLE) where follow-up of positive samples by more specific tests (anti-double-stranded DNA antibodies (anti-dsDNA Abs)) occurs.

Cut-off point

The cut-off point for any assay is the point above which results are considered positive. It must be set so that the minimum number of patients with disease are tested negative (false negative) and as few as possible individuals without disease are tested positive (false positive).

Laboratory test categories

◆　Quantitative assays measure concentrations and numbers, for example, complement or immunoglobulin (Ig) levels in g/L or mg/ml; numbers of cells in a given volume. International reference material with a known concentration or number of the analyte/cell being measured is available for standardisation of many tests within and between laboratories.
◆　Semi-quantitative assays define a range of values between which the unknown sample value falls. The results may be expressed as a titre or as classes, for example, negative, weak, moderate or strong positive, if a known standard has been used for comparison.

♦ Titres – Many laboratory tests are carried out at an optimal serum dilution selected to maintain assay sensitivity and specificity. In assays used to detect circulating autoantibodies, such as indirect immunofluorescence (IIF) and agglutination assays, the amount of antibody present is indicated by titration of a positive serum by serial dilution. The titre is defined as the reciprocal of the last dilution where a positive reaction is seen, that is, the endpoint. Defining the endpoint of a titration is usually highly subjective. Whenever a titre is reported, the accuracy is assumed to be plus or minus one dilution. For example:

— ANAs are detected by IIF
— A common screening dilution for ANAs is 1/40
— If serum is positive for ANA at 1/40, then serial doubling dilution is performed to obtain the serum dilutions 1/80, 1/160, 1/320
— The last point at which positive fluorescence is observed is 1/160
— Therefore, the ANA titre is 160
— In practise, the titre may be reported as the dilution or as the reciprocal of the dilution.

♦ Qualitative assay results are usually expressed in the following terms: negative, positive; normal or abnormal; present or absent. International reference material may not be available. Determination of the cut-off point requires extensive clinical validation and is dependent on the sensitivity and specificity required.

INTERPRETATION

The correct interpretation of laboratory tests requires some knowledge of the test performance parameters described above. However, in all cases tests should only be interpreted in the context of the clinical presentation. Treat the patient not the test.

CROSS REFERENCE
Section 3   Section 3.1 is relevant to all sections of Part 3

Antibodies are Essential Tools in the Clinical Immunology Laboratory

An extensive range of assays have been developed that can yield quantitative or qualitative measurement of antigen (e.g. protein chemistry) or antibody (e.g. detection of autoantibodies). Many of these assays utilise customised antibodies (Table 3.2.1).

Antibodies that are used as tools in the clinical immunology laboratory may be raised in animals. Immunisation using the antigen of interest induces production of antibodies that can be isolated for use in immunoassays.

Table 3.2.1 A summary of methodologies that use antibodies as tools in the clinical immunology laboratory

APPLICATION	METHOD	ANTIBODY TOOL	EXAMPLE
Autoimmune and infectious disease serology	IIF	FITC-labelled anti-human Ig antibody	ANA Syphilis testing – FTA
	DIF	FITC-labelled anti-human Ig/complement antibody	Deposition of Ig and complement in tissue
	ELISA	Enzyme-labelled anti-human Ig antibody	Anti-dsDNA antibody HIV screening
	RIA	Radio-labelled antibody	AchR antibody
	Immunoblotting	Enzyme- or radio-labelled antibody	Confirmatory HIV serology
Cell numbers and function	Flow cytometry	FITC-labelled monoclonal antibody to cell surface marker	CD4+ and CD8+ T cell numbers
Protein chemistry	Nephelometry Radial immunodiffusion	Antibody against protein in question	Concentration of C3, C4, IgG, IgG or IgM

Note: Antibodies are polyclonal unless otherwise stated.

- The antigen may be a protein such as a human complement component; antibodies to complement components are used to measure complement levels by nephelometry or by radial immunodiffusion (RID).
- Human antibody is a foreign antigen to other species: antibodies that recognise human immunoglobulins are used to detect antibodies (against autoantigens or infectious organisms) in patient's serum.

Antibodies are used as primary reagents to detect antigen levels where antibody/antigen immune complex formation is detected by precipitation assays such as RID or nephelometry.

Antibodies may also be labelled with a fluorescent dye, enzyme or radioisotope to facilitate the detection and/or measurement of antigen or antibody using a range of immunoassays.

POLYCLONAL AND MONOCLONAL ANTIBODIES ARE USED AS LABORATORY TOOLS

Polyclonal antibodies

In response to foreign antigens, animals make polyclonal antibodies, that is, a mixture of antibodies produced by different clones of B cells, each having its own specificity for different epitopes on the same injected antigen. Each antibody has a different variable

Figure 3.2.1 Diagram of monoclonal antibody production.

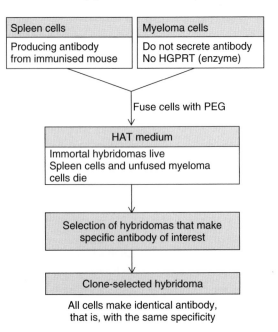

region. The majority of antibodies are raised in mice and rabbits, although other animals may also be used. Antibody is purified from animal serum usually by affinity chromatography. Different batches of polyclonal antibody may not behave in an identical manner in an assay.

Some human antigens are poorly immunogenic in animals as a result of a high degree of homology (similarity). Use of animals with distinct antigenic differences (e.g. guinea-pig, chicken, etc.) may overcome this problem.

Monoclonal antibodies

Monoclonal antibodies are the product of a single B cell clone and its progeny. Each of these antibodies have identical variable regions and react with identical epitopes. Spleen cell suspensions from immunised mice contain numerous secreting B cells from different clones many of which recognise the antigen of interest. These B cells are fused with cells from a non-secreting myeloma line to form hybrids: the spleen cell provides the ability to make specific antibody while the myeloma cell provides the ability to grow indefinitely in culture and secrete immunoglobulins continuously.

After fusion, the hybrid cells are selected using drugs that kill the myeloma parental cell, while the unfused parental spleen cells have a limited life-span and die. Only the hybrid myeloma cell lines or hybridomas survive. Hybridomas producing antibody of the desired specificity are identified and cloned by regrowing cultures from single cells. The affinities of the antibody as well as cross-reactivity patterns are used to select the most useful antigen-specific clone. It is important to appreciate that while all monoclonal antibodies are identical, this does not guarantee that they will be monospecific. Unfortunately many mono-clonal antibodies are of relatively low affinity and cross-react with proteins other than the analyte of interest (Figure 3.2.1).

CROSS REFERENCE

Section 4.5   Therapeutic Antibody Production

SECTION 3.3

Detection of Antibodies and Antigen

DETECTION OF ANTIBODY – AUTOANTIBODIES

The hallmark of many autoimmune disorders is the presence of specific autoantibodies circulating in the blood and/or deposited in the affected tissue. Organ-specific and non-organ specific autoimmunity results in a multitude of overlapping clinical disorders. The detection of autoantibodies provides diagnostic and prognostic information and is useful in monitoring disease activity.

Some autoantibodies are directly involved in disease pathogenesis making them highly specific for the disease (e.g. anti-GBM antibody and Goodpastures syndrome). Other autoantibodies are epiphenomena, either produced incidentally or arising as a consequence of the tissue damage associated with a disease process. Although not directly pathogenic, such autoantibodies may be useful serological markers of disease. Many autoantibodies are found in healthy subjects, particularly in older people. When interpreting the clinical significance of autoantibodies, the clinical history, examination and other laboratory information should be considered.

DETECTION OF ANTIGEN – MEASUREMENT OF PROTEIN LEVELS

Many of the methods used for the detection and measurement of autoantibodies are also used to measure the concentration of proteins including many involved in the immune response. This is important in the investigation of immunodeficiency and inflammatory markers.

IMMUNOASSAY TECHNIQUES

Precipitation assays

These assays depend on the formation of insoluble immune complexes when antibody and antigen concentrations reach equivalence.

Radial ImmunoDiffusion (RID)   Wells are cut into agarose containing antibody to the analyte of interest. A series of standards of known analyte (antigen) concentration and unknowns (patient sera) are placed into the wells. The antigen diffuses radially from the well and a ring of precipitate forms around the well at the antigen–antibody equivalence (precipitin ring). The diameter of the ring is proportional to the concentration of analyte in the well since the antibody concentration in the agarose remains constant. Using standards of known analyte concentration, a calibration curve is generated by plotting the square of the diameter against concentration. The calibration curve is used to determine the concentration of analyte in test sera (Figure 3.3.1).

Nephelometry or turbidimetry   When immune complex formation takes place in the liquid phase, the light absorbing/scattering properties of the solution change and can be measured. Nephelometry measures the amount of light scattered at a defined angle to the incident beam. Turbidimetry measures the reduction of incident light due to absorption. Patient serum is diluted and incubated with antibody against the component of interest; this may be

Figure 3.3.1 RID and nephelometry.

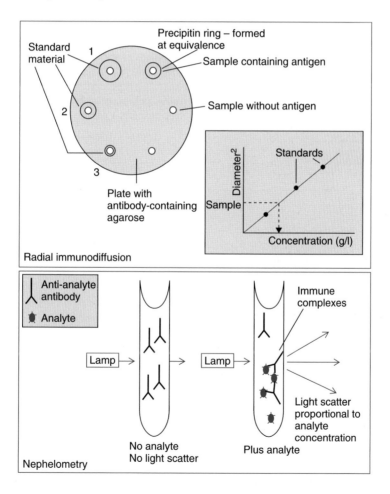

a protein, such as a complement component. Alternatively, when measuring antibody concentration, patient serum is incubated with antigen. Formation of antibody–antigen complexes leads to an increase in the light scattering or turbidity of the solution. This process may be measured at equilibrium or during complex formation using a nephelometer or turbidimeter. In the presence of a constant amount of antibody, the concentration of the component of interest may be measured. Inaccuracies can arise if the antigen of interest is present in excess concentration relative to the detecting antibody–antigen excess. Further dilution of test serum allows accurate measurement to be made. Lipaemic or haemolysed samples interfere with the optical properties of the solution and are not suitable for analysis.

Double diffusion   Antigen and antibody solutions are placed in wells cut into an agarose gel and allowed to diffuse for several days. Preciptin lines form in the gel where antigen and antibody reach equivalence. Precipitating antibodies to specific antigens in patients' sera can be detected using this method, where antigen is placed in a central well, and control or patients' sera are placed in surrounding wells (Figure 3.3.2).

Counter-current immunoelectrophoresis   Antigens and antibodies are electrophoresed towards each other in an agarose gel made up in a suitable buffer. Patients' and reference sera are placed in a line of wells cut into the agarose, and antigen is placed into a trough or line of wells parallel to this. Negatively charged antigens will move towards the anode (+) and antibodies will move towards the cathode (−). If the patient's serum contains a relevant antibody, a precipitin line is formed between the wells. After electrophoresis, precipitin lines may visualised by drying the agarose gel and staining with Coomassie Blue stain. The specificity of the antibody can be ascertained by comparing precipitin lines formed by patient sera with control sera. Formation of a line of identity (both precipitin lines merge imperceptibly) between patient and control sera allows antibody specificity to be identified. Counter-current immunoelectrophoresis (CCIE) is used to detect anti-ENA antibodies (see Figure 3.4.3).

Figure 3.3.2 Double diffusion.

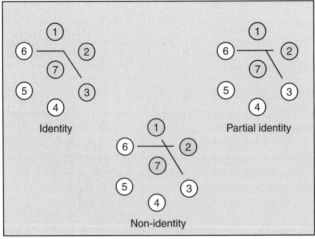

Wells 1 and 4   Known positive control serum
Wells 2, 3, 5 and 6 Test sera
Well 7   Antigen

Notes on RID and nephelometry

- ◆ Both of these methods may be used to measure the concentration of complement components, immunoglobulins, protease inhibitors, acute-phase proteins, transport proteins and coagulation proteins.
- ◆ RID is sensitive, but interpretation is subjective; it takes several days for the reaction to reach equivalence so that results are delayed.
- ◆ Nephelometry gives greater precision than RID and facilitates greater speed, automation and objectivity; it is suitable for large throughput tests.
- ◆ Standard preparations, which have been calibrated against International WHO standards, are available for most common analytes.

Agglutination assays

Antigen is coated onto an inert carrier particle such as gelatin, latex beads or red blood cells (RBCs). Serum containing specific antibody agglutinates antigen-coated particles. Agglutination results in the formation of a 'carpet' of particles at the base of a round-bottomed reaction well (microtitre plate). If no antibody is present in the serum, the particles will form a tight 'button'. The endpoint titre is the last serum dilution where agglutination is still 50% greater than the serum incubated with non-coated particles. Agglutination assays are not class-specific and detect all agglutinating antibody; IgM pentamers are more efficient at agglutinating antigen-coated particles/RBCs. Agglutination is used to detect anti-thyroid antibodies and rheumatoid factors. Agglutination is the basis for the Direct Coombs' test for detection of anti-RBC antibodies (Figure 3.3.3).

Figure 3.3.3 Agglutination.

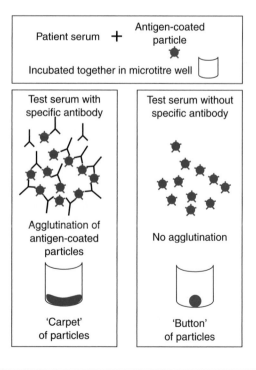

Some serum components may react non-specifically with gelatin particles or RBCs in agglutination assays and this may interfere with the detection of antibodies. If present such heterophile antibodies must be fully adsorbed prior to use of a particle agglutination assay.

Enzyme linked immuno-sorbent assay (ELISA)

ELISA for the detection of antibody   Test serum is incubated in microtitre plates that have been coated with purified antigen. After washing to remove unbound serum constituents, an enzyme-labelled anti-immunoglobulin antibody is incubated with the bound antibody. After washing to remove unbound conjugated antibody, enzyme-labelled antibody is visualised by the addition of a chromogenic enzyme substrate. Colour development is proportional to the concentration of antibody in the test serum and is measured spectrophotometrically. Using known positive sera, a standard curve is generated to determine the antibody levels (expressed in arbitrary units or International Units (IU) if the assay is calibrated against an international standard). ELISAs are sensitive and specific assays. Antigen purity determines the specificity of the assay. ELISAs are readily automated and with increasing availability of purified or recombinant antigens are commonly used to detect antibodies (Figure 3.3.4).

Sandwich ELISA   Serum containing the analyte (antigen) is incubated in a microtitre plate coated with a capture antibody. A second enzyme-labelled antibody, which recognises a different antigenic site on the antigen of interest, is added. Following incubation, unbound antibody is removed by washing. After addition of a chromogenic enzyme substrate, colour development is proportional to the concentration of antigen in the test serum and is measured spectrophotometrically. This type of ELISA is suitable for

Figure 3.3.4   Enzyme linked immunosorbent assay (ELISA).

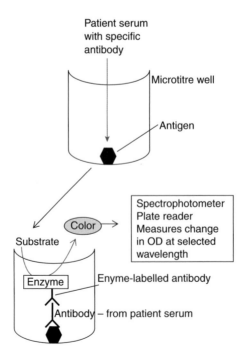

measuring analytes other than antibodies. Modifications of this technique can increase the sensitivity, allowing very low concentrations of analyte be measured (e.g. cytokines).

Radioimmunoassay

Radioimmunoassays (RIAs) are laboratory tests in which either antigen or antibodies are radiolabelled. RIAs designed to measure antibody levels utilise excess radiolabelled antigen, which is incubated with patient serum, as well as a series of standard antibody preparations. The antigen bound to antibody is then precipitated either with a specific precipitating second antibody or by a non-specific protein precipitant (e.g. ammonium sulphate). Precipitated antigen (quantified using a beta counter) is proportional to the antibody concentration (Figure 3.3.5).

The use of RIAs in the clinical immunology laboratory is largely restricted to the detection of high-affinity anti-dsDNA antibodies (Farr assay), anti-AChR and anti-TSH receptor antibodies. RIA is sensitive and specific. It is limited in use because of the hazards associated with dealing with radioactive isotopes (I^{125}) and the short shelf life of RIA reagents.

ELISA is more sensitive but often less specific than RIA. ELISA detects both high- and low-affinity antibodies, while RIA detects only high-affinity antibodies;

Figure 3.3.5 Competitive radioimmunoassay (RIA).

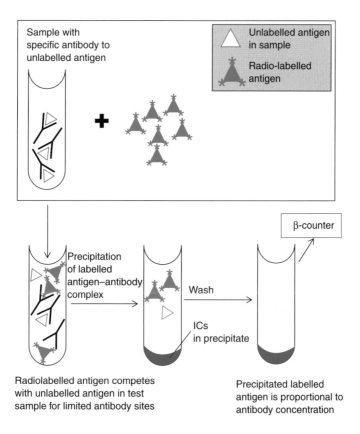

high-affinity antibodies are often more closely disease associated. ELISA reagents are less hazardous than radioactivity and usually last longer.

Indirect and direct Immunofluorescence

Indirect immunofluorescence (IIF) is a commonly used technique that detects autoantibodies in serum when they bind antigens in an appropriate substrate (rodent, primate or human antigen-expressing tissue sections or cultured cells). Bound antibody is stained with a fluorescein (FITC)-labelled anti-immunoglobulin antibody, and visualised using ultraviolet (UV) fluorescence microscopy. Antibody specificity may be inferred from the pattern of staining observed, however confirmatory objective tests are generally used when available. Titration gives a semiquantitative estimate of the amount of autoantibody present in serum. Human serum contains heterophile antibodies that react with non-human animal tissues but not with human tissues. These must be distinguished from patterns produced by true autoantibodies on rodent tissues. It is essential to use serum not plasma for IIF as fibrinogen causes non-specific fluorescence (Figure 3.3.6).

Direct immunofluorescence (DIF), is used to demonstrate antibody and complement deposition in patients' tissues. Fresh tissue, usually from a skin or renal biopsy is snap frozen in liquid nitrogen and sectioned (7 μm sections) onto glass slides. These sections of tissue are incubated with FITC-conjugated antisera against complement components (C3 and C4), Igs (IgA, IgG and IgM) and fibrin. This allows visualisation of the deposited antibody or complement components in a distinctive pattern with a fluorescence microscope. The pattern of deposition of these components in tissue (e.g. skin or kidney) may be diagnostic of several diseases. Tissue-bound antibody may be present in the absence of circulating autoantibody.

Figure 3.3.6 Indirect immunofluorescence (IIF) and direct immunofluorescence (DIF).

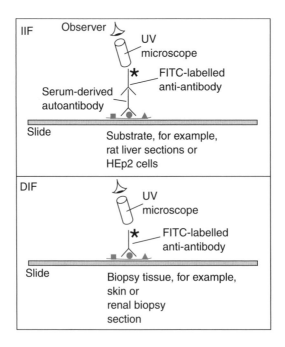

Flow cytometry

Flow cytometry can be used to analyse single particles, where specific molecules (e.g. cluster of differentiation (CD) markers) or functions (e.g. calcium release) can be indicated using fluorescent techniques. In diagnostic immunology, the most common applications are measurement of lymphocyte subpopulations after staining with fluorescence-labelled antibodies, and characterisation of leukaemias and lymphomas. Using flow cytometry the percentage of a cell population expressing a particular marker, as well as the intensity of expression can be objectively measured in thousands of individual cells within a short time. Flow cytometry can also be used to measure antibody in serum, using antigen(s) of interest immobilised on fluorescent beads or donor cells (see Section 3.15).

Additional applications include measurement of any cell function for which a fluorescent probe is available such as Ca^{++} flux, reactive oxygen intermediate production and intracellular cytokine production.

Cell marker studies

For cell marker studies, aliquots of fresh anti-coagulated whole blood are incubated with fluorescence-labelled monoclonal antibodies. This is followed by red cell lysis and usually fixation of cells. The cell suspension is aspirated into the flow cytometer and cells pass in single file past a laser beam, which excites the fluorescent probes. Light sensors detect light scatter emitted by each individual cell. Cell populations vary in size and granularity,

Figure 3.3.7 Flow cytometry and examples of data display.

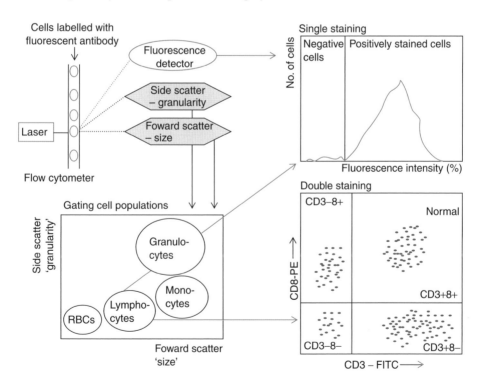

affecting the forward and side scatter properties of the light. Specified limits on light scatter can be used to 'gate' on the cell population of interest, often supplemented by analysis of fluorescence with anti-CD45 (all white cells) and anti-CD14 (monocytes). Further analysis of cell markers can be limited to the gated population.

Light emitted by excited fluorescent dye on the cell surface is detected by sensors, amplified by photomultipliers and analysed by computer software. The instrument may have a number of detectors for a number of different fluorescent dyes (FITC, phycoerythrin (PE)) – this is essential for double labelling of cells (known as two-colour analysis). Routine applications involve up to four-colour analysis, allowing four parameters in addition to light scatter to be measured for each cell. The data may be displayed as single parameter histograms; dot plots where two parameters are compared, or even three-dimensional plots (Figure 3.3.7).

If absolute counts are required a known volume of a bead suspension (where the count per ml is known) is added to the stained cell suspension. When the appropriate number of

Figure 3.3.8 Immunoblotting.

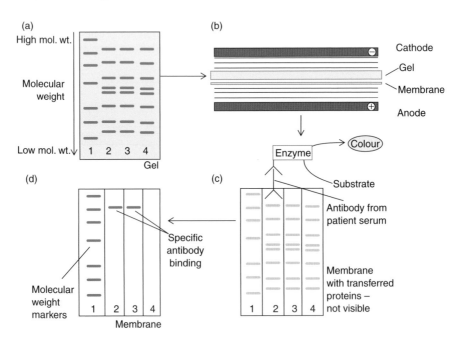

Notes: Immunoblotting can be used for the detection of specific antibodies in patient sera. Gel electrophoresis of a standard antigen preparation separates proteins according to their size (molecular weight). At the same time a mixture of proteins of known molecular weights is also run. These separated proteins are transferred to another matrix (e.g. nitrocellulose membrane), which is suitable for subsequent immunodetection methods. The membrane is cut into separate strips and incubated with control or patient sera. Specific antibody binds protein on the membrane strip and unbound serum components are removed by washing. Bound antibody is detected with an enzyme-labelled antibody and visualised by the addition of a suitable substrate.

(a) Separation of proteins by electrophoresis: lane 1, molecular weight markers; lanes 2–4, standard antigen preparation, (b) electroblotting to transfer separated proteins to membrane, (c) immunoassay to detect specific antibody: lane 1, stained molecular weight markers; lane 2, positive control; lanes 3–4, patient 1 and 2 and (d) membrane strips showing the presence of specific antibody in patient 1 (lane 3).

gated events has been acquired by the flow cytometer, the ratio of beads to cells of interest is compared and the absolute cell count derived mathematically. For analysis of lymphocyte subtypes, results expressed in absolute numbers rather than percentages are more meaningful.

Immunoblotting of antibodies/antigens

Immunoblotting (also know as Western blotting) is a multistage procedure where proteins are separated by electrophoresis, transferred to a semipermeable membrane and probed with antibody (Figure 3.3.8). Bound antibody is visualised using an appropriate detection system. This system may be used to investigate the presence of specific antibody in patients' sera, or characterised antibody can be used to investigate the presence of proteins of interest in biological samples. In addition to its value in routine diagnostics, immunoblotting can be used to begin to identify previously unknown antibody specificity in patient's serum. Detection of ANA specificities by immunoblotting is illustrated in Figure 3.4.4.

Immunoblotting is a powerful tool for detection of antibodies that recognise linear epitopes (dependent on the amino acid sequence alone) as the process of electrophoresis frequently denatures proteins. Immunoprecipitation may be required to detect antibodies that bind conformational epitopes (composed of amino acids from different parts of a folded protein), however details of this technique are outside the scope of this text.

CROSS REFERENCE

Sections 3.4–3.17   Applications of methodologies in clinical immunology

---

REFERENCES

Catty, D. (ed.) (1988) *Antibodies. A Practical Approach*. Oxford University Press, Oxford.
Rose, N. R., deMacario, E. C., Folds, J. D. *et al.* (eds) (1997) *Manual of Clinical Laboratory Immunology*. ASM Press, Washington, D.C.

Autoantibody Profiles in Connective Tissue Diseases and Rheumatoid Disease

RHEUMATOID DISEASE

Rheumatoid factors (RFs) are autoantibodies directed against the Fc portion of IgG. RF may be IgM, IgA or IgG but IgM is most commonly measured. The presence of IgM RF is included in the American Rheumatological Association (ARA) clinical criteria for diagnosis of rheumatoid arthritis (RA).

Clinical indications

Suspected rheumatoid disease.

- Inflammatory, symmetrical polyarthropathy (hands and feet especially)
- Periarticular bony erosions on X-ray
- Features of extra-articular rheumatoid disease, including:
  — Sjögrens syndrome
  — Lymphadenopathy
  — Scleritis and episcleritis
  — Cutaneous vasculitis and ulceration
  — Skin and lung nodules
  — Pleural effusions, alveolitis, bronchiolitis obliterans
  — Pericarditis, endocarditis
  — Splenomegaly (often neutropaenia)
  — Myositis, mononeuritis multiplex, cord compression from spinal involvement.

Principle of the test

RFs are routinely detected by particle agglutination or nephelometry. Nephelometry gives quantitative data with high precision and accuracy.

Latex agglutination test – latex particles coated with human IgG agglutinate when incubated with serum containing RF.

In nephelometry, serum is diluted and incubated with RF antigen (aggregated human IgG) resulting in complex formation. The rate of light scatter is proportional to the concentration of RF in the serum sample.

Interpretation

- RF is present in up to 90% of patients with RA, but is not specific for RA. Negative RF does not exclude disease.
- Strongly positive RF is suggestive of rheumatoid disease. A high RF level in rheumatoid disease is a poor prognostic factor. Extra-articular features, such as rheumatoid nodules and vasculitis are more common.
- Strongly positive RF may also be found in Sjögren's syndrome and cryoglobulinaemia.
- RF levels do not vary significantly with changes in disease activity; CRP is a better indicator of activity.

RF may also occur in a wide variety of conditions including connective tissue diseases, infections and lymphoproliferative conditions. Infection-induced RF usually disappears following adequate treatment. The presence of RF becomes more common with increasing age (over the age of 70 years, 5–10 % of the healthy population will have detectable RF).

Frequency of IgM RFs (varies with assay technique)

- RA   50–90%
- Sjögrens syndrome   70–80%
- SLE   15–35%
- Juvenile RA   7–10%
- Polymyositis   5–10%
- Chronic infection   up to 50% (usually weak).

Pitfalls

- The levels of RF may fluctuate with the use of disease-modifying drugs such as gold and salazopyrine, but this is not a reliable guide to response to therapy.
- RFs may occur in a variety of situations where it does not necessarily indicate disease and therefore it is important to interpret RF results in the context of the clinical setting.
- Frequently, relatives of patients with RA are weakly RF positive; this does not indicate disease.

CROSS REFERENCES

Section 1.13   Immunoglobulin Structure
Section 2.22   Rheumatoid Disease and Spondylarthropathies
Section 3.3   Detection of Antibodies and Antigen

AUTOANTIBODIES ASSOCIATED WITH CONNECTIVE TISSUE DISEASES (CTDs)

Anti-nuclear antibody (ANA) – also known as anti-nuclear factor (ANF)

ANAs are autoantibodies directed against a variety of constituents of cell nuclei including DNA, RNA and nuclear proteins. ANAs directed against double-stranded DNA (dsDNA), centromeric proteins and the extractable nuclear antigens (ENAs) are the most clinically significant. ENAs include antibodies to Ro, La, Sm, RNP, Jo-1 and Scl-70. Other ANA specificities of interest include anti-histones, anti-PM-Scl, anti-Ku, and anti-Mi-2 antibodies. Antibodies to Ro, Jo-1, ribosomal-P protein and signal recognition protein (SRP) bind cytoplasmic antigens, but are also of interest in diagnosing CTDs. Despite their cytoplasmic location Ro and Jo-1 are loosely termed ENAs in clinical practice.

Clinical indications

- Suspected CTDs – SLE, Sjögrens syndrome, mixed connective tissue disease (MCTD), scleroderma, CREST syndrome (calcinosis, Raynaud's phenomenon, oesophageal dysmotility, sclerodactyly and telangiectasiae), polymyositis/dermatomyositis.
- Autoimmune hepatitis (ANA only).
- Investigation of autoimmune haemolytic anaemia (AIHA) or immune thrombocytopaenia (ITP) to exclude associated CTD (SLE).

Principle of the test

ANA is usually detected by IIF on HEp-2 cells, a cell line containing large nuclei. Rodent liver is also used as a substrate. ANAs react with nuclear antigens including dsDNA and ENAs. ANA reactivity is clarified by additional methods including ELISA, RIA and immunoblotting.

The main staining patterns observed include homogenous, speckled, centromere and nucleolar. The staining patterns are distinguished by evaluation of resting and dividing cells. They are a poor guide to antibody specificity.

- Homogenous pattern – in resting cells, the nucleus stains evenly throughout. In dividing cells the condensed chromosomal region is positive while the surrounding cytoplasm is negative (Figure 3.4.1(a)).
- Speckled pattern – in resting cells, there are speckles of fluorescence throughout the nucleus. Mitotic (or dividing cell) chromosomes are negative (Figure 3.4.1(d)).
- Centromere pattern – in resting cells, discrete uniform points of fluorescence throughout the nucleus are observed. In mitotic cells, the speckles cluster in the chromosome mass giving the classical centromere pattern (Figure 3.4.1(c)).
- Nucleolar pattern – in resting cells the nucleolus is stained (Figure 3.4.1(b)).
- Mixed patterns occur when a patient's serum contains more than one type of ANA.

Strong positive ANAs should be investigated further to identify significant autoantibody specificities (anti-dsDNA and anti-ENA antibodies).

Important notes on ANA testing by IIF

- Only IgG-ANAs are of proven clinical value.
- Antibodies have a long circulating half-life and therefore frequent measurement of ANA is unhelpful.
- The use of human epithelial cell line (HEp-2) cells rather than rodent liver has several advantages:

    — Nuclei are large, allowing easier pattern recognition
    — More sensitive assay
    — Required for anti-centromere antibody identification.

Figure 3.4.1 ANA patterns of staining by IIF on HEp-2 cells: (a) homogenous, (b) nucleolar, (c) centromere, (d) speckled and (e) IIF on *C. luciliae* – kinetoplast (K) and nucleus (N) are shown. See Plate Section for colour reproduction of these images.

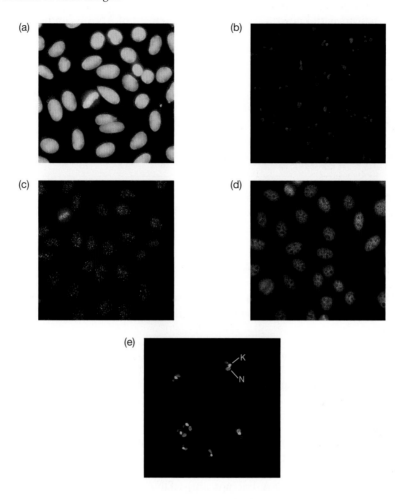

Interpretation

- Interpretation of ANAs is dependent on the clinical situation, and the age and sex of the patient. Strongly positive ANAs are associated with CTDs and autoimmune liver disease.
- Weak ANA is often a non-specific finding, seen more commonly in women and the elderly, and in many inflammatory disorders (including infection). However, if clinical suspicion of a CTD is strong, then anti-dsDNA and anti-ENA antibody follow-up testing should be performed.
- A negative ANA result, using a sensitive test system, makes SLE or CTD very unlikely.
- A wide variety of drugs may induce ANAs (often associated with anti-histone antibodies). Drug-induced ANA usually disappears within 6 months of drug withdrawal.
- In practice, speckled or homogenous patterns are poor indicators of antibody specificity and both anti-dsDNA and anti-ENA antibodies may be associated with either pattern.

- ◆ Anti-centromere antibody is found in CREST syndrome, in about 10% of patients with scleroderma, as well as 13% of patients with primary biliary cirrhosis (PBC).
- ◆ Nucleolar ANAs are associated with scleroderma and autoimmune liver disease, but are not specific for these conditions.
- ◆ In patients with known CTDs serial measurement of ANA is not helpful at monitoring disease activity.

Pitfalls

When HEp-2 cells are used for ANA detection, the increased sensitivity results in many weak false positives (approximately 20% of women over the age of 60 years are positive unrelated to disease). Care must be taken with interpretation.

CROSS REFERENCES

Section 2.23   Connective Tissue Diseases
Section 3.3   Detection of Antibodies and Antigen

ANTI-DOUBLE STRANDED DNA (dsDNA) ANTIBODY

Anti-dsDNA antibodies (Abs) are useful in diagnosis and monitoring of SLE. As dsDNA is found in cell nuclei, anti-dsDNA antibodies will result in staining of nuclei by IIF, regardless of substrate.

Clinical indications

Diagnosis and monitoring of SLE.

Principle of the test

Three assays for the detection and/or measurement of anti-dsDNA antibodies are in routine use: the Farr assay, IIF and ELISA. Antigen quality is pivotal in ensuring the quality of both Farr and ELISA assays. DNA exists in three forms: dsDNA, z-DNA and single-stranded DNA (ssDNA). Anti-dsDNA but not anti-ssDNA is relatively specific for SLE. Helical DNA treated with S1 endonuclease removes ssDNA, improving assay specificity.

Farr assay   High-affinity anti-dsDNA antibodies are detected in this quantitative RIA. I^{125}-labelled dsDNA is added to the test serum and bound by anti-dsDNA antibodies, if present. Precipitation using ammonium sulphate brings down anti-dsDNA antibodies bound to labelled dsDNA, leaving unbound dsDNA in solution. Antibody-bound-I^{125}-labelled dsDNA is measured using a scintillation counter. The amount of anti-dsDNA antibody present is proportional to the amount of recovered radioactivity (Figure 3.4.2).

IIF   *Crithidiae luciliae* is a parasitic haemoflagellate, in which the kinetoplast contains pure dsDNA. Anti-dsDNA antibody staining of this specialised organ is detected by IIF. Staining of the nucleus is not specific for anti-dsDNA antibodies (Figure 3.4.1(e)).

ELISA   Measurement of anti-dsDNA antibodies by ELISA detects both high- and low-affinity antibodies. Quantification of antibody by ELISA is straightforward and precise, and makes follow-up straightforward. ELISA also avoids the use of radio-nucleotides.

Notes on the use of different assays to measure anti-dsDNA antibodies

♦ Detection of anti-dsDNA antibodies by IIF on *Crithidia luciliae* is highly specific but is less sensitive than the Farr assay or ELISA. IIF is less useful for monitoring disease activity.

♦ ELISA methods show high sensitivity but reduced specificity, possibly related to detection of low-affinity antibodies or antibodies that bind contaminating ssDNA (ssDNA can be removed by S1 endonuclease treatment).

Interpretation

♦ High levels of anti-dsDNA antibodies are suggestive of SLE. As many as 80% of sufferers are positive depending on the assay used. Anti-dsDNA antibodies may also be found in autoimmune hepatitis.

♦ Some SLE patients may be negative when first tested but if clinical suspicion is high, should be retested in 3–6 months.

♦ Quantitative measurement of anti-dsDNA antibody levels is used for monitoring disease activity in patients with SLE. However, since the half-life of IgG is 3 weeks, it is not helpful to measure levels more frequently than this unless a patient is undergoing

Figure 3.4.2 Farr assay for the measurement of anti-dsDNA antibodies.

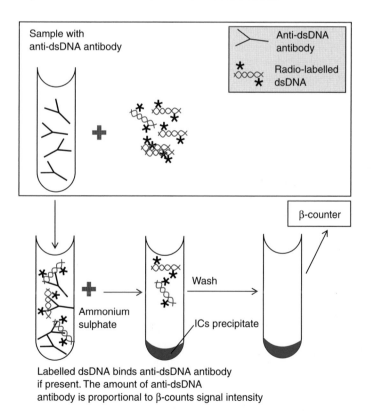

plasmapheresis. Levels of anti-dsDNA usually rise before a clinical relapse or flare, however occasionally levels may fall precipitously before a flare, as anti-dsDNA is incorporated into immune complexes which lodge in tissues causing the clinical flare.

Pitfalls

- The presence of RF (IgM) may cause interference in ELISAs that detect both IgG and IgM anti-dsDNA antibodies (IgG anti-dsDNA are more clinically relevant). This should be considered when a strongly positive anti-dsDNA antibody is seen with a negative ANA.
- False negative results may be seen when cryoglobulinaemia complicates SLE, as the anti-dsDNA antibody may be lost in the cryoprecipitate.

CROSS REFERENCES

Section 2.23 Connective Tissue Diseases
Section 3.3 Detection of Antibodies and Antigen

ANTIBODIES TO ENAs – ANTI-Ro, La, RNP, Sm, Jo-1, Scl-70 ANTIBODIES

Antibodies to ENAs bind saline-extracted cellular antigens, and usually are associated with a positive ANA detected by IIF. Anti-ENAs which are routinely measured are directed against the following targets: Ro, Sm, RNP (ribonucleoproteins), La (nuclear phosphoprotein), the enzymes Jo-1 (histidyl-tRNA-synthetase) and Scl-70 (topisomerase-1).

Clinical indications

- Suspected CTD – including SLE, discoid lupus erythematosus (DLE) and subacute cutaneous lupus; Sjögren's syndrome, scleroderma, polymyositis, MCTD.
- Strong positive ANA.

Principle of the test

ELISA ELISA may be used to screen for and identify the precise anti-ENAs present using microtitre plates that have been coated with purified antigens (Ro, La, Sm, RNP, Scl-70, Jo-1) either alone or in combination. A two-stage procedure is often used: an initial screen of patient's serum with a mixture of four or six antigens; followed by an identification ELISA with individual antigens which is performed on screen positive sera.

Counter current immunoelectrophoresis (CCIE) This assay is carried out in two stages: an initial screen of sera for reactivity to antigen extract is followed by an identification step where positive sera are run with reference sera of known specificity to identify specific antibodies. The antigen preparation now most commonly used is calf thymus. However, due to concerns about prion disease, this antigen source is rarely used. Human spleen extract is a rich source of Ro antigen, however due to concerns about HIV and difficulty with obtaining consent, this is no longer in routine use. Jo-1 and Scl-70 can only be detected in freshly extracted thymus, and as repeated extraction is impractical, ELISA is more commonly used to detect antibodies to these antigens (Figure 3.4.3).

Interpretation

♦ Anti-Sm antibodies

— Found in 30% of patients with SLE
— Specific for SLE.

♦ Anti-RNP antibodies

— MCTD (overlap of SLE, polymyositis and scleroderma)
— Also found in SLE (anti-dsDNA antibodies also present)
— Weakly positive anti-RNP antibodies may be found in other CTD.

♦ Anti-Ro antibodies

— Many patients with Sjögren's syndrome
— 30% of patients with SLE
— Subacute cutaneous lupus erythematosus (SCLE)
— Neonatal lupus
— Majority of babies with congenital heart block (transplacental transfer of maternal anti-Ro which damages the foetal cardiac conducting system)
— Lupus associated with C2 deficiency
— Anti-Ro antibodies are often associated with photosensitivity in SLE.

Figure 3.4.3 Counter current immunoelectrophoresis (CCIE).

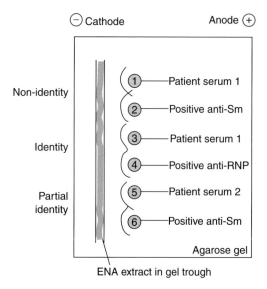

Notes: Patient sera and positive reference sera are placed in a line of wells cut into the agarose: wells 1, 3 and 5, patient sera; wells 2 and 6, positive anti-Sm; well 4, positive anti-RNP. ENA extract is placed in the trough parallel to these wells. Antibodies and antigen are electrophoresed towards each other and if the patient's serum contains anti-ENA antibodies, a precipitin line is formed. Precipitin lines indicate the presence (identity) or absence (non-identity) of specific antibody: in this example, patient serum 1 is positive for anti-RNP antibodies and negative for anti-Sm antibodies.

- Anti-La antibodies

  — Usually found in association with anti-Ro antibodies
  — Rarely found alone
  — 30% of patients with Sjögren's syndrome
  — 10% of patients with lupus.

- Anti-Jo-1 antibodies

  — 30% of patients with polymyositis
  — Anti-synthetase syndrome (interstitial lung disease, Raynaud's phenomenon and thickened sausage shaped fingers).

Anti-Jo-1 (histidyl-tRNA synthetase) antibodies are part of a group of antibodies directed against aminoacyl-tRNA synthetases associated with polymyositis and dermatomyositis including Jo-1, PL-7, PL-12, EJ and OJ.

- Anti-Scl-70 antibodies

  — 30% of patients with scleroderma
  — Strong positive Anti-Scl-70 antibodies are specific for this disease
  — Presence of this antibody may pre-date clinical signs of the disease
  — Poor prognostic marker.

Detection of anti-ENA antibodies is useful in diagnosis, but not follow-up of patients. Most well-established assays are qualitative, however anti-ENA antibody levels have never been shown to reflect disease activity. In view of the obstetric implications, it is reasonable to repeat anti-ENA tests when a patient with SLE or other CTD becomes pregnant (Table 3.4.1).

Pitfalls

- Most patients that are anti-ENA antibody positive also have a positive ANA. However, Ro and Jo-1 are predominantly cytoplasmic in location and this may result in a negative ANA. Hence anti-ENA antibodies should be specifically requested when there are suggestive clinical features despite a negative ANA.
- CCIE is moderately sensitive, but is specific for most antigen types. As a result of increased sensitivity, the use of ELISAs may give false positives thus reducing disease specificity.
- Poor antigen purity may result in false positive results on ELISA. This should be considered if antigens not usually found in combination are detected.

Table 3.4.1 Anti-ENAs and disease associations

ANTI-ENA SPECIFICITY	DISEASE ASSOCIATION	INCIDENCE (%)
Ro	Sjögren's syndrome	>70
	SLE	30
La	Sjögren's syndrome	30
	Lupus	10
Sm	SLE	30
RNP	MCTD	100
Jo-1	Polymyositis	30
Scl-70	Scleroderma	30

- Most studies on the clinical relevance of anti-ENAs were performed using CCIE. It remains unclear whether extrapolation of these findings to results of more sensitive ELISAs is appropriate.

CROSS REFERENCES

Section 2.23 Connective Tissue Diseases
Section 3.3 Detection of Antibodies and Antigen

OTHER CTDs – ASSOCIATED ANTIBODIES

Anti-ribosomal-P-protein and anti-histone antibodies

- Anti-histone antibodies are directed against histones (DNA binding proteins) that are classified into different subtypes (H1, H2A, H2B, H3, H4).
- Anti-ribosomal-P protein antibodies are directed against phosphoproteins (P0, P1, P2) found in ribosomes. These appear to be SLE specific.

Anti-PM-Scl, anti-Ku, anti-Mi-2, anti-SRP antibodies (anti-ENAs)

Anti-PM-Scl, anti-Ku, anti-Mi-2 and anti-SRP antibodies are autoantibodies directed against ENAs. These are associated with autoimmune myositis.

Details of these additional ANAs, their target antigens and disease associations are summarised in Table 3.4.2.

Clinical indications

These tests are usually ordered by specialised request only, following discussion with the rheumatology or immunology teams.

- Anti-ribosomal P – strong suspicion of SLE with negative routine serology
- Anti-histone – drug-induced lupus, Felty syndrome
- Anti-Mi-2, Anti-SRP – polymyositis/dermatomyositis
- Anti-PM-Scl – scleroderma/polymyositis overlap.

Principle of the test

Methods in use for detection of these antibodies include double diffusion, ELISA and immunoblotting. These assays are usually carried out in a reference laboratory (Figure 3.4.4).

Interpretation

- Anti-ribosomal-P-protein antibodies

  — Found in 10–15% of patients with SLE, sometimes in the absence of anti-dsDNA antibodies.

281

Table 3.4.2 Unusual nuclear antibodies

AUTOANTIBODY SPECIFICITY	TARGET ANTIGEN	DISEASE ASSOCIATIONS
Ribosomal-P-protein	Ribsomal-P-protein	10–15% SLE
Histones	H2A, H2B, H3, H4	18–50% SLE 95% drug-induced lupus Felty syndrome
PM-Scl	Complex of around 11 proteins found in the nucleolus	25% polymyositis/ scleroderma overlap 8% mysositis alone 3% scleroderma alone
Ku	86 kDa DNA-binding protein	SLE, MCTD, Sjögren's syndrome, scleroderma (often with polymyositis)
Mi-2	220 kDa nuclear antigen	15–30% dermatomyositis
SRP	54 kDa protein complexed with RNA	Polymyosistis/ dermatomyositis

Figure 3.4.4 Western blotting for the detection of specific ANAs using HEp-2 cell antigen.

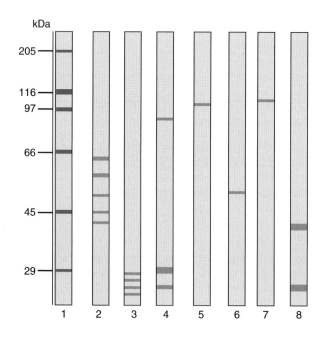

Notes: HEp-2 antigens are separated by electrophoresis and blotted onto nitrocellulose. This membrane is cut into strips, which are incubated with patient sera for the detection of specific anti-nuclear antibodies present. Lane 1: stained molecular weight markers; lanes 2–8: autoantibodies detected using different patient sera. Lane 2: SS-A (60 kDa), SS-A (52 kDa), SS-B; lane 3: Sm; lane 4: RNP; lane 5: Scl-70; lane 6: Jo-1; lane 7: PM-Scl; lane 8: ribosomal-P-protein.

♦ Anti-histone antibodies
— Found in 18–50% of patients with SLE
— 95% of patients with drug-induced lupus (procainamide, hydralazine)
— Felty syndrome (RA, neutropaenia, splenomegaly).

♦ Anti-PM-Scl antibodies (anti-ENA)

— 25% of patients with the polymyositis/scleroderma overlap syndrome
— 8% of patients with myositis alone
— 3% of patients with scleroderma alone
— Possible increased risk of renal involvement in overlap patients.

♦ Anti-Mi-2 antibodies (anti-ENA)

— Highly specific for dermatomyositis
— Found in 15–30% of these patients
— Antibody positive patients are usually steroid responsive.

♦ Anti-SRP antibodies

— Polymyositis/dermatomyositis.

Pitfalls

These tests are not widely available and are usually only performed in specialised laboratories. Clinical validation data are limited.

CROSS REFERENCES

Section 2.23   Connective Tissue Diseases
Section 3.3   Detection of Antibodies and Antigen

AUTOANTIBODIES ASSOCIATED WITH THE ANTIPHOSPHOLIPID SYNDROME

Anti-cardiolipin antibodies and lupus anticoagulant

Anti-cardiolipin antibodies (ACA) are directed against cardiolipin (a phospholipid), in the presence of a protein co-factor β_2-glycoprotein 1.

Related anti-phospholipid antibodies include lupus anti-coagulants, and antibodies to other phospholipids (phosphatidylserine, phosphatidylcholine, phosphatidylethanolamine, phosphatidylinositol). Anti-cardiolipin antibodies may give rise to false positive syphilis serology (VDRL).

Lupus anti-coagulants are antibodies that interfere with the clotting process *in vitro*. Paradoxically this autoantibody results in thrombosis *in vivo*.

Current diagnostic criteria for anti-phospholipid syndrome (APS) recognise anti-phospholipid antibodies detected by the following assays:

♦ Anti-cardiolipin antibody (IgG or IgM class)
♦ Lupus anti-coagulant.

Clinical indications

- ◆ Suspected APS

  — Arterial or venous thrombosis
  — Pregnancy associated morbidity – second or third trimester pregnancy loss; three first trimester losses; early delivery for severe pre-eclampsia or intrauterine growth retardation
  — SLE (particularly women who wish to become pregnant)
  — Thrombocytopaenia
  — Livedo reticularis
  — Sneddon's syndrome (cerebral events and livedo)
  — Budd–Chiari syndrome.

Principle of the test

ELISA Anti-cardiolipin antibodies (IgG and IgM) – anti-cardiolipin antibodies bind cardiolipin in the presence of the serum co-factor β_2-glycoprotein 1 (Apolipoprotein H). It is thought that when β_2-glycoprotein 1 binds cardiolipin, it exposes a conformational epitope on cardiolipin, which the antibody recognises. Patient sera are incubated in microtitre wells that have been coated with cardiolipin and β_2-glycoprotein 1 as substrate.

Detection of lupus anticoagulants (plasma required) Lupus anti-coagulants cause a prolonged activated partial thromboplastin time (APTT), kaolin clotting time (KCT) and dilute Russell viper venom test (DRVVT). International Society on Thrombosis and Haemostasis guidelines for demonstration of lupus anti-coagulant require:

- ◆ Prolonged phospholipid-dependent coagulation demonstrated on two of three screening tests
- ◆ Failure to correct the prolonged coagulation time by mixing with platelet-poor plasma
- ◆ Exclusion of other coagulopathies as appropriate.

Interpretation

- ◆ Anti-cardiolipin antibodies:

  — Are reported semiquantitatively as weak, moderate or strong positive. Laboratory criteria for diagnosis of APS require detection of moderate or strong positive IgG or IgM ACA on two or more occasions at least 6 weeks apart, measured by standardised ELISA for β_2-glycoprotein 1-dependent anti-cardiolipin antibodies. Nintey per cent of patients with APS have detectable ACA.
  — Weak positive antibodies may be non-specific, associated with infection or other inflammatory conditions.

- ◆ Lupus anti-coagulant – for diagnosis of APS, lupus anti-coagulant must be present in plasma on two or more occasions at least 6 weeks apart. This antibody is detected in 60% of APS patients.

Pitfalls

- ◆ Cardiolipin antibodies and lupus anti-coagulant recognise different phospholipid specificities, therefore it is important to test for both, as either may be present independently of the other and present with similar clinical problems.

◆ Lack of standardisation is significant. ACA are low-affinity highly heterogeneous antibodies; assay design is complex and good quality reference material is not readily available.

ANTI-β_2-GLYCOPROTEIN 1 ANTIBODIES

These autoantibodies are directed against the phospholipid binding protein β_2-glycoprotein 1. This is a serum co-factor that binds anionic phospholipids *in vivo* and its normal function is to inhibit coagulation and platelet aggregation. Clinically significant anti-cardiolipin antibodies bind cardiolipin only in the presence of β_2-glycoprotein 1, however some patients also have antibodies to β_2-glycoprotein 1 alone. These antibodies are currently not accepted as diagnostic laboratory criteria for APS.

Clinical indications

Suspected APS.

Principle of the test

◆ Anti-β_2-glycoprotein 1 antibodies are detected by ELISA.

Interpretation

Anti-β_2-glycoprotein 1 – the role of these antibodies is currently under investigation. They may be useful in patients suspected of having APS but are negative for ACA and lupus anti-coagulant. It is positive in 80% of affected individuals.

CROSS REFERENCES

Section 3.3   Detection of Antibodies and Antigen
Section 2.16   Immune-mediated Haematological Conditions

Autoantibodies Associated with Vasculitic Syndromes and Renal Diseases

ANTI-NEUTROPHIL CYTOPLASMIC ANTIBODIES

Anti-neutrophil cytoplasmic antibodies (ANCAs) are autoantibodies directed against cytoplasmic components of neutrophils and monocytes. Clinically, the most significant ANCAs are those directed against the cytoplasmic enzymes proteinase-3 (PR3) and myeloperoxidase (MPO). Other minor ANCA specificities include bactericidal permeability increasing protein (BPI), catalase, cathepsin G, elastase, lysozyme, lactoferrin and α-enolase.

Clinical indications

- Suspected vasculitis – primary systemic small vessel vasculitides including Wegener's granulomatosis, microscopic polyangiitis
- Glomerulonephritis, especially rapidly progressive (RPGN)
- Pulmonary haemorrhage
- Cutaneous vasculitis with systemic features
- Chronic destructive disease of the upper airways
- Pulmonary infiltrates or cavitating lesions
- Retro-orbital mass
- Long-standing sinusitis or otitis (especially with blood-stained discharge)
- Subglottic tracheal stenosis
- Mononeuritis multiplex or other peripheral neuropathy (especially if painful).

Principle of the test

ANCA is detected by indirect immunofluorescence (IIF) on human peripheral blood neutrophils. Two patterns of fluorescence are seen most commonly – cytoplasmic or C-ANCA and perinuclear or P-ANCA. ANCA bind different cytoplasmic antigens including PR3 and MPO. These two main ANCA specificities PR3-ANCA and MPO-ANCA, and other minor ANCAs are confirmed by ELISA.

Figure 3.5.1 ANCA patterns of staining by IIF on ethanol fixed neutrophils: (a) C-ANCA and (b) P-ANCA. See Plate Section for colour reproduction of these images.

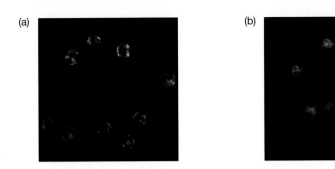

ANCA – indirect immunofluorescence (IIF)

Ethanol-fixed normal human peripheral blood neutrophils are used as a substrate. The staining patterns observed by IIF include C-ANCA, P-ANCA and atypical ANCA. P-ANCA is distinguished from C-ANCA when ethanol is used as the cell fixative. P-ANCA is an artifactual pattern that results from the re-distribution of these negatively charged cytoplasmic antigens during ethanol fixation (Figure 3.5.1 (a) and (b)).

- C-ANCA pattern refers to classical cytoplasmic granular fluorescence with central interlobular accentuation. This pattern is most commonly produced by the antigen PR3, a granule enzyme.
- P-ANCA produces perinuclear fluorescence with nuclear extension. Multiple antigens produce this pattern including MPO.
- Atypical ANCA refers to staining patterns other than C-ANCA or P-ANCA and may comprise a combination of cytoplasmic and perinuclear fluorescence. These patterns of fluorescence may also be divided into C-ANCA (atypical), P-ANCA (without nuclear extension) and atypical ANCA.

Notes on ANCA testing by IIF

- IIF should be performed on serum samples from all new patients.
- Optimal serum dilution for ANCA screening is 1/20.
- IgG-ANCA is the most clinically significant class of ANCA detected.
- The endpoint titre is required when ANCA levels are monitored by IIF, however antigen-specific ELISAs are more accurate methods for quantifying antibody levels.

ANCA – ELISA

ANCA positive sera (including C-ANCA, P-ANCA and atypical ANCA) are tested for PR3 and MPO reactivity using ELISA. Serial measurement of ANCA levels by quantitative ELISA is helpful for patient monitoring. IIF-ANCA positive sera that are negative for PR3-ANCA and MPO-ANCA when tested by ELISA, may be further characterised by additional ELISAs, however this is not performed routinely.

Interpretation

- C-ANCA occur in over 70% of patients with Wegener's granulomatosis (more frequently in active generalised untreated disease, less frequently without renal involvement) and in 30% of those patients with microscopic polyangiitis. Most of these are PR3-ANCA.

♦ P-ANCA with MPO specificity occur in 50–80% of patients with active microscopic polyangiitis (may be renal limited) and in up to 25% of patients with Wegener's granulomatosis. Occasional ANCA positive patients with RPGN also have anti-GBM antibodies.

♦ Atypical-ANCA occur in some patients with IBD, sclerosing cholangitis, RA, SLE, chronic active hepatitis and in chronic infections such as cystic fibrosis and bronchiectasis.

Pitfalls

♦ ANA fluorescence may interfere with ANCA IIF. ELISA testing for PR3-ANCA and MPO-ANCA allows exclusion of vasculitis-associated ANCA despite the presence of ANAs.

♦ Occasionally, C-ANCA occurs with MPO specificity and P-ANCA occurs with PR3 specificity.

CROSS REFERENCES

Section 2.24   Vasculitis
Section 3.3   Detection of Antibodies and Antigen

REFERENCES

Savige, J. *et al.* (1999) 'International consensus statement on testing and reporting of Antineutrophil Cytoplasmic Antibodies (ANCA)', *Am. J. Clin. Pathol.*, 111: 507–13.

AUTOANTIBODIES ASSOCIATED WITH RENAL DISEASE

Anti-glomerular basement membrane (GBM) antibody

These are autoantibodies directed against the α-3-chain of type IV collagen found in glomerular and alveolar basement membranes. GBM antibodies are pathogenic. They induce Type II hypersensitivity resulting in anti-GBM disease, a rare but important cause of acute renal failure.

Clinical indications

♦ Suspected anti-GBM disease

— Pulmonary haemorrhage
— Acute renal failure
— Pulmonary renal syndrome.

Principle of the test

IIF   Anti-GBM antibodies can be detected in serum by IIF using human or monkey kidney as substrate. The presence of these antibodies generates a typical linear glomerular staining pattern, similar to that seen by direct immunofluorescence (DIF) on renal biopsies.

Rapid screening and ELISA   Early diagnosis of anti-GBM disease is essential and a rapid screening test has been produced commercially. In 5 min the presence of anti-GBM antibodies can be detected. ELISA may be used to screen for or quantitate the levels of anti-GBM antibodies in serum. Serial measurement of GBM antibodies by quantitative ELISA is essential for monitoring patients' response to therapy.

Notes on anti-GBM antibody tests

♦ IIF is insensitive, and is not suitable for monitoring antibody removal.
♦ DIF on renal biopsy remains the gold standard for establishing the diagnosis of anti-GBM disease.

Interpretation

♦ Anti-GBM antibodies are found in almost all cases of recent onset Goodpasture's disease. Even in the absence of treatment, these antibodies will disappear over a 6–24 month period.
♦ Serial measurement of anti-GBM antibodies by quantitative ELISA is valuable for monitoring the response to plasmapheresis as well as long-term response to immunosuppression.
♦ Some patients with anti-GBM antibodies may also have P-ANCA (MPO-ANCA) and this group may respond to aggressive therapy, even when dialysis-dependent at presentation.

CROSS REFERENCES
Section 2.21   Immune-mediated Renal Disease
Section 3.3   Detection of Antibodies and Antigen

Autoantibodies Associated with Liver and Gastrointestinal Diseases

AUTOANTIBODIES ASSOCIATED WITH AUTOIMMUNE LIVER DISEASE

Anti-mitochondrial antibody

Anti-mitochondrial antibodies (AMAs) are directed against a number of antigenic structures of the mitochondria. At least nine subtypes of AMA have been identified to date, termed M1–M9. The most important is M2, directed against the E2 component of pyruvate dehydrogenase complex.

Clinical indications

- Suspected primary biliary cirrhosis (PBC)
    - Pruritus
    - Clinical/laboratory evidence of chronic liver disease
    - Raised IgM.
- Associated autoimmune disease.

Principle of the test

- IIF – AMA is detected by IIF on a composite block of rodent liver, kidney and stomach (LKS). Staining must be observed in the liver, kidney and stomach to define the staining pattern as AMA (Figure 3.6.1). Several AMA subtypes may be detected by IIF (M1, M2, M5, M6), but distinguishing these subtypes by immunofluorescence is difficult.
- Confirmatory follow-up testing (by ELISA or immunoblotting) is helpful to confirm the presence of the M2 subtype.

Notes on AMA testing

- AMA may also be detected by IIF on HEp-2 cells where granular cytoplasmic staining is observed. IIF on rat LKS should be performed for confirmation.

Figure 3.6.1 Anti-mitochondrial antibody staining by IIF on a composite block of rat LKS: (a) rat stomach and (b) kidney (low power), (c) rat kidney and liver (high power) and (d) rat stomach (high power). See Plate Section for colour reproduction of these images.

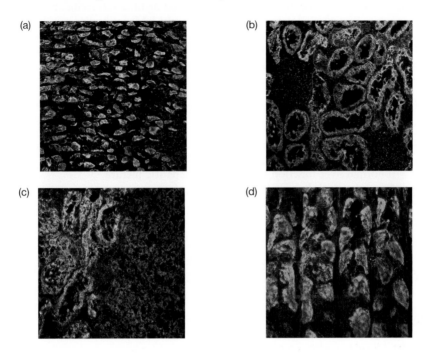

Interpretation

AMA (M2 subtype) are found in the following:

- 95% of patients with PBC
- PBC / autoimmune hepatitis overlap
- Autoimmune disease associated with PBC (thyroiditis, Sjögren's syndrome)
- Occasionally in overlap connective tissue diseases.

Non-M2 AMAs are found in the following:

- Myocarditis and cardiomyopathy
- SLE
- Syphilis
- Some cases of drug-induced hepatitis.

Pitfalls

AMA staining on LKS must be distinguished from anti-LKM antibodies, anti-ribosomal-P protein antibodies and anti-SRP antibodies.

ANTI-SMOOTH MUSCLE ANTIBODY AND ANTI-LIVER KIDNEY MICROSOMAL (LKM) ANTIBODY

Anti-smooth muscle antibodies (SMAs) are directed against intracellular microfilaments, including actin, vimentin, desmin and tubulin. Anti-LKM antibodies are directed against microsomes in the cytoplasm of hepatic cells and proximal renal tubular cells. Three types of LKM antibodies have been described, of which LKM-1 antibodies, directed against cytochrome p450, are the most important (Figure 3.6.2).

Clinical indications

◆ Suspected autoimmune hepatitis

— Chronic liver disease, jaundice
— Profound malaise and fatigue
— Abnormal liver function tests (LFTs) – hepatitic picture
— Hypergammaglobulinaemia (IgG and IgA)
— Associated autoimmune diseases.

Principle of the test

IIF – SMA and LKM antibodies may both be detected by IIF using a composite block of rodent LKS as substrate (Figure 3.6.2).

Figure 3.6.2 SMA and anti-LKM antibody staining by IIF on a composite block of rat LKS: (a) SMA staining of smooth muscle (low power) and (b) high power, (c) rat liver (anti-LKM) and (d) rat kidney (anti-LKM). See Plate Section for colour reproduction of these images.

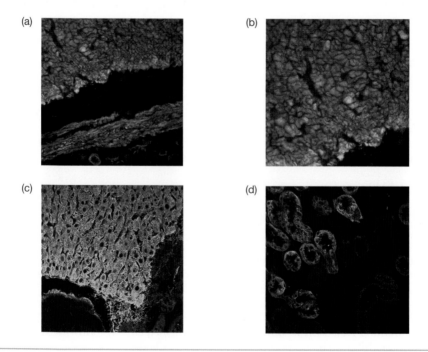

Table 3.6.1 Classification of autoimmune hepatitis by autoantibody profile

HEPATITIS	AUTOANTIBODIES
Type I (lupoid)	
Mean age of onset (35 years)	SMA 50–70%
Female predominance	ANA and anti-dsDNA Abs 25%
High frequency of extrahepatic symptoms	
Type II	
Onset in childhood – 50%	Anti-LKM-1 antibodies 80%
Female predominance	
Frequent extrahepatic symptoms	
Rapid damage to liver	
Type III	
Onset – 35 years	Anti-SLA (soluble liver antigens)
Female predominance	antibodies 25%
No extrahepatic features	

- SMA stains the muscle fibres in artery walls, intergastric gland fibres and muscle layers of the stomach.
- LKM antibodies produce fine granular staining in the liver and proximal renal tubules, with no staining in the gastric parietal cells (GPCs). LKM antibodies can be distinguished from AMAs by the differential staining of renal tubules and lack of staining in the stomach.

Confirmatory Testing – follow-up testing for anti-LKM-1 antibodies can be performed by immunoblotting or ELISA using purified P450 cytochrome.

Interpretation

- High titre SMAs are detected in 50–70% of patients with chronic active hepatitis
- Lower titre SMAs may be detected in patients with PBC, and after an infection
- SMAs may also be found in 5–15% of normal individuals (low titre)
- Anti-LKM antibodies are found in type II autoimmune hepatitis, and in some patients with Hepatitis C. These antibodies are of no known prognostic significance in Hepatitis C (Table 3.6.1).

Pitfalls

Anti-LKM antibodies may resemble AMA, particularly when anti-GPC antibody is also present. LKM antibodies may be found in patients who are Hepatitis C positive.

CROSS REFERENCES	
Section 2.17	Autoimmune Liver Diseases
Section 3.3	Detection of Antibodies and Antigen

AUTOANTIBODIES ASSOCIATED WITH GI DISEASE

Anti-endomysial antibody and anti-tissue transglutaminase antibody

Anti-endomysial antibody (EMA) and anti-tissue transglutaminase (tTG) antibody are directed against the same target antigen, tTG. Coeliac disease is usually associated with EMA or anti-tTG antibodies of IgA-class, but IgG-EMA or IgG-anti-tTG antibodies may be significant in patients with IgA deficiency.

Clinical indications

- Suspected gluten sensitive enteropathy
  - Coeliac disease (malabsorption, diarrhoea, etc.)
  - Dermatitis herpetiformis (DH) (itchy, blistering rash).

- Incidental detection of R1 type anti-reticulin antibody by IIF on composite block of rat LKS.

Principle of the test

- IIF – IgA-EMAs are detected using monkey oesophagus as substrate and FITC-labelled anti-IgA. EMAs produce a distinctive staining pattern – a network of thin irregular lines around individual smooth muscle fibres in the muscularis mucosa, producing a 'lacework' pattern (Figure 3.6.3).
- ELISA – Anti-tTG antibodies are detected by ELISA. Human tTG gives better sensitivity.

Interpretation

- Detection of EMA is consistent with a diagnosis of coeliac disease. The diagnosis is confirmed by jejunal biopsy, which shows villous atrophy.

Figure 3.6.3 Endomysial antibody staining by IIF on monkey oesophagus: (a) low power and (b) high power. See Plate Section for colour reproduction of these images.

(a)

(b)

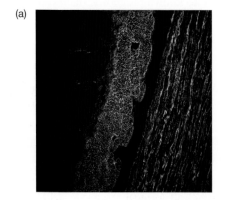
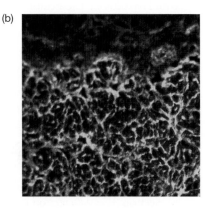

♦ IgA-EMAs are found in 90–100% of patients with coeliac disease and 50–70% of those with DH, with high specificity (90–100%) (Table 3.6.2).

♦ Removal of gluten from the diet results in the gradual disappearance of this antibody from the circulation (over months to years).

Pitfalls

♦ One in thirty patients with coeliac disease have selective IgA deficiency. IgA deficiency should be excluded in all patients undergoing coeliac screening using IgA based assays only. IgG-EMA should be measured routinely in IgA deficient patients.

♦ A false negative result may also be obtained when a patient is on a gluten-free diet.

♦ The characteristic staining (IIF) associated with EMAs may be obscured in the presence of a smooth muscle antibody.

♦ Antibody binding to tTG in ELISA systems is critically dependent on the calcium concentration of the buffer solutions.

ANTI-GLIADIN ANTIBODY AND ANTI-RETICULIN ANTIBODY

Anti-gliadin antibodies (AGAs) are directed against α-gliadin, a water insoluble fraction of gluten, which is found in wheat, barley and rye.

Antibodies directed against reticulin, a component of connective tissue are of five different types and are detected by IIF. IgA antibodies to the R1 type of reticulin are closely associated with coeliac disease.

Clinical indications for AGA testing

Suspected gluten sensitive enteropathy.

Principle of the test

AGAs (both IgA and IgG) are measured by ELISA. Anti-reticulin antibody (IgA) is detected by IIF using a composite block of rodent LKS. The antibody shows a distinctive linear staining pattern around the tubules in the kidney, together with staining of the intergastric glands in the submucosa and blood vessels. R1 reticulin antibodies may be distinguished from other reticulin antibodies by their staining pattern in the kidney.

Interpretation

♦ AGA – Significantly positive IgA-AGA is found in coeliac disease and in DH. Weak levels are not specific for these disorders. IgG-AGAs may be found in bowel disease associated with increased mucosal permeability, but are also useful in patients with IgA deficiency. In cases where there is a positive IgG-AGA but a negative IgA-AGA, IgA deficiency should be excluded (Table 3.6.2).

♦ IgA-AGA are also found in the following patients who carry a risk of developing CD

— Adults and children with diabetes mellitus (DM) (type I)
— First-degree relatives of patients with coeliac disease
— Patients with Down syndrome.

♦ IgA and IgG AGAs may be useful for monitoring compliance with a gluten-free diet.

Table 3.6.2 Specificity and sensitivity of coeliac disease-associated antibodies

COELIAC DISEASE	SENSITIVITY (%)	SPECIFICITY (%)
EMA-IgA	95–100	100
Anti-tTG-IgA	90–100	100
AGA-IgA	95	100
AGA-IgG	50	60
Anti-reticulin antibody	25–30	59–100

ANTI-RETICULIN ANTIBODIES

IgA anti-R1 reticulin antibodies are fairly specific but insensitive markers for coeliac disease. IgG anti-reticulin, as well as other patterns of IgA anti-reticulin are not specific for coeliac disease. However, when a reticulin antibody is detected during autoantibody screening, testing for anti-endomysial antibody is worthwhile.

CROSS REFERENCES

Section 2.17   Autoimmune Liver Diseases
Section 2.18   Immune-mediated Gastrointestinal Disorders
Section 2.20   Immune-mediated Skin Disease
Section 3.3   Detection of Antibodies and Antigen

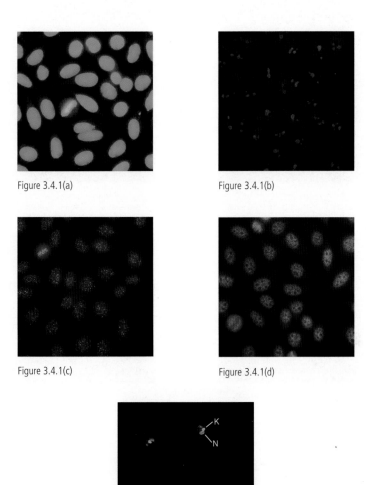

Figure 3.4.1(a)

Figure 3.4.1(b)

Figure 3.4.1(c)

Figure 3.4.1(d)

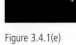

Figure 3.4.1(e)

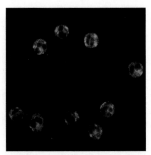

Figure 3.5.1(a)

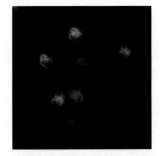

Figure 3.5.1(b)

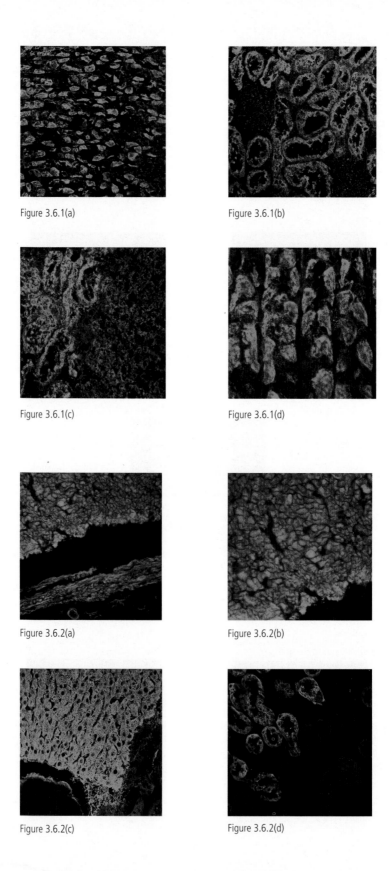

Figure 3.6.1(a)

Figure 3.6.1(b)

Figure 3.6.1(c)

Figure 3.6.1(d)

Figure 3.6.2(a)

Figure 3.6.2(b)

Figure 3.6.2(c)

Figure 3.6.2(d)

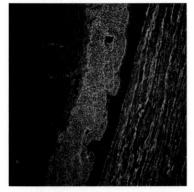

Figure 3.6.3(a)

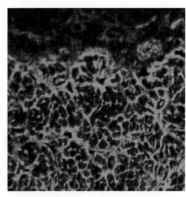

Figure 3.6.3(b)

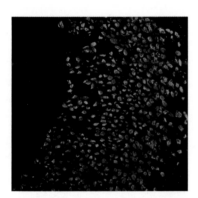

Figure 3.7.1(a)

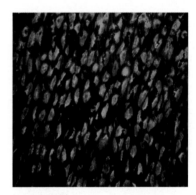

Figure 3.7.1(b)

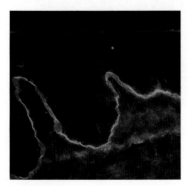

Figure 3.8.1(a)

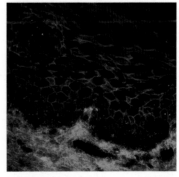

Figure 3.8.1(b)

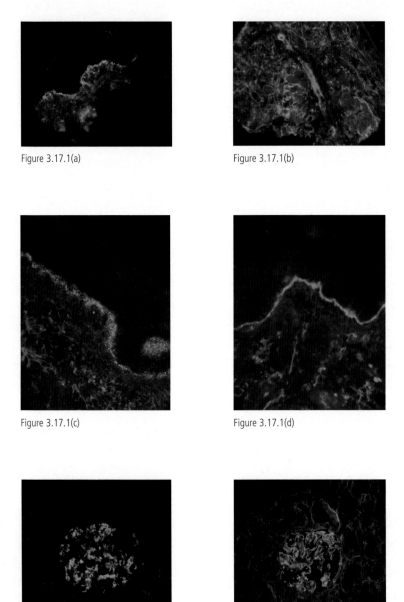

Figure 3.17.1(a)

Figure 3.17.1(b)

Figure 3.17.1(c)

Figure 3.17.1(d)

Figure 3.17.1(e)

Figure 3.17.1(f)

Autoantibodies Associated with Endocrine Diseases and Pernicious Anaemia

ANTI-GASTRIC PARIETAL CELL ANTIBODY AND ANTI-INTRINSIC FACTOR ANTIBODY

Anti-gastric parietal cell (GPC) antibodies are directed against the α and β subunits of the $H^+ K^+$-ATPase (proton pump) of the GPC.

Vitamin B_{12} is absorbed from the intestine in complex with intrinsic factor (IF). Anti-IF antibodies are of two main types:

◆ Blocking antibody – prevents IF from binding to B_{12}
◆ Binding antibody – binds free IF and IF–B_{12} complex preventing absorption.

Clinical indications

Suspected pernicious anaemia

◆ Symptoms of anaemia
◆ Paraesthesia (neuropathy)
◆ Sore tongue
◆ B_{12} deficiency, macrocytosis
◆ Subacute combined degeneration of cord
◆ Dementia.

Principle of the test

Anti-GPC antibodies produce granular staining of the GPCs by IIF using a substrate of composite block of rodent liver, kidney and stomach (Figure 3.7.1). Anti-IF antibodies may be detected using ELISA or RIA.

Notes on testing for anti-GPC antibody

There is no correlation between the titre of GPC antibodies and disease, therefore titration is not necessary.

Figure 3.7.1 Anti-GPC antibody staining by IIF on rat stomach: (a) low power and (b) high power. See Plate Section for colour reproduction of these images.

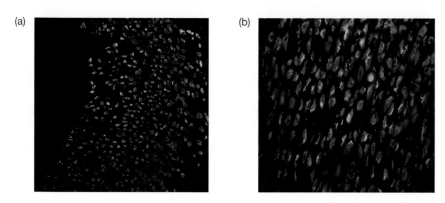

Interpretation

♦ Anti-GPC antibody is positive in 90% of patients with pernicious anaemia (PA). IF antibodies are less sensitive (present in 50–70%) but are highly specific for this condition.

♦ Anti-GPC antibodies may be found in asymptomatic patients with gastric atrophy some of whom will develop PA. They are found in 2–10% of normal individuals.

♦ PA is strongly associated with autoimmune thyroid disease (50% of patients with PA have anti-thyroid antibodies), while 30% of patients with thyroiditis have anti-GPC antibodies.

♦ PA may also be associated with autoimmune polyglandular syndrome (APGS). GPC antibodies may be found in APGS types I and III.

Pitfalls

Heterophile antibodies (which usually also stain the renal brush border) must be differentiated from anti-GPC antibodies.

ANTI-THYROID MICROSOMAL (TM) ANTIBODY AND ANTI-THYROGLOBULIN ANTIBODY

Anti-thyroid microsomal (TM) antibodies are directed against thyroid microsomal peroxidase (TPO) found in thyroid microsomes. Anti-thyroglobulin (TG) antibodies are directed against the thyroid antigen thyroglobulin.

Clinical indication

♦ Suspected Graves' disease, Hashimoto's thyroiditis or subacute thyroiditis syndromes

— Thyrotoxicosis and diffusely enlarged thyroid gland (goitre)
— Exophthalmos and thyroid acropachy
— Abnormal thyroid function tests (TSH, T3, T4).

♦ Chronic urticaria.

Table 3.7.1 Thyroid autoantibodies in thyroid disease

AUTOANTIBODY	INCIDENCE
Anti-TM (high titre)	Autoimmune thyroid disease
	Graves disease 80%
	Hashimoto's thyroiditis 95%
	Primary myxoedema 90%
Anti-TM (low titre)	Thyroid carcinoma 25%
	Normal individuals 5–15%

Principle of the test

Anti-TM and anti-TG antibodies can be detected by agglutination techniques (using red blood cells, gelatin or other particles coated with TPO or TG, respectively) or using ELISA.

Interpretation

- Anti-TM antibodies are found in 99% of patients with autoimmune thyroid disease (Table 3.7.1). Many patients are also positive for anti-TG, however anti-TG are rarely found alone.
- The presence of these antibodies in asymptomatic individuals may be predictive of future hypothyroidism.
- Anti-thyroid antibodies during pregnancy indicate a risk of post-partum thyroiditis, which can be associated with post-partum depression.
- Anti-thyroid antibodies may be found in patients with other autoimmune diseases including pernicious anaemia, Addisons disease, and Sjögren's syndrome.
- Anti-TG should be measured in patients with follicular carcinoma of the thyroid gland if thyroglobulin levels are used as a tumour marker – measurement of TG is unreliable in antibody positive subjects.

Pitfalls

Some serum components may react non-specifically with gelatin particles or RBCs in agglutination assays and this may interfere with the detection of thyroid antibodies. If present, such heterophile antibodies must be fully adsorbed prior to use of a particle agglutination assay.

ANTI-ISLET CELL ANTIBODY AND ANTI-GAD ANTIBODY

These autoantibodies are directed against islet cells of the pancreas, the main target antigen being glutamic acid decarboxylase (GAD). GAD is involved in the release of insulin from secretory granules, and is also found in the GABAminergic neurones involved in the control of muscle tone. Distinct isoenzymes are found at both sites.

Clinical indication

- Suspected diabetes mellitus (DM) type I (insulin-dependent DM (IDDM))
- Identification of first-degree relatives at risk of developing DM
- Stiff Man syndrome (painful muscular rigidity).

Principle of the test

- IIF – Anti-islet cell antibodies are detected using human pancreatic tissue as substrate.
- Immunoblotting – Anti-GAD antibodies may be detected by immunoblotting. There are two types of GAD autoantibody: one binds conformational epitopes and is associated with IDDM, while the other binds linear epitopes and is associated with Stiff Man syndrome. Only the anti-GAD antibodies that recognise linear epitopes (i.e. associated with Stiff Man syndrome) are routinely detected by immunoblotting.

Interpretation

- Anti-islet cell antibodies are present in 65–85% of newly presenting IDDM, but disappear within 1–2 years. A small group of patients with multiple autoimmune endocrine diseases maintain their antibody levels.
- Anti-islet cell antibodies are seen in first-degree relatives of patients (2–5%) with IDDM who have a high risk of developing the disease: the presence of these antibodies increases the risk of developing diabetes 75-fold.
- 10% of patients with non-insulin dependent diabetes (type II) will have islet cell antibodies and have a higher risk of progression to insulin-dependence.
- Type I DM is clinically associated with coeliac disease, so patient's serum should also be screened for anti-EMAs.
- Anti-GAD antibodies have been described in IDDM (conformational epitope antibodies) and in 60% of patients with the very rare Stiff Man syndrome (linear epitope antibodies).

ANTI-ADRENAL ANTIBODY

Anti-adrenal antibodies are autoantibodies directed against the adrenal cortex. The major target antigens are 21-hydroxylase and 17α-hydroxylase.

Clinical indications

- Clinical or laboratory evidence of adrenal insufficiency
- Type I or type II autoimmune polyglandular syndrome (APGS)
- Other organ-specific autoimmune endocrine disease.

Principle of the test

Anti-adrenal antibodies are detected by IIF using monkey adrenal gland as the substrate. The staining pattern results from these antibodies reacting with microsomes of the zona glomerulosa, zona fasiculata and zona reticularis.

Interpretation

Anti-adrenal antibodies are found in:

- 50% of patients with Addisons disease in the presence of other autoimmune diseases
- Minority of patients with autoimmune adrenalitis alone
- Rarely present in patients with tuberculous adrenal destruction
- <5% of normal individuals.

Autoimmune adrenal disease is closely related to organ-specific autoimmune disease and at least 40% of patients have at least one other autoimmune endocrinopathy and should undergo appropriate antibody screening.

Multiple autoimmune endocrinopathies can occur together or sequentially in patients – these conditions are described as autoimmune polyglandular syndromes. Non-endocrine organ-specific autoimmune conditions frequently accompany these syndromes, which are described in Section 2.15.

CROSS REFERENCES

Section 3.3   Detection of Antibodies and Antigen
Section 2.15   Autoimmune Endocrinopathies

Other Organ-specific Autoimmunity

TESTS ASSOCIATED WITH AUTOIMMUNE CYTOPAENIAS

Anti-platelet antibody

Anti-platelet autoantibodies are directed against a variety of platelet antigens.

Clinical indications

- Suspected autoimmune thrombocytopaenia (ITP) – primary, or secondary to drugs, CTDs or infection.
- Alloimmune thrombocytopaenia.

Principle of the test

Flow cytometry using typed platelets from several donors.

Interpretation

Anti-platelet antibodies are found in:

- Over 90% of patients with primary ITP.
- Secondary immune thrombocytopaenia associated with HIV, CTD, heparin-induced thrombocytopaenia, common variable immunodeficiency (CVID) and B cell malignancy.

Pitfalls

- ◆ Detection of anti-platelet antibodies is difficult and this test should be performed in a specialised laboratory.
- ◆ It is important to distinguish between anti-platelet autoantibodies and alloantibodies, including anti-HLA antibodies that bind platelets.

ANTI-ERYTHROCYTE (RED BLOOD CELL) ANTIBODIES

Anti-red blood cell (RBC) antibodies may be classified as warm antibodies or cold antibodies (cold agglutinins).

Warm antibodies are specific for a particular RBC antigen or a mixture of RBC surface antigens (a major target is the Rhesus system); they are usually IgG class.

Cold agglutinins are autoantibodies that reversibly agglutinate RBCs in the cold causing small vessel obstruction in the skin of the extremities. The main antibody specificities are anti-i, anti-I and anti-Pr (RBC cell surface antigens); they are usually IgM, and may be monoclonal.

Clinical indications

- ◆ Suspected autoimmune haemolytic anaemia (AIHA)

  — Anaemia
  — Jaundice or laboratory evidence of haemolysis
  — Raynauds phenomenon.

Principle of the test

Anti-RBC may be detected bound to RBC (direct Coomb's test), or unbound antibody may be detected in serum (indirect Coomb's test). Warm antibodies are detected at 37°C, while cold antibodies are detected at 4°C. Anti-RBC antibodies are investigated for the temperature of maximal activity, specificity, complement binding and agglutinating or haemolytic activity.

Direct Coomb's test   Antibodies and complement components are detected on the surface of red cells by means of an 'anti-globulin agent' that contains anti-immunoglobulin (Ig) and anti-C3 antibody. This reacts with Igs and C3 but cannot distinguish between specific antibodies directed against the red cells, and immune complexes firmly adsorbed onto the red cell surface. Specific antibodies to IgG, IgM and C3 can be used at different temperatures to type the antibody.

Indirect Coomb's test   In patient's serum, circulating autoantibodies to RBCs can be detected by incubating the serum with red cells. After washing, the red cells are washed and incubated with 'anti-globulin agent'.

Interpretation

AIHA is categorised according to the temperature at which haemolysis takes place.

- ◆ Warm antibodies are found in 50% of patients with AIHA – warm AIHA. Warm AIHA may be idiopathic or secondary to SLE, CLL, lymphomas or viral infection.
- ◆ Cold agglutinins may be associated with infection or lymphoproliferative disease.

Pitfalls

- ◆ Cold agglutinins bind red cells in the cold. They are distinct from cryoglobulins, which are immunoglobulins that precipitate in the cold.
- ◆ Incorrect collection and transport of the blood sample will render it unsuitable for the assay.

AUTOANTIBODIES ASSOCIATED WITH AUTOIMMUNE SKIN DISEASE

Anti-basement membrane zone antibody

Anti-basement membrane zone (anti-BMZ) autoantibodies are directed against keratinocyte hemidesmosomal proteins. The specific antigens recognised in bullous pemphigoid (BP) are BP230 and BP180.

Anti-epidermal intercellular substance antibody

Anti-epidermal intercellular substance (anti-ICS) antibodies recognise the intercellular substance of the epidermis and the main target antigens are desmoglein-1 and 3 (intercellular adhesion molecules), and under some circumstances desmoplakin-1 (a desmosomal protein).

Clinical indications

- ◆ Blistering skin disease +/− mucosal lesions with suspicion of autoimmune cause

  — Bullous pemphigoid, herpes gestationis, epidermolysis bullosa acquisita
  — Pemphigus vulgaris, pemphigus foliaceus, paraneoplastic pemphigus.

Principle of the test

IIF – These antibodies may be detected in serum by IIF using monkey oesophagus, human skin or other epithelial substrates. Anti-BMZ antibodies produce linear staining along the basement membrane zone between the epithelial layer and submucosa. Anti-ICS produce a typical chickenwire staining pattern in the epithelium (Figure 3.8.1).

Usually a skin biopsy will also be taken and sent for histology and direct immunofluorescence (DIF) which detects antibody deposited in the patient's skin. Patterns seen on DIF are similar to those detected by IIF.

Interpretation

- ◆ BMZ antibodies are detectable in the serum of 70–90% of BP patients. This antibody is also detected in a small number of patients with epidermolysis bullosa acquisita (10%) and herpes gestationis (25%). The titre of anti-basement membrane antibodies in serum does not correlate with disease activity and antibody may still be found in serum during disease remission.
- ◆ Intracellular substance antibodies are present in 70–90% of cases of pemphigus vulgaris. The titre of anti-ICS antibody in serum correlates well with disease activity. Low titres of anti-ICS antibody have also been detected in SLE, myasthenia gravis with thymoma, burns and some cutaneous infections (leprosy).

Figure 3.8.1 Skin antibody patterns by IIF on monkey oesophagus: (a) anti-BMZ antibody and (b) anti-intercellular substance antibody. See Plate Section for colour reproduction of these images.

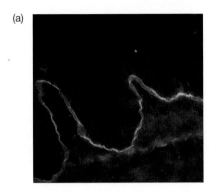
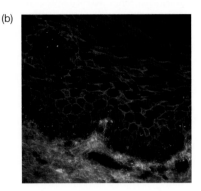

(a)   (b)

Pitfalls

A complete investigation of the bullous skin diseases should include both IIF to detect circulating antibodies, and DIF on skin biopsy, and results should be interpreted with full clinical and histological information.

CROSS REFERENCES

Section 3.3   Detection of Antibodies and Antigen
Section 3.17   Direct Immunofluorescence
Section 2.20   Immune-mediated Skin Disease

AUTOANTIBODIES ASSOCIATED WITH NERVOUS SYSTEM DISEASES

Anti-neuronal antibodies – anti-Hu, Yo or anti-Ri antibodies

Anti-neuronal nuclear antibodies (ANNA-1 and ANNA-2) are autoantibodies directed against the neuronal cell nuclei and are also known as anti-Hu and anti-Ri antibodies. Purkinje cell cytoplasm antibodies (PCCAs) are also known as anti-Yo antibodies. The antigen for anti-Yo antibodies is thought to be CDR34, which is expressed on epithelial tumours as well as on neuronal tissue. Anti-Yo, Hu and Ri are thought to be cross-reactive anti-tumour antibodies.

Clinical indications

- Suspected paraneoplastic neurological syndromes

  - Paraneoplastic cerebellar degeneration, ataxic sensory neuropathy or encephalomyelitis particularly in association with carcinoma of the breast, ovary and small cell lung carcinoma.

Principle of the test

IIF and immunohistochemistry – anti-Hu and anti-Yo antibodies are detected by IIF or immunohistochemistry using cerebellum as the substrate.

- Anti-Hu antibodies produce homogenous staining of neuronal nuclei in the granular layer of cerebellum.
- Anti-Yo antibodies stain cytoplasm of the Purkinje cells (at the junction of granular and molecular layers of the cerebellum).
- Anti-Ri antibodies stain neuronal nuclei; confirmatory testing is required for definitive identification.
- Immunoblotting, using cerebellar lysates, may be used to confirm the presence of anti-Hu, anti-Yo and anti-Ri antibodies detected by IIF screening. This technique is also useful for characterisation of novel antigens when unusual patterns of staining are detected by IIF screening.

Notes on testing for anti-Hu, Yo and Ri antibodies

- In IIF using primate tissue substrate, sensitivity is improved by using anti-human antibodies which have been adsorbed to removed reactivity to primate tissue, reducing non-specific binding.
- May be present in cerebrospinal fluid (CSF) and serum.
- May disappear following removal of the tumour.

Interpretation

- Anti-Hu antibodies are associated with small cell carcinoma of the lung and paraneoplastic syndromes; sensory neuropathies and encephalomyelitis.
- Anti-Yo antibodies are found in patients with paraneoplastic cerebellar degeneration associated with ovarian cancer or Hodgkin's disease.
- Anti-Ri antibodies have been detected in women with breast cancer together with ataxia, myoclonus and opsoclonus.
- A positive result (Hu, Yo or Ri antibodies) should initiate further investigations for underlying malignancy. Tumours may be small and if no tumour is found, investigations should be repeated after several months.

Pitfalls

Anti-Hu antibodies must be carefully distinguished from non-neurone specific anti-nuclear antibodies on immunofluorescence.

ANTI-ACETYLCHOLINE RECEPTOR ANTIBODY

Autoantibodies (IgG) directed against the acetylcholine receptor (AChR) found on skeletal muscle cells are associated with myasthenia gravis (MG). Anti-AChR may:

- Bind the receptor at sites distinct from the binding site for acetylcholine
- Block the neurotransmitter binding site on the receptor
- Cause the accelerated degradation of AChR.

Clinical indications

- Suspected MG
  - — Fatigue of voluntary muscles with weakness which increases with activity
  - — Thymoma; thymic hyperplasia.

Principle of the test

Double antibody immunoprecipitation radioimmunoassay (RIA) – α-bungarotoxin binds specifically and firmly to the AChR protein, which is isolated from detergent – solubilised skeletal muscle. Radiolabelled AChR-toxin complexes are incubated with patient serum. The IgG–AChR–toxin complexes are separated from non-bound AChRs by a precipitation step using a second antibody to human IgG. The level of precipitated radioactivity is a measure of the antibody activity. Results are expressed as nmol/L of α-bungarotoxin binding activity.

Interpretation

- These antibodies are found in 80–90% of patients with MG. However, a negative result does not exclude this diagnosis. In ocular MG, antibodies are only detected in 60% of patients.
- These antibodies are absent in healthy individuals, and in patients with other neurological disorders.
- These antibodies (IgG isotype) can be transferred across the placenta and cause neonatal myasthenia.

GANGLIOSIDE ANTIBODIES

Sialylated glycolipids form part of the myelin sheath. In Guillain–Barré syndrome (GBS) and immune-mediated neuropathies, autoantibodies including anti-GM1, GD1b, GQ1b, GT1a and LMI antibodies are seen. These antibodies react with epitopes in carbohydrate domains of molecules and there is a high frequency of cross-reactions with other carbohydrate-rich molecules including bacterial capsular lipopolysaccharides, for example, *Campylobacter jejuni*.

Clinical indications

- Suspected GBS and the Miller–Fischer variant
- Chronic inflammatory demyelinating polyneuropathy (CIDP)
- Paraprotein associated neuropathies.

Principle of the test

These autoantibodies are detected by immunoblotting or ELISA.

Interpretation

- Antibodies to GM1 and other gangliosides including LM1 and GD1b have been associated with GBS.
- Antibodies to GQ1b have been associated with the Miller–Fischer variant of GBS (in 90–100% of cases).

- Anti-GM1, LM1 and GD1b antibodies can also be found in patients with CIDP and multifocal motor neuropathy.
- In paraproteinaemic neuropathies, anti-GM1 antibodies may be the main specificity of the paraprotein (usually IgM).

CROSS REFERENCES

Section 3.3   Detection of Antibodies and Antigen
Section 2.19   Immune-mediated Neurological Disease

Measurement of the Acute Phase Response

Alterations in plasma proteins occurring in response to tissue injury are useful in detection and monitoring of inflammation. Direct measurement of specific reactants (e.g. CRP, α-1 acid glycoprotein), or indirect measures (e.g. ESR), are used. The clinical utility of individual tests varies depending on the nature of the underlying disorder.

CLINICAL INDICATIONS

- Infections – Acute and chronic; especially relevant in bacterial sepsis, including atypical organisms and TB
- Inflammatory arthritis – RA; SLE; other connective tissue diseases (CTDs)
- Systemic inflammation – Systemic CTDs; systemic vasculitides
- Malignancy – Lymphoreticular; renal cell cancer. Also, may be elevated if infective complications arise
- Possibly atherosclerosis – high sensitivity assay required.

PRINCIPLE OF THE TEST

CRP – measured by nephelometry

This is the most accurate indicator of the acute phase response. Highly sensitive assays are available and of possible value in cardiovascular medicine. High sensitivity assays are not required to monitor most inflammatory states where large increases in CRP occur.

ESR

A negative charge on the surface of red blood cells (RBCs) inhibits aggregation. Acute phase proteins, most especially fibrinogen, but also α_2-macroglobulin and immunoglobulins, reduce electrical charge. As a result of this, RBCs sediment. The rate of sedimentation of fresh, anti-coagulated blood in a vertical column over 1 h is measured.

INTERPRETATION

CRP

Basal concentrations are extremely low. Increases are detectable within 6–8 h of the triggering stimulus. The half-life of CRP is short and concentrations fall again within a few hours of response. Huge increases (up to a thousandfold) can occur in severe inflammatory states. CRP is the most accurate assay available for the assessment of acute inflammatory activity.

- Levels are normal (<4 mg/l) in most viral states and in degenerative arthritis.
- Modest increases (up to 100 mg/l) are seen in inflammatory arthritic conditions, as well as in certain viral illnesses (EBV, CMV, adenovirus), and in malignant disease.
- Levels of >100 mg/l occur in systemic vasculitis, systemic bacterial infection and sometimes in lymphoid malignancies.
- Gross elevations (>300 mg/l) usually indicate serious bacterial infection or very severe vasculitis.

Extremely sensitive modified nephelometric methods can identify minor variation in CRP levels, even if the absolute level is still within the normal population range. Such differences appear to be relevant in risk stratification of patients with ischaemic heart disease, and are thought to be a marker for inflammation within atherosclerotic plaques. Such high-sensitivity assays are also required for monitoring inflammation in neonates, where the basal level and peak level are much lower than in adults.

ESR

Some elevation in the ESR occurs in most inflammatory states. Gross elevations (>100 mm/h) are most often related to:

- Tuberculosis
- Multiple myeloma
- Giant cell arteritis/polymyalgia rheumatica
- Lymphoma
- Severe inflammatory synovitis
- Severe systemic bacterial infection.

Fibrinogen has a slower rate of production, in comparison to CRP, in response to inflammatory stimuli. It also has a long half-life. Significant lag phases between onset and resolution of inflammatory stimuli and subsequent variation in the ESR can occur. ESR is a very good indicator of chronic inflammation.

PITFALLS

- CRP is often normal in active SLE. The ESR is a better indicator of activity in this condition. Elevation of CRP may result from superimposed infection. Severe serositis or synovitis may also cause CRP to rise in SLE.
- CRP levels vary with age. Age-matched reference ranges are essential for correct interpretation.
- ESR is elevated with anaemia, increasing age, female gender and oestrogen-rich states (pregnancy, use of combined oral contraceptives (OCPs)) even if inflammation is quiescent. These confounding factors can make interpretation difficult.

- Drugs such as aspirin which carry a negative charge, can reduce the ESR, even in the absence of resolution of inflammation.
- The lag phase between alteration in the ESR and changing intensity of inflammation limits the usefulness of this assay in day-to-day monitoring of inflammatory states. Nonetheless, it remains a very useful indicator of chronic inflammation over extended periods.

CROSS REFERENCES

Section 1.6   Innate Immune Responses III – Other Soluble Factors
Section 1.26   Consequences of an Immune Response
Section 3.3   Detection of Antibodies and Antigen

Complement

MEASUREMENT OF COMPLEMENT COMPONENTS

Complement components C3 and C4 are routinely measured to diagnose and monitor autoimmune disease. Other complement components can be measured, although this is usually only necessary when complement deficiency is suspected. The pattern of abnormality in CH50 and AP50 complement function tests indicates which components should be measured (see Section 3.11).

Clinical indications

- SLE, immune complex glomerulonephritis and vasculitis – diagnosis and monitoring
- Angioedema without urticaria
- Follow-up investigation of absent CH50 or AP50.

Principle of the test

Complement components can be measured by nephelometry or RID. Nephelometry is usually used for C3 and C4, as these components are frequently measured in large numbers. RID is used in most laboratories for measuring other complement components.

Notes on the measurement of complement levels

- Normal ranges for C4 are very wide because C4A and C4B null alleles occur frequently in the normal population.
- Serum should be frozen as rapidly as possible to prevent *ex vivo* C3 or C4 cleavage which results in artificially high levels for these components if measured by RID.
- International standard available: Certified Reference Material for Plasma Protein Analysis (CRM 470).

Table 3.10.1 Complement changes in disease

LEVELS OF COMPLEMENT

C3	C4	ACTIVATION PATHWAY	EXAMPLES
↓	↓	Classical	SLE, vasculitis
↓	N	Alternative	C3 nephritic factor (autoantibody) MPGN II; partial lipodystrophy
N	↓	Classical (early)	Hereditary angioedema (C1-Inh deficiency)
↑	↑	Increased synthesis of components	Acute and chronic inflammation

Interpretation

Low C3 and C4 suggest that activation of the classical pathway has occurred. Normal C4 levels with low C3 levels suggest that the alternative pathway has been activated in isolation. Low C4 with normal C3 indicates early classical pathway activation, which results from fluid phase activation (Table 3.10.1).

Serial measurement of C3 and C4 is useful in monitoring disease activity in immune complex disease, including SLE and cryoglobulinaemia. Low levels of C3 and C4 usually return to normal in remission.

C3 and C4 levels are generally raised in pregnancy, therefore low normal levels in a pregnant patient with SLE may reflect worsening disease activity.

C4 levels must be interpreted carefully. There are two C4 genes, *C4A* and *C4B*. An individual's normal serum concentration of C4 depends on the number of expressed and 'null' alleles which they possess. By performing a number of C4 measurements, the normal level for an individual can be established and this facilitates interpretation of changes in C4 levels.

In patients with angioedema or crampy abdominal pain a low C4 may indicate C1 inhibitor deficiency. C4 remains reduced between attacks of angioedema.

A persistently low C3 may be indicative of the presence of a C3 nephritic factor. In infective endocarditis, low or reduced C3 levels may indicate glomerulonephritis.

Pitfalls

Complement components are acute phase reactants, and raised levels of C3 and C4 are frequently seen during an acute phase response. When inflammation results from immune complex disease complement consumption may be masked by the increased rate of complement synthesis due to the acute phase response. In these cases the measurement of C3 breakdown products may be helpful.

COMPLEMENT ACTIVATION PRODUCTS

Only intact native C3 can be detected in normal plasma provided blood is immediately put into ethylene diamine tetra acetic acid (EDTA). C3 breakdown *in vivo* results in a number of breakdown products, of which C3dg has the longest half-life. C3a is unstable and rapidly degraded, however if intact C3, C3b and C3c are removed from the plasma, available assays can accurately measure C3dg. An example of such a technique is double-decker rocket electrophoresis.

Complement activation may also be demonstrated by measuring plasma levels of multimolecular activation complexes including C1r:C1s:C1-Inh, C3bBbP and C5b-9 (by sandwich ELISA).

Interpretation

C3dg levels are increased due to complement activation, and are not masked by the acute phase response.

C3dg levels correlate with disease activity in SLE and are also elevated in patients with severe diffuse cutaneous disease associated with systemic sclerosis.

AUTOANTIBODIES TO COMPLEMENT COMPONENTS – C3-NEPHRITIC FACTOR

C3-nephritic factor is an autoantibody that binds and stabilises the alternative pathway C3 convertase enzyme. This prevents the natural destruction of this enzyme by the regulatory proteins factor H and factor I. The presence of C3-nephritic factor results in continuous C3 breakdown and depletion.

Clinical indications

*   Unexplained low C3 in kidney disease or lipodystrophy
*   Type II membranoproliferative glomerulonephritis.

Principle of test

C3-nephritic factor is detected by its ability to cause C3 cleavage in normal serum. The cleavage of intact native C3 molecules results in the generation of smaller molecules of C3 including C3a, C3b, C3c and C3dg, which have different electrophoretic mobilities. The addition of patient serum (with C3-nephritic factor) to normal serum causes C3 cleavage. After incubation, the presence of the autoantibody may be inferred by examination of subsequent changes to C3 mobility on electrophoresis followed by immunofixation, or crossed immunoelectrophoresis (also called a Laurell plate) (Figure 3.10.1). Native and cleaved C3 may be detected simultaneously by using antisera to C3c or C3dg.

Interpretation

C3-nephritic factor is associated with type II, dense deposit, membranoproliferative glomerulo nephritis and partial lipodystrophy. It is reported as 'present' or 'absent' and may be IgG or IgM class. Typically, patients with MPGN will be 'nephritic' with haematuria, hypertension and oliguria.

Patients with partial lipodystrophy and C3-nephritic factor are at significant risk of developing renal disease. Partial lipodystrophy is present in less than 50% of patients with nephritic factor.

Pitfalls

Normal serum used in these assays must be handled carefully in order to minimise spontaneous C3 cleavage. The measurement of C3-nephritic factor is a specialised test, only available in expert laboratories.

ANTI-C1q ANTIBODIES

Anti-C1q antibodies have recently been described in patients with SLE and hypocomplementaemic vasculitis. These autoantibodies bind to C1q resulting in complement activation. Assays for these antibodies are not widely available currently, but are likely to become so in the next few years.

Figure 3.10.1 Crossed immunoelectrophoresis (Laurell plate) for the detection of C3-nephritic factor.

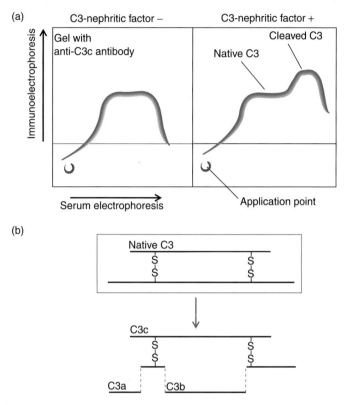

Notes: (a) Patient serum is incubated with normal serum. The presence of C3-nephritic factor in patient serum causes C3 cleavage in normal serum. Native and cleaved C3 may be detected by crossed immunoelectrophoresis (also called a Laurell plate): serum electrophoresis followed by immunoelectrophoresis into an anti-C3c antibody containing gel. (b) Native C3 is cleaved into smaller molecules C3a, C3b and C3c.

CROSS REFERENCES

REFERENCES

International Federation of Clinical Chemistry and Laboratory Medicine: www.ifcc.org/iffc.asp
Walport, M. (2001) 'Advances in immunology: complement', N. Engl. J. Med., 344: 1058–66, 1140–4.

Immunodeficiency

COMPLEMENT DEFICIENCY

Deficiencies of complement components may be genetic (primary) or acquired (secondary to another disease). Genetic deficiencies of all complement components except factor B have been described, including the inhibitors C1-Inhibitor (C1-Inh), Factor I, Factor H, DAF and CD59.

Clinical indications

- Recurrent pyogenic infections
- Recurrent neisserial infections – especially meningitis
- Lupus-like disease; glomerulonephritis
- Family or personal history including combinations of these findings.

Principle of the tests

The diagnosis of a complement deficiency is performed in two stages:

- Complement function assays to assess the functional integrity of the classical, alternative and terminal pathways of complement activation.
- Measurement of individual complement component levels (as indicated by functional assays) to identify the missing components.

Assays of complement function

Total haemolytic complement – CH50   The total haemolytic complement assay measures the functional integrity of the classical complement pathway C1, C2, C3, C4 and the late components C5–C9. Patient serum, which should provide a source of complement, is added to sheep red blood cells (RBCs) sensitised with anti-RBC antibody (an immune complex). An intact classical pathway results in RBC lysis, which is measured with a spectrophotometer. The amount of serum (complement) required to cause 50% lysis is known as a CH50 unit.

Alternative pathway haemolytic complement – AP50   The alternative pathway total haemolytic complement assay (CH50) measures the functional integrity of the alternative pathway, C3, Factor B, Factor D and properdin and the late components C5–C9. Patient serum is added to guinea pig RBCs, which are susceptible to direct lysis by the alternative pathway. The assay is performed in the presence of Mg-EGTA, which chelates calcium preventing classical pathway activation. An intact alternative pathway results in RBC lysis, which is measured with a spectrophotometer. The amount of serum (complement) required to cause 50% lysis is called an AP50 unit.

Gel-based assays   Patient serum diffuses from a well into agarose-containing sensitised sheep RBCs (for measurement of CH100), or guinea pig RBCs (for measurement of the AP100). Activation of complement leads to RBC lysis, which is evident as a clear zone around the well. The diameter of this clear zone is dependent on functional complement activity in serum. This is a semiquantitative assay, however it is a useful screen to exclude complement deficiency.

Measurement of individual complement components (see Section 3.10)

Figure 3.11.1 Complement function assays: CH100-classical pathway and AP100-alternative pathway.

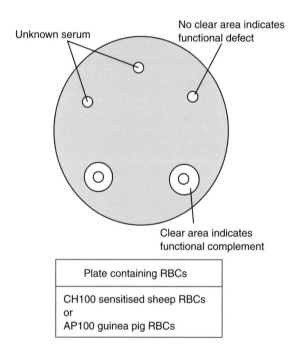

Interpretation

The results of complement haemolytic assays and the possible complement deficiencies are summarised in Table 3.11.1.

Complement consumption *via* the classical or alternative pathways may be so marked that the CH50 and AP50 are reduced. However, a normal CH50 or CH100 does not exclude significant complement consumption.

Table 3.11.1 Complement haemolytic assay results and complement deficiency

COMPLEMENT FUNCTION ASSAY	POSSIBLE DEFICIENCY
Reduced CH50	C1–C9
Reduced CH50 and normal AP50	Early classical components (C1, C2 or C4)
Reduced AP50 and normal CH50	Alternative pathway Factor B, properdin, Factor D
Reduced AP50 and CH50	Terminal attack complex (C5–C9) or C3

Table 3.11.2 Deficiencies of complement regulatory proteins and receptors

DEFICIENCIES	ASSOCIATED DISORDER
Regulatory proteins	
C1-Inh	Hereditary or acquired angioedema
Factor I, Factor H	Pyogenic infections, vasculitis (Factor H – glomerulonephritis and haemolytic uraemic syndrome (HUS)), Familial HUS
DAF	Paroxysmal nocturnal haemoglobinuria
CD59	Paroxysmal nocturnal haemoglobinuria
Complement receptors	
CR3	Leucocyte adhesion deficiency
CR1	? significance ?defective immune complex handling and possible SLE

Factor I or Factor H deficiencies may result in reduced levels of C3, which may in turn result in reduced CH50s and increased susceptibility to bacterial infections (secondary).

Deficiencies of regulatory complement proteins and receptors are associated with the following disorders (see Table 3.11.2).

Pitfalls

◆ Complement proteins are labile and therefore samples for functional assays must be processed and frozen at −80°C rapidly, and repeated freeze-thawing avoided.

◆ Haemolytic activity of either pathway may be absent because of *in vivo* or *ex vivo* consumption of complement as well as deficiency.

◆ Patients with an acute illness may show abnormal complement function and should be tested 3–4 weeks after the infection has resolved.

CROSS REFERENCES
Section 1.5 Innate Immune Responses II – The Complement System
Section 2.11 Complement Deficiency
Section 3.3 Detection of Antibodies and Antigen

MEASUREMENT OF LYMPHOCYTES – B CELLS AND T CELLS

Lymphocyte deficiencies may be primary, as a result of an intrinsic defect in the immune system, or secondary to drug therapy or infection. B and T cells cannot be identified morphologically, however they can be distinguished based on expression of different 'markers' (termed CD – cluster of differentiation – antigens). Common markers used when measuring lymphocyte subtypes include:

* CD3   All T cells
* CD19, CD20 or CD23   All B cells
* CD4   Helper T cells
* CD8   Cytotoxic T cells.

Clinical indications

* Suspected T cell immunodeficiency
* Hypogammaglobulinaemia – to differentiate causes and exclude B cell malignancy
* Lymphopaenia in a child (lymphocytes $<2 \times 10^9/L$) – suspected SCID
* Chronic lymphopaenia in an adult (lymphopaenia is common during acute illness and does not require further investigation).

Principle of the test

* Flow cytometry – quantitation of lymphocyte numbers is carried out by flow cytometry using a panel of fluorochrome-labelled-monoclonal antibodies against different lymphocyte surface markers. By highlighting ('gating') the lymphocyte population, the percentage of lymphocytes positive for each marker is measured. A suspension of beads of known concentration is added to allow conversion of these percentages to an accurate quantitative measurement of absolute cell counts (Figure 3.11.2).

Figure 3.11.2 Flow cytometric readout of CD4 T cells in normal and deficient individuals.

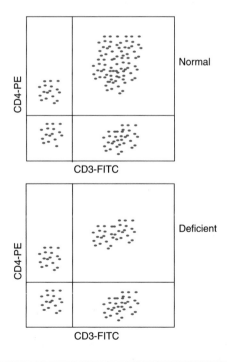

Interpretation

Interpretation is based on the absolute cell counts rather than percentages of each cell subtype.

The numbers of T and B cells present assist in the diagnosis of primary T and B cell immunodeficiencies. Patients' results must be compared with age-related normal ranges. Interpretation is complex and should be carried out by the immunologist supervising the testing.

Abnormal lymphocyte profiles are also seen in viral infections (HIV, EBV and CMV), acute bacterial infections, SLE, lymphoma, malignancy, chronic fatigue syndromes, drugs, toxins (alcohol and cigarettes), protein-losing enteropathy and splenectomy.

Reduced lymphocyte levels are usual during long-term immunosuppressive therapy.

Pitfalls

- Monoclonal antibody therapy may mask antigens producing artificially low counts. For example, in patients receiving OKT3, use of anti-CD3 antibodies that bind the same CD3 epitope as the therapeutic antibody, gives erroneously low results.
- Lymphopaenia is common when patients are acutely ill. Where possible lymphocyte subsets should be measured when patients are in chronic stable state.
- While awaiting analysis, specimens should be stored at room temperature, and never refrigerated.

CROSS REFERENCES

Section 2.8   Defects in Antibody-mediated Immunity
Section 2.9   Defects in T Cell-mediated Immunity
Section 3.3   Detection of Antibodies and Antigen

HIV DIAGNOSIS AND MONITORING

Diagnosis of HIV depends on the detection of anti-HIV antibody, HIV antigen or HIV genomic material. Sequential measurement of CD4+ T cell numbers and the viral load are used to monitor disease progression and the need for and response to therapy.

Clinical indications and principles of tests

- *Diagnosis of HIV infection* – Anti-HIV antibodies are detected by ELISA, and their presence is confirmed by immunoblotting. Occasionally, PCR may be useful in diagnosis of infection, particularly in neonates. CD4 T CELL COUNTS PLAY NO ROLE IN DIAGNOSIS OF HIV.
- *Monitoring of HIV infection* – The viral load or concentration of HIV-RNA in blood is measured by quantitative PCR. Accurate measurement of helper T cell numbers is performed using flow cytometry, measuring dual-stained CD3+ CD4+ lymphocytes.

Interpretation

The antibody response to HIV appears after a lag phase of up to 3 months. During this 'window phase' infected patients may appear negative by antibody-based screening tests. Exclusion of HIV infection after a risk exposure requires a second test after 6 months to allow time for seroconversion.

During seroconversion illness, there is a fall in the absolute CD4+ T cell count and an increase in CD8+ T cell count. Rarely, levels of CD4+ T cells may fall so low that opportunistic infections occur and this is a poor prognostic indicator. CD4+ T cell counts then return to normal or near normal, following on which there is a slow decline of CD4+ T cells over several years. Disease progression is characterised by the development of new symptoms and a rapid fall in CD4+ T cell numbers.

Persistent lymphopaenia after seroconversion illness is a poor prognostic factor, particularly with a high viral load, and indicates the need for highly active anti-retroviral therapy (HAART).

Pitfalls

Less than 2% of lymphocytes are present in peripheral blood. Significant changes in the immune system can occur with minimal perturbation of peripheral blood counts (but massive depletion of CD4+ T cells in lymphoid organs occurs during the latent phase of HIV infection).

A decrease in CD4+ T cells and an increase in CD8+ T cells is not specific for HIV infection and is seen in most acute viral infections. Therefore, the measurement of T cell subsets can never replace anti-HIV antibody testing or PCR in the diagnosis of HIV infection.

CROSS REFERENCES

Section 2.13   Human Immunodeficiency Virus
Section 3.3   Detection of Antibodies and Antigen

LYMPHOCYTE FUNCTION ASSAYS

Immunodeficiency results when T or B cells are unable to function normally, even when they are present in normal numbers. Lymphocyte function may be tested *in vivo* (delayed hypersensitivity skin tests) or using *in vitro* proliferation assays.

Clinical indications

- ◆ Suspected T cell immunodeficiency
- ◆ Clinical features suggestive of abnormal cell-mediated immunity.

Principle of the tests

- ◆ *In vitro* tests of T and B cell function – lymphocytes are purified from whole blood by density gradient centrifugation. When stimulated in culture, resting lymphocytes respond by proliferating, which is a measure of functional ability. Proliferation assays may be combined with measurement of T cell products, such as cytokines, in culture supernatants.

  — *T cell function – proliferation assays* – T cell proliferation assays are performed by stimulating cells in culture using antigens, mitogens, monoclonal antibodies or phorbol ester and calcium ionophore. The incorporation of tritiated thymidine into the DNA of replicating cells is a measure of proliferation. Results are expressed as the stimulation index – SI, that is, the ratio of counts in stimulated cells compared to unstimulated cells. A control sample from an age-matched healthy volunteer is used as control for assay variation as well as age-related variations (see Table 3.11.3).

T cell function may also be assessed by flow cytometry to measure the surface expression of activation markers following stimulation (CD25, CD69, CD71 and intracellular cytokines).

— *B cell function* – may be tested by exposing mononuclear cells to the following stimulating agents in culture:

Pokeweed mitogen (PWM)
Anti-IgM + IL-2
Staphylococcus strain A Cowan (SAC)
EBV
After seven days, the production of IgM, IgG and IgA in the cell supernatant are measured by ELISA.

◆ *In vivo* tests of T and B cell function

— *T cell function* – tested *in vivo* by assessing delayed type hypersensitivity reactions. Appropriate antigens are injected intradermally and 72–96 h later a positive reaction results in a cellular infiltrate that is palpable with overlying erythema (wheal formation). The most useful antigens are Purified Protein Derivative (PPD), Candida, mumps and tetanus, which are available as single antigens. Responses depend on prior exposure.
— *B cell function* – the best assay of B cell function is the measurement of antibody production *in vivo*, which is described later in this section.

Interpretation

◆ *In vitro* T cell function
Absent response to mitogens

— SCID

Poor responses to mitogens and antigens

— CVID
— Hyper IgM syndrome (X-linked and autosomal); defective expression of CD40L
— X-linked lymphoproliferative disease (Duncan's syndrome)
— DiGeorge syndrome
— Wiskott–Aldrich syndrome
— Ataxia telangiectasia.

Table 3.11.3 Stimulating agents used in lymphocyte proliferation assays

STIMULATING AGENT	EXAMPLE	ACTIVATION PATHWAY
Antigen (prior exposure)	Purified protein derivative of *M. tuberculosis* (PPD) Tetanus Candida	TCR
Mitogen	Phytohaemagglutinin (PHA)	Several including TCR–CD3 complex
Monoclonal antibody	Anti-CD3 (mimics antigen)	TCR–CD3 complex
Phorbol ester and calcium ionophore	Phorbol myristate acetate (PMA) and ionomycin	Direct activation of protein kinase C without receptor involvement

Poor T cell proliferative response may also be seen in secondary immunodeficiency states including viral infections (CMV, rubella, influenza virus), bacterial infections (bacterial endocarditis), malignancy and immunosuppressive drug therapy.

♦ *In vivo* T cell function assay – poor responses are seen in primary T cell defects, combined defects and in some patients with CVID. They are also found in leukaemias, lymphomas and other malignant diseases, renal failure and during some chronic infections (e.g. HIV).

♦ *In vitro* B cell function assay – these tests are not commonly indicated however, the anti-IgM + IL-2 system may be used to identify subgroups of CVID.

Pitfalls

♦ *In vitro* tests are performed in specialised referral laboratories with tissue culture facilities. Prior discussion is essential to choose the most informative tests.

♦ It is essential to exclude HIV before performing lymphocyte proliferation assays, as culture of HIV-infected lymphocytes is so hazardous that it can only be safely performed in Category 3 laboratories.

♦ Batch variability and lack of standards, make interpretation and comparison between laboratories difficult.

♦ *In vivo* tests are dependent on previous exposure to the test antigen.

CROSS REFERENCES

Section 2.9   Defects in T Cell-mediated Immunity
Section 3.3   Detection of Antibodies and Antigen

MEASUREMENT OF IMMUNOGLOBULINS, IgG SUBCLASSES AND SPECIFIC ANTIBODY LEVELS

Immunoglobulins (Ig) are also called antibodies or gammaglobulins (migrate to gamma-region during electrophoresis). IgG, IgA and IgM are the three major Ig classes detected in serum. IgE is present at very low levels in serum (see Section 3.14). IgD is rarely present in secreted form. There are four main subtypes or subclasses of IgG that are distinguishable structurally and functionally. The term 'specific antibodies' in clinical immunology refers to measurement of antibodies against specific microbial antigens or against blood group antigens.

MEASUREMENT OF IgG, IgA AND IgM

Clinical indications

♦ Repeated infections – essential investigation in patients presenting with recurrent bacterial infections of the upper or lower respiratory tract, as well as the GIT, skin, joints or central nervous system (CNS).

♦ Known primary immunodeficiency states – baseline essential in all patients with known immunodeficiency states.

♦ IgG monitoring in patients receiving replacement Ig therapy to assess adequacy of treatment.

♦ Lymphoproliferative conditions – chronic lymphocytic leukaemia (CLL); non-Hodgkin's lymphomas; plasma cell malignancies, for example, multiple myeloma, Waldenström's macroglobulinaemia.

Table 3.11.4 Causes of hypogammaglobulinaemia

IMMUNOGLOBULIN REDUCTION	CONDITION	COMMENT
IgA only	IgA deficiency Primary immunodeficiency; other defects in immunity; coeliac disease; RA; CTDs; allergy	1/500 Population Asymptomatic in many If history of infection – assess IgG subclass and specific antibody status. May represent a sub-group of patients with CVID – in evolution
IgG, IgA, IgM	Primary hypogammaglobulinaemia XLA (Bruton's agammaglobulinaemia). Usually detectable but very low IgG, A and M	Onset >3 months of age. Males only No mature B cells detected
	Hyper-IgM syndrome (CD40L deficiency)	Onset early; Males; IgM may be very high. T cell defects also common
	CVID – IgG usually <2g/l; IgA also very low, IgM variable	Onset – any age. Males and females affected B and T cells present in blood but numbers and function often abnormal Clinically – T cell related defects, autoimmune and malignant features in some patients
	Trasient Hypogammaglobulinaemia of infancy	Resolves with age. Monitor serial values
	Rare – Thymoma	Usually >50 years
	Transcobalamin II deficiency	
	Secondary hypogammaglobulinaemia Lymphoproliferative conditions Light chain multiple myeloma Other types of myeloma; CLL; NHL	All Igs deficient Monoclonal increase in one Ig with reduction in all other Igs
	Protein – losing states Nephrotic syndrome Protein-losing enteropathies	IgM normal, low IgG, Albumin low
	Drugs	Cytotoxics; anticonvulsants

♦ Chronic liver disease – chronic inflammatory states and cirrhosis.
♦ Other chronic inflammatory states – HIV infection; Sjögren's syndrome; RA and other connective tissue diseases; sarcoidosis and chronic infections, for example, TB.

Principle of the tests

Levels of IgG, IgA and IgM are most often measured by nephelometry, which is rapid and automated. RID can also be used. Reference ranges for each of the immunoglobulin classes are defined on the basis of the values obtained in age- and sex-matched, normal control populations.

Other methods using enzyme-, chemiluminescent- or fluorescent-probes can be used to measure Ig levels, but the high sensitivities achieved are not routinely necessary.

Table 3.11.5 Causes of hypergammaglobulinaemia

IMMUNOGLOBULIN INCREASE	CONDITION	COMMENT
Single immunoglobulin class	Monoclonal	
	Single heavy chain (class) and light chain (κ or λ) expansion, that is IgGκ, IgMλ	Covered in Section 3.12
	Lymphoproliferative conditions	
	Amyloidosis	
	Paraprotein-related neuropathies	
	POEMS	
	Polyclonal	
	Single heavy chain (class) and combined κ and λ expansions	Causes are as for polyclonal rises in all Ig classes but expansion of one isotype may dominate – see below for comments
All immunoglobulin classes	Chronic liver diseases	All Ig classes but IgM especially in primary biliary cirrhosis; IgA in alcoholic liver disease; IgG in chronic active hepatitis
	CTDs/chronic inflammatory disorders	RA; SLE; Sjögren's syndrome (typically IgG1 rise is dominant); sarcoidosis
	Chronic infections	TB; bronchiectasis; cystic fibrosis
	Viral infections	Polyclonal rise in Igs may be massive in
	HIV	HIV, but functional antibody deficiency
	EBV, CMV	is common in children – measure specific antibodies

Interpretation

Immunoglobulin concentrations below the 95% confidence limits of an age- and sex-matched control population is defined as hypogammaglobulinaemia (Table 3.11.4).

Elevation in Ig levels is called hypergammaglobulinaemia. The rise in immunoglobulins may be monoclonal – meaning a single B cell population is causing the increase. This is covered further in Section 3.12. Polyclonal rises in immunoglobulins are the result of many different specificities of antibody being over-produced. Polyclonal rises may be class-specific or involve more than one class of immunoglobulin (Table 3.11.5).

Pitfalls

- Precipitation assays are accurate only if the detecting antibody is present at constant concentration in excess of the 'antigen' (antibody excess). Very high concentrations of immunoglobulin may be underestimated if antigen excess occurs, an error which can be avoided by interpreting immunoglobulin results in combination with electrophoresis.
- Turbidity (cloudiness) of serum as occurs in haemolysed or lipaemic samples may also interfere with accuracy of results using nephelometry.
- RID is labour-intensive and slow.
- Abnormal immunoglobulin molecules (e.g. monoclonal IgM) or presence of immune complexes may interfere with diffusion and precipitation leading to inaccuracies in quantitation.
- Normal total immunoglobulin levels do not equate with normal antibody-mediated immunity (see IgG subclass and specific antibody measurements).

CROSS REFERENCES
Section 2.8   Defects in Antibody-mediated Immunity Section 3.3   Detection of Antibodies and Antigen

IgG SUBCLASSES

Clinical indications

Repeated infections – suspected primary immunodeficiency: IgG subclasses should be measured even if the total immunoglobulin levels are normal. Combined IgG subclass (IgG2 and IgG4 typically) and IgA deficiency may represent a type of CVID and some patients subsequently develop full-blown immunoglobulin deficiency.

Principle of the test

IgG subclasses, like total Igs are measured by precipitation assay. RID is currently used most commonly but nephelometry is also used.

Interpretation

IgG1 is the most abundant of the four IgG subclasses in serum. Deficiency usually results in low levels of total IgG. Clinically, patients with significant reductions in IgG1 behave as CVID.

Deficiency of one or more of the other IgG subclasses may occur without reduction in total IgG levels. Major reductions in IgG2, IgG3 and IgG4 either alone or in combination (usually IgG2 and IgG4) occur in perfectly healthy individuals.

IgG subclass levels vary with age, sex and race. Accurate interpretation requires comparison with reference ranges drawn up from a matched control population.

IgG subclass levels may be disturbed in a variety of conditions, for example, polyclonal rise in IgG1 with suppression of IgG2, IgG3 and IgG4 in Sjögren's syndrome; IgG3 deficiency in a subgroup with asthma; IgG3 deficiency in some children with intractable epilepsy and complete IgG4 deficiency in some patients with bronchiectasis. There is no clear indication of what these deficiencies mean or how they should be managed and at the moment IgG subclass analysis is not indicated in such conditions.

Pitfalls

Normal IgG subclass measurements must not be taken to mean that antibody-mediated immunity is normal. Total Ig levels may even be high in patients with IgG subclass deficiency.

IgG1, IgG3 and IgG4 typically occur in responses to protein antigen challenges (e.g. viruses, tetanus, diphtheria). IgG2 production characteristically occurs on challenge with polysaccharide antigens (capsules of pyogenic bacteria). However, total IgG2 levels correlate badly with responsiveness to polysaccharide vaccines (e.g. Pneumovax®). Polysaccharide – specific IgG of other subclasses is highly protective. Normal IgG subclass levels do not exclude defective specific antibody production.

SPECIFIC ANTIBODIES

It is possible to measure antibodies specific for certain pathogens either commonly encountered in the community (e.g. *Pneumococcus*) or encountered as part of the standard immunisation schedule (*Tetanus*, *Haemophilus influenzae B* (*HiB*), *Meningococcus* strain C). Baseline levels of specific antibody, and levels before and after challenge with immunisation, are measured. If baseline values are low, this provides an excellent test of antibody function *in vivo*. Natural antibodies, for example, blood group antibodies have been used as indicators of antibody function but microbial antibody testing has taken over in this area.

Clinical indications

♦ *Suspected primary immunodeficiency* – measurement of microbial antibodies (most commonly *Pneumococcus* and *HiB*) is indicated in patients with repeated bacterial infections typically involving the respiratory tract even if immunoglobulin and IgG subclass levels are normal. Response to test immunisation with the relevant vaccine is indicated if baseline levels are low. Specific antibody deficiency syndromes are increasingly recognised.

♦ *Secondary immunodeficiency* – HIV infection, especially in children; post-bone marrow transplant; splenectomised patients.

♦ *Vaccine failure* – clinical infection after immunisation, for example, *Haemophilus* meningitis or septicaemia post *HiB*-conjugate vaccine; Hepatitis B vaccine failure. Vaccine failure is less clear-cut with *Pneumococcus* because of the huge variety of strains and limited strain coverage of existing vaccines.

Principle of the test

Total IgG antibody directed against specific microbial antigens is usually measured by ELISA. Reference ranges of antibody concentrations must be age-matched. Less is known about normal post-immunisation responsiveness and ranges obtained in immunisation studies using similar assay conditions are often adopted.

Standardisation of assays is difficult. International standard sera with known concentrations of specific antibody for *HiB* and *Tetanus* toxoid are available. Bacterial antigens used in assays vary, with some laboratories using preparation of crude *pneumococcal* polysaccharides and other using *pneumococcal* cell wall polysaccharide-depleted preparations. The latter are thought to measure truly protective antibodies only. Strain-specific *pneumococcal* antibody assays are not widely used as a test of immune function. They are most useful in the context of assessing vaccine efficacy in clinical trials.

Interpretation

Low levels of specific antibodies may indicate lack of exposure or impaired immune function. Levels of polysaccharide-specific antibodies are normally low until 5 years of age.

If levels are low, immunisation with the relevant vaccine(s) followed by post-challenge testing at 3–4 weeks is indicated. Normal responsiveness is generally interpreted as a twofold or greater increase and antibody levels rising to the normal range.

Pitfalls

Difficulties interpreting these assays include:

♦ Failure to compare test results with age-matched controls (especially important for polysaccharide antibodies).

♦ Protection does not always equate with responsiveness. Levels of specific antibodies conferring protection are known for tetanus and *HiB*. This is not the case for pneumococcus.

♦ Some patients make adequate antibody responses to challenge antigens but lose the antibodies quickly – for example, in splenectomised patients. Late follow-up of antibody levels are indicated if this is suspected.

Patients should not be revaccinated for the purpose of immune function testing unless microbe-specific antibodies are low. Inadvertent administration of vaccines to patients with high levels of antibodies is associated with a higher incidence of adverse reactions.

CROSS REFERENCES

Section 1.13 Immunoglobulin Structure
Section 2.8 Defects in Antibody-mediated Immunity
Section 2.31 Plasma Cell Diseases
Section 3.3 Detection of Antibodies and Antigen
Section 3.12 Abnormal Immunoglobulins

NEUTROPHIL FUNCTION TESTS

In order to adequately protect us, neutrophils must be present in normal numbers, and must be able to:

- Adhere to endothelium, using a variety of adhesion molecules, at the site of inflammation.
- Traverse the endothelium and follow a gradient of chemoattractant to the site of inflammation.
- Phagocytose organisms/cellular debris causing inflammation.
- Undergo a respiratory burst, generating toxic chemicals to kill ingested pathogens.

Clinical testing of neutrophil function attempts to test each of these functions.

Clinical indications

- Recurrent skin infections, soft tissue infections and abscesses
- Infections with *Staphylococcus aureus* and/or *Burkholderia cepacia*
- Family history of a neutrophil disorder
- Failure of separation of the umbilical cord.

NB: Neutrophil function testing is difficult and time consuming, and these tests should never be performed without detailed discussion with a clinical immunologist. Neutrophil defects are extremely rare, however several factors may interfere with the assays giving misleading results. These factors include intercurrent infection and drug therapy. Additionally, common causes of the above infections including diabetes should be excluded initially.

Principle of the test

Quantification of neutrophils   Neutrophils are routinely quantified in the five-part white cell differential count obtained from haematology analysers. An apparently low neutrophil count should always be confirmed by examining a blood film.

Prior to considering neutrophil function testing, a blood film should be performed to assess neutrophil morphology, as neutrophils that appear abnormal rarely function normally. Rare genetic abnormalities of neutrophil granulation as well as myelodysplasia (a premalignant condition in which neutrophil development and function is abnormal) can readily be recognised on a blood film. In these conditions formal neutrophil testing rarely adds to the management of the patient.

Adhesion Measurement of key neutrophil adhesion molecules, using standard flow cytometry techniques, is commonly used. The adhesion molecules which may be measured in this way include CD15 – sialyl Lewis x, CD11a, CD11b, CD11c and CD18.

Neutrophil adhesion assays involve allowing neutrophils to adhere to plastic, fibronectin coated glass or cultured endothelium. Unbound neutrophils are washed away and the adherent neutrophils quantified either by microscopy or measurement of a neutrophil specific protein such as myeloperoxidase.

Chemotaxis Neutrophil chemotaxis (migration in response to chemotactic stimuli) may be measured under agarose. Wells cut into agarose are filled with neutrophils, chemoattractant or control saline, and the numbers of cells migrating after a defined period are counted. A control is always included and the results are compared with age-matched controls. Alternatively, specialised Boyden chambers may be used.

Phagocytosis Phagocytosis of organisms is measured using latex particles or stained organisms incubated with patient cells. The percentage of cells that have ingested particles and the number of particles ingested is compared to controls. If fluorescent particles are used, phagocytosis can be measured by flow cytometry. In both assays distinguishing adherent particles on the cell surface from those that have been phagocytosed is difficult.

Respiratory burst The nitroblue tetrazolium (NBT) test relies on reduction of NBT to formazan by oxygen radicals produced by stimulated neutrophils. Neutrophils are incubated with colourless NBT, appropriately stimulated and the presence of formazan is assessed visually using a microscope or by spectrophotometry. Intracellular dyes, which become fluorescent after reduction by reactive oxygen intermediates, have led to flow cytometric equivalents of the NBT test.

Interpretation

Interpretation of neutrophil function tests is difficult and requires an interpretive report by the supervising immunologist.

Repeated absence of the neutrophil respiratory burst is seen in chronic granulomatous disease (CGD). Partial reduction may be seen in carriers of this condition.

Absence of neutrophil adhesion molecules or significant reduction compared with age-matched controls is seen in leucocyte adhesion deficiency (LAD).

Pitfalls

- Neutrophil function testing should be performed when patients are well, as intercurrent infections and a variety of drugs can impair neutrophil function.
- These tests are highly variable, even within the normal population. Additionally normal values are age-related in many assays. Hence establishing a normal range is difficult.
- Neutrophil function changes progressively after venepuncture and purification of neutrophils. Therefore, blood must be sent directly to the testing laboratory.
- Usually if tests are abnormal, repeat testing will be suggested as well as confirmatory protein or genetic testing.

NK CELLS

NK cells are part of the innate immune response to viral infections. In routine practice assessment is usually limited to quantification of these cells, however assays of NK cell function are well described although not widely available.

Clinical indications

NK cell deficiency states are extremely rare. Patients who have been described have recurrent viral infections, particularly caused by herpes viruses. Infections are extremely severe in the first few days, but subsequently resolve (as the adaptive cellular response takes over).

Principle of the test

NK cell numbers are measured by flow cytometry after staining for CD16 (an FcR expressed on all NK cells) often in combination with other NK markers such as CD56 or CD57 (each of which stain a subset of NK cells). Cell numbers, however, do not correlate well with activity.

NK cell activity is only measured in rare cases. An erythroblastic cell line K562 is susceptible to lysis by NK cells. Prelabelling these cells with ^{51}Cr allows the degree of target cell death to be assessed by chromium release.

Interpretation and pitfalls

Age-related ranges for assessment of NK cell numbers are available. As NK cell numbers fluctuate, low measurements should be tested repeatedly to exclude artifactual reductions.

NK cell function assays are not well established. The significance of any abnormal findings must be cautiously interpreted in the light of repeated testing of several controls.

Abnormal Immunoglobulins

Proliferation of a single population (clone) of B cells may result in excessive production of immunoglobulin (Ig) of a single specificity. The resulting Ig product is a monoclonal protein, also known as a paraprotein. Paraproteins may be fragments of or intact Ig. Monoclonal Ig light chain in urine is known as Bence–Jones protein (BJP). Marked activation of a small number of B cell populations may result in the production of more than one paraprotein and is described as an oligoclonal response.

DETECTION AND MONITORING OF PARAPROTEINS

Clinical indications

This is important in B cell lymphoproliferative conditions. These include:

- Plasma cell dyscrasias

    — Multiple myeloma – essential for diagnosis, and monitoring of therapeutic response and progress.
    — Waldenström's macroglobulinaemia – essential for diagnosis and monitoring therapeutic interventions.
    — Plasmacytoma – 50% have a paraprotein in serum. Serial monitoring required as 50% progress to multiple myeloma.
    — AL Amyloid – light chain or primary amyloidosis.
    — Plasma cell leukaemia.
    — Heavy chain diseases – rare disorders where monoclonal heavy chain only – usually IgA – is secreted.

- Other lymphoproliferative conditions associated with paraproteins include:

    — Chronic lymphocytic leukaemia
    — Lymphoma – both Hodgkin's and non-Hodgkin's
    — POEMS syndrome
    — Paraprotein-associated neuropathies.

Detection of paraprotein in these conditions is supportive of the diagnosis provided other typical features are present.

- ◆ Monoclonal gammopathy of uncertain significance (MGUS) – is diagnosed only if other causes of paraprotein are excluded. Monitoring is essential as some evolve into multiple myeloma.
- ◆ Small paraproteins arise in a variety of states associated with immune activation. They include:
    - — Connective tissue diseases (CTDs)
    - — Severe infections
    - — Post bone marrow transplantation (BMT).

Monoclonal or oligoclonal paraproteins are seen, especially when there is underlying immunodeficiency. Measurement of paraprotein while not essential is informative of the degree and pattern of immune activation.

Principle of the test

Detection of paraproteins

Electrophoresis Electrophoresis (in an appropriate support medium) separates proteins in body fluids according to surface charge. Application of protein-binding dyes to electrophoresed material allows visualisation of separated proteins. Besides paraprotein detection, electrophoresis is useful in many other conditions where variation in protein levels can be qualitatively demonstrated (e.g. hypo- and hypergammaglobulinaemia, acute phase response, protein-losing states such as nephrotic syndrome and protein-deficiency states such as α-1-antitrypsin deficiency) (Figure 3.12.1).

All immunoglobulin molecules have a common structure, but minor variations in size and electrical charge distinguish immunoglobulin molecules of one specificity from immunoglobulins of all other specificities. Immunoglobulin molecules normally move to the negative pole – the gamma (γ) region – under standard electrophoresis conditions. The minor variations in charge of different immunoglobulins results in a 'smear' in the γ-region representing the huge number of differing specificities of immunoglobulin in normal individuals. However, in situations where a single B cell clone is producing excessive amounts of monoclonal immunoglobulin, a band results. This is how paraproteins are most commonly identified.

Densitometry This technique is used to measure the amount of paraprotein present. The absorbance of transmitted light by the dye–protein complexes on the electrophoretic strip is directly proportional to the amount of protein present in each region. Measurement of total protein allows the concentration of the paraprotein to be calculated.

Immunofixation This is the method most commonly used to 'type' paraproteins (Ig heavy/light chain composition). Serial lanes of electrophoresed material are overlaid with isotype and light chain specific anti-sera. Following a washing step, only protein bound by antisera remains. Visualisation is as for standard electrophoresis.

Other tests in paraproteinaemic states:

- ◆ Serum β$_2$-microglobulin is a valuable indicator of myeloma tumour burden and can be measured by a variety of immunochemical methods. Renal impairment reduces the rate of β$_2$-microglobulin excretion so levels should be adjusted to take account of this.
- ◆ Hyperviscosity is a feature of some paraproteinaemic states, especially Waldenström's macroglobulinaemia (IgM paraprotein), but also some IgA and IgG3 multiple myelomas. Viscosity is measured using a capillary tube system (viscometer) in which

Figure 3.12.1 Electrophoresis–immunofixation of monoclonal band.

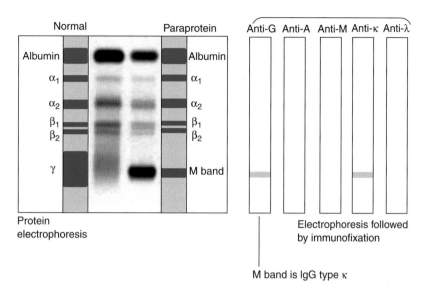

the time taken for serum to fall a given distance is compared with the time taken for water to fall the same distance. The value is expressed in terms of the ratio of serum to water fall. The normal range is 1.4–1.9 and patients with values >4 are especially at risk of hyperviscosity-related complications.

Interpretation

The prevalence of serum paraprotein detection increases with age. This finding occurs in <0.1% of young adults, 3% of 70 year olds and 10% of 80 year olds. The critical issue is to differentiate paraproteins associated with malignant conditions such as multiple myeloma from MGUS and benign conditions.

The significance of a serum paraprotein is assessed using these indicators.

♦ Amount – small concentrations of paraproteins (<10g/l) are typical of non-malignant conditions such as MGUS, infection, CTDs and post-BMT, and in these conditions the concentration of paraprotein rarely increases progressively. Larger amounts of para-proteins occur in malignant conditions like multiple myeloma and Waldenström's macroglobulinaemia.

♦ Other immunoglobulins – suppression of the non-paraprotein immunoglobulins (immunoparesis) is a characteristic feature of malignant paraprotein states but rarely occurs in MGUS (<5% of cases).

♦ Urinary monoclonal light chain bands (Bence–Jones proteins (BJPs)) – BJPs are character-istic of malignant paraprotein states, particularly multiple myeloma. This finding is rare in non-malignant conditions.

♦ Other features – haematological (Hb, bone marrow findings), biochemical (renal parameters, serum calcium), and X-ray findings (osteoporosis and lytic changes) should be taken into account when assessing the likely cause of a paraprotein.

♦ Immunoglobulin-related abnormalities – hyperviscosity (due to physico-chemical char-acteristics of the paraprotein) occurs in malignant paraprotein states but not in MGUS.

Pitfalls

- Urinary paraproteins do not react with protein-detecting urine dip-sticks. Negative urinalysis for protein does not rule out the presence of BJPs.
- Paraproteins may lie anywhere on the electrophoretic strip but are usually in the β or γ regions.
- Serum, not plasma should be used. Fibrinogen in plasma forms a band in the β region. Other protein bands (complement components and CRP) can also mimic paraproteins.
- The sensitivity of some electrophoretic techniques used for urine paraprotein detection will require that concentrated urine (an early morning sample) or a 24-h collection is provided. Check local arrangements.
- Some paraproteins polymerise resulting in a few rather than a single band on electrophoresis. This is especially common with IgA and IgM proteins.
- Light chains only are produced in 15% of multiple myeloma cases. Serum paraproteins are rarely detected in such cases as the low-molecular weight light chains are readily excreted in urine. Therefore, paired serum and urine specimens are required for myeloma screening.
- Detection of monoclonal light chain only in serum requires immunofixation for IgD and IgE heavy chains to detect these rare myelomas. If only heavy chains are found on immunofixation, different light chain anti-sera should be used in an attempt to identify monoclonal light chains. Addition of McClelland reagent (dithiothreotol) may unfold paraproteins (particularly IgA) of abnormal conformation, allowing access of the light chain antiserum to a previously masked light chain. Myeloma with unusual light chains that bind poorly to standard light chain antisera is far more common than heavy chain diseases.
- Immunoglobulin concentrations calculated using densitometry are not directly comparable with those calculated using immunochemical methods. Estimation of the concentration of non-paraprotein Ig of the same isotype as the paraprotein must not be calculated by subtracting the densitometry result from the immunochemical result.
- Some conditions such as paraprotein-related neuropathies are associated with very low levels of paraprotein. The more sensitive technique of immunofixation is indicated in such cases even when paraprotein is not evident on electrophoresis.

DETECTION AND MEASUREMENT OF CRYOGLOBULINS

Immunoglobulins that precipitate in the cold are called cryoglobulins. Cryoglobulins that precipitate at higher temperatures are more likely to cause clinical problems.

Clinical indications

- Cutaneous vasculitis
- Glomerulonephritis associated with normal C3 and reduced C4 levels
- Cold-related symptoms such as Raynaud's phenomenon, especially if there is evidence of vasculitis
- Cold-induced inflammatory states
- Vasculitis in the presence of known precipitant of cryoglobulin formation (e.g. Hepatitis C virus; B cell malignancy).

Principle of the test

Correct handling of blood is critical. Blood should be taken using a pre-warmed syringe, put into a pre-warmed plain tube, transported to the laboratory, and allowed to clot at

37°C. Serum is then placed in a series of clear tubes that are left at ambient temperatures of 4°C (cold room), 20°C (room temperature) and 37°C (warm room or warm water bath) for 2–3 days. Most cryoglobulins of clinical significance will precipitate and be evident to the eye within 24 h but some form more slowly. Cryoglobulins formed at room temperature and 4°C are more likely to be of clinical significance than those that form at 4°C only.

Cryoprecipitate is quantified by centrifugation of the precipitate-containing serum in a graduated tube at 4°C and the ratio of precipitate to serum (cryocrit) is calculated.

Typing requires definition of clonality and reactivity of the cryoglobulin. The precipitate is washed and re-dissolved in warmed buffer. Clonality is identified using electrophoresis and immunofixation at 37°C. Immunoglobulin isotype and rheumatoid factor (RF) activity must be measured at 37°C. Manual RID and agglutination methods are often used as nephelometry is difficult to perform at a defined temperature.

Interpretation

Cryoglobulins are classified as follows:

- Type 1 – monoclonal cold-precipitating immunoglobulin (Ig), found in B cell malignancies (multiple myeloma, Waldenström's macroglobulinaemia and B cell lymphoma/leukaemias).
- Type 2 – cryoglobulinaemic monoclonal component that binds and precipitates polyclonal immunoglobulins – mixed cryoglobulin, usually with RF activity. It is seen in B cell malignancies, chronic infections – especially hepatitis C, chronic bacteraemic states and in connective tissue diseases (CTDs).
- Type 3 – cold-precipitating Ig with polyclonal RF activity. These occur in chronic infections and CTDs.

Pitfalls

- Failure to maintain the specimen at temperature of 37°C may result in loss of cryoglobulin from serum giving a false negative result.
- Serum should be left at 4°C for at least 3 days before reporting absence of a cryoglobulin.
- Cryoglobulins are not the same as cold agglutinins. The latter are antibodies that bind to red blood cells at low temperatures and that target bound cells for haemolysis.

DETECTION OF OLIGOCLONAL BANDS IN CSF

In health, the blood brain barrier prevents leakage of high-molecular weight proteins into the CSF, and immunoglobulin is not synthesised within the CSF. Intrathecal synthesis of immunoglobulin may occur in patients with multiple sclerosis (MS) as well as a variety of inflammatory CNS conditions.

Clinical indications

Suspected multiple sclerosis (MS) – intrathecal oligoclonal immunoglobulin bands are useful in diagnosis and prognosis.

Principle of the test

Highly sensitive methods such as nephelometry are required to measure levels of IgG and albumin in CSF, as concentrations are low.

Intrathecal Ig synthesis is confirmed by isoelectric focusing (IEF). IEF is an electrophoretic technique where proteins are separated based on their isoelectric points, using gels containing ampholytes that form a pH gradient during electrophoresis. Proteins are sharply focused at the point in the gel where the pH equals their isoelectric point. The proteins are then transferred to nitrocellulose and detected using antisera to human IgG (immunoassay similar to immunoblotting). Serum and CSF are run together, and the presence of bands in the CSF, which are not detectable in serum, demonstrates intrathecal IgG synthesis.

Interpretation

Albumin in the CSF reflects the passage of this protein from the blood to the CSF and levels increase if the blood brain barrier is leaky. CSF IgG may reflect passage of serum-derived protein across the blood brain barrier or may indicate local intrathecal production. CSF IgG to albumin ratio is increased to >22% in patients with increased intrathecal production.

The detection of oligoclonal bands supports a diagnosis of MS, but is also found in other neuro-inflammatory conditions.

Pitfalls

* Raised CSF IgG and CSF oligoclonal bands are not specific for MS. They are also seen in CNS sarcoidosis, neurosyphilis, bacterial meningitis and viral encephalitis.
* CSF oligoclonal bands are only considered positive when similar bands are absent in serum.
* Oligoclonal bands cannot be interpreted in blood-stained CSF.

CROSS REFERENCES

Angioedema: C1-Inhibitor Disorders

C1-Inhibitor (C1-Inh) is a plasma protease inhibitor of the first component (C1) of the classical pathway of complement activation. It is also an important control protein for coagulation, fibrinolytic and kinin pathways. Low levels of C1-Inh allow uncontrolled C1 activation resulting in consumption of C2 and C4 (reduction in levels). In fluid phase activation of C1s, levels of C1s, C3 and C5–C9 remain normal. Measurement of C1-Inh and C4 levels may be used to monitor disease activity.

C1-Inh deficiency may be hereditary or acquired and results in angioedema. Diagnosis is made by demonstrating low levels of C1-Inh, functionally or antigenically.

Clinical indications

- ◆ Recurrent bouts of acute local oedema of skin and mucosa, regardless of age.
- ◆ Recurrent bouts of crampy abdominal pain, if the C4 is low.
- ◆ Family history of hereditary angioedema (HAE).
- ◆ Monitoring response to treatment in patients with known C1-Inh deficiency.

Principle of the test

The diagnosis of, and distinction between, different types of hereditary and acquired angioedema can usually be established by measuring antigenic levels of C1-Inh, C1q, C3 and C4 together with the clinical history.

In a patient with angioedema:

- ◆ C1-Inh deficiency is unlikely in the absence of a reduced level of C4.
- ◆ Substantial reduction of C1-Inh levels, with reduced C4, reduced or normal C1q and normal C3, establishes the diagnosis of C1-Inh deficiency. Minor reductions in C1-Inh level may be due to complement consumption in immune complex disease.

- A low C4 and normal levels of C3 should trigger measurement of C1-Inh function, even in the presence of normal or high antigenic levels of C1-Inh. This assay detects Type II HAE.
- A low C1q but normal C1-Inh level should lead to consideration of acquired anti-C1-Inh autoantibodies.

Measurement of C1q, C4, C3 and C1-Inh levels

The individual complement components are measured by RID or nephelometry.

C1-Inh function assay

C1-Inh function is assayed by measuring inhibition of the hydrolysis of amino acid esters by a standard preparation of C1s (an enzyme subunit of C1). Purified activated C1s catalyses the chromogenic conversion of appropriate substrates, and this is measured by spectrophotometry. Functionally active C1-Inh (normally present in fresh plasma or serum) inhibits C1s reducing the amount of colour produced. Results are expressed as a percentage of C1s activity remaining in normal plasma.

Detection of anti-C1-Inh antibody

Measurement of these antibodies is not routinely performed, however when suspected based on complement studies, they can be demonstrated by immunoblotting or ELISA.

Interpretation

- Hereditary angioedema Type I (85% of cases) – functionally normal C1-Inh present in reduced amounts. C4 is low; C1q may be normal or low.
- Hereditary angioedema Type II (15% of cases) – normal or elevated levels of inactive C1-Inh, but low C1-Inh activity. C4 is low, C1q may be normal or low.
- Acquired angioedema Type I – levels of C1-Inh are reduced because of increased consumption, associated with lymphoproliferative disorders or connective tissue disease. C1-Inh, C1q and C4 are reduced.
- Acquired angioedema Type II – characterised by the presence of an autoantibody directed against C1-Inh. This may prevent binding of C1-Inh to its substrate or facilitate C1-Inh cleavage (inactivation) by proteinases activated in the inflammatory response including C1, plasmin and kallikrein. C1-Inh levels are variable (low or normal), with low levels of C1q and C4.

Pitfalls

- C1-Inh is a labile protein and samples should be separated as soon as possible to avoid artifactual reduction.

- *In vitro* C1 activation may occur in poorly stored specimens, which will result in reduced functional activity of the inhibitor.
- Serum levels of C1-Inh are increased by exogenous androgens and related steroids, and reduced by exogenous oestrogens including oral contraceptives.

CROSS REFERENCES

Section 1.5   Innate Immune Responses II – The Complement System
Section 2.11   Complement Deficiency
Section 3.3   Detection of Antibodies and Antigen

Allergy and Hypersensitivity

Both laboratory and clinical testing procedures are used to investigate allergy and hypersensitivity disorders. The most frequently performed investigations are aimed at determining the cause of allergies, and do not need to be performed when symptoms are present. Measurement of mast cell tryptase and urinary methylhistamine during reactions helps to differentiate mast cell degranulation (usually due to Type I hypersensitivity) from other causes of ill health.

TOTAL IgE LEVELS

Clinical indications

- Suspected allergic disease
- Confirmation of atopic tendency
- Useful in interpreting levels of allergen specific IgE.

Principles of the test

IgE is present in nanogram quantities in serum, and unlike other immunoglobulin isotypes cannot be detected by nephelometry. Solid phase assays using sensitive detection systems such as radioimmunoassays, enzyme immunoassays or fluorescence-based assays are used. IgE is captured by solid-phase bound anti-IgE, and after incubation and washing labelled anti-IgE is added followed by appropriate development or detection steps.

Interpretation

Reference ranges for total IgE levels are age-related. Elevated IgE is most commonly associated with atopy, but may also be seen in parasitic infections and Churg–Strauss syndrome.

Pitfalls

Confirmation of an atopic tendency does not prove that symptoms are due to allergic disease. Severe allergy (usually to a single or few allergens) may be seen even with a normal or low total IgE.

ALLERGEN-SPECIFIC IgE LEVELS

Clinical indications

Assessment of IgE-mediated allergy to specific allergens, suggested by history.

Principles of the test

Most laboratories use a similar system to that used to measure total IgE. However, the solid phase is coated with the allergen under investigation rather than anti-IgE.

Interpretation

Comparison of positive results with total IgE is useful. Most test systems report grades of positivity from 0 (negative) to 5 or 6 (strongly positive). Strongly positive results suggest significant sensitisation and are usually associated with symptoms. Negative results make clinical sensitivity unlikely, but do not absolutely exclude allergy. Intermediate grades must be interpreted with the total IgE and history.

Pitfalls

- Weak positives to many allergens are common in patients with grossly elevated total IgE.
- Tests are expensive, and therefore it is usually only feasible to test for a limited range of allergens.
- Range of allergens available is limited – particularly for investigation of drug allergy.
- False negative results occur when major allergens are labile, or metabolites rather than a parent compound, or become denatured during coupling to solid phase.
- Negative results do not absolutely exclude allergy – challenge tests remain necessary.

ALLERGY SKIN TESTS

Skin prick tests (SPTs) are widely used allergy investigations performed in the clinic. There are two main types – skin prick tests and intradermal tests. SPTs are more commonly used, as they are more comfortable for the patient, safer, quicker and easier to perform. Intradermal tests require injection of the allergen, which must be sterile. They are painful for the patient, carry a higher risk of provoking an allergic reaction and are more cumbersome to perform. However, they are more sensitive than SPTs and are used in specialist clinics particularly to investigate drug allergy.

Clinical indications

Investigation of allergic symptoms – a broad range of suspected allergens may be assessed. Results are read 15 min later, allowing immediate counselling of patients.

Principle of the test

A drop of allergen solution is placed on the forearm, or injected into the skin. Negative control (diluent) and a positive control (histamine solution) are also used. For SPTs the drop of control or allergen is pricked with a lancet. Thus a small amount of allergen is introduced into the skin. If mast cells carrying allergen-specific IgE are present they are activated and degranulate, releasing histamine. Histamine causes a wheal and flare reaction. The diameter of the wheal is measured, and compared with controls.

Interpretation

Allergens producing a wheal 2–3 mm larger than the negative control are considered positive. Positivity indicates sensitisation to the allergen, but may not be associated with clinical symptoms. Larger reactions are more likely to be associated with symptoms. Positive results should be carefully reviewed together with the history to assess their clinical significance.

Pitfalls

- SPTs assess sensitisation, and do not imply clinical allergy to an allergen.
- SPTs may miss sensitisation to labile allergens, or allergy to metabolites of a parent compound, which is often important in drug allergy. SPTs for labile components may be performed using a prick–prick technique, where a fresh fruit is pricked with the lancet, which is then used to prick the skin – however this technique is poorly standardised.
- A negative SPT does not exclude allergy.
- It may not be possible to carry out SPTs if the patient cannot stop antihistamines (which interfere with the tests), has extensive skin disease, has dermographism (where skin trauma induces a wheal) or where the risk of anaphylaxis is considered unacceptable.

ALLERGEN CHALLENGES

The gold standard in allergy diagnosis is the double-blind placebo-controlled allergen challenge (DBPCAC). This is most commonly used to investigate food and drug allergy, but may also be used to assess inhaled allergens. Where symptoms are subjective it is essential that challenges are performed in a double blind fashion. However, when objective signs predominate in the allergic reaction under investigation an open challenge may be appropriate.

Clinical indications

Assessment of specific allergy to staple foodstuff or essential drug. Performed under specialist supervision only, with appropriate resuscitation equipment. Risk of anaphylaxis must be considered acceptable.

Principle of the test

Escalating doses of allergen and placebo are prepared by dietician or pharmacist. Allergist performing test is unaware of contents. Numbered doses are administered to patient, and effects noted. Test is stopped if significant symptoms/signs of allergy emerge. Test results are unblinded and discussed with patient.

Interpretation

Symptoms/signs resulting from placebo suggest psychogenic reaction. Reproducible symptoms/signs resulting from allergen prove allergy.

Pitfalls

- ◆ Carries significant risk of anaphylaxis
- ◆ Can only be performed in patient who could tolerate severe reaction (no significant cardiac or respiratory disease, not on β-blockers)
- ◆ Test is time consuming and requires specialised day care facilities and full resuscitation facilities
- ◆ Co-factors such as infection, exercise, alcohol, etc. are not present – allergen may be missed.

MAST CELL TRYPTASE

Clinical indications

Demonstration of mast cell degranulation in a patient – often useful to differentiate allergy to anaesthetic agent from other anaesthetic mishap.

Principle of the test

Mast cell degranulation is associated with release of mast cell tryptase. Elevated levels may be seen from 1 to 12 h after a systemic allergic reaction. Tryptase is measured using solid phase enzyme or radio-immunoassay. Pre-reaction serum when available should be analysed for comparison.

Interpretation

Elevated levels compared to baseline indicate mast cell degranulation. This is usually due to IgE-mediated reactions, however mast cell degranulation resulting from other stimuli cannot be excluded.

Pitfalls

Elevated tryptase is seen infrequently in allergic reactions due to food allergy. Failure to detect elevated tryptase does not exclude allergy. Appropriately timed samples are required for analysis. Test does not distinguish between allergy and other causes of mast cell degranulation.

PRECIPITATING ANTIBODIES

The majority of patients with extrinsic allergic alveolitis (EAA) form precipitating antibodies to the allergen. The lung damage resulting from this condition results from both Type III and Type IV hypersensitivity.

Common precipitating antibodies measured include antibodies to avian proteins (bird fanciers lung), *Micropolyspora faenii* (farmers lung) and aspergillus (allergic bronchopulmonary aspergillosis, ABPA).

Clinical indications

- Suspected EAA (interstitial lung disease in exposed individual; fever, dyspnoea and/or cough on exposure to allergen).
- Suspected ABPA (asthma, pulmonary infiltrates, bronchiectasis usually with eosinophilia).

Principle of the test

Antibodies to suspected allergen may be demonstrated by double diffusion (Ouchterlony plate) or by counter current immunoelectrophoresis (CCIE).

Interpretation

Positive test indicates sensitisation. Clinical significance must be interpreted in light of the history.

Pitfalls

Positive results support but do not establish the diagnosis of EAA. Positive results are common following antigen exposure, even in the absence of disease. Tests are not 100% sensitive. CCIE is more sensitive than double diffusion.

CROSS REFERENCES	
Section 1.30	Atopy and Allergic Inflammation
Sections 2.1–2.6	Various allergic diseases
Section 4.13	Management of Acute Allergic Reactions

Transplantation

Tests used in transplantation include HLA typing of donor and recipient, detection and identification of anti-HLA antibodies and cross-matching which is the final test of compatibility between an individual recipient and a particular donor.

HLA-TYPING

HLA-typing is performed on both donor and recipient before most types of transplantation. The number of HLA loci typed and the resolution required varies with the type of transplantation. For example in unrelated bone marrow transplantation high resolution typing of six loci (HLA-A, B, C, DR, DP and DQ) is routinely performed. In renal transplantation only three loci (HLA-A, B and DR) have routinely been typed, although recent data suggest that matching donor and recipient at more loci may improve outcome.

There are many alleles of most *HLA* genes, some of which are very closely related, where the corresponding HLA protein differs by only one or a small number of amino acids. Traditional serological HLA-typing techniques are 'low resolution' and can only identify the broad HLA-types. Molecular techniques are required to delineate a 'high resolution' type in which many of the 'splits' of HLA antigens can be defined. Some alleles are so alike that routine molecular techniques cannot distinguish them – in these cases sequencing of the variable portion of the *HLA* genes may be necessary to fully resolve the HLA-type. Some *HLA* genes can only be reliably typed using molecular techniques (e.g. HLA-DP).

Methods of HLA-typing

Serology was the first method described, and is still in use today. Sera containing antibodies to defined HLA-types are placed in wells in multiwell trays. Cells from the subject to be typed are added and incubated, following which guinea pig complement and later vital dyes are added. The dyes aid distinction of living and dead cells under the microscope. Each well is read and scored for the percentage of cells killed. By comparing the results from hundreds of wells, the HLA type can be deduced. Problems with this technique include limited availability of well-characterised sera, intensive labour requirements and subjective nature of interpretation. In comparison with more recently available molecular techniques, a significant error rate was identified, particularly typing HLA-DR. Additionally, failure to detect a weakly expressed second antigen leads to an erroneous assignment of a homozygous type, and on occasion a Class II type cannot be obtained using peripheral blood.

Molecular typing techniques rely on PCR to amplify the DNA encoding the variable portion of *HLA* genes. Two main methods are used:

Sequence-specific oligonucleotides (SSOs)   PCR primer pairs are specific for the gene to be typed, but not individual alleles. Following amplification PCR product is probed with several DNA probes and the HLA-type is determined by the pattern of probe binding. This technique is slow, but useful for typing several samples. It is useful for typing potential recipients and family members, in advance of a potential organ becoming available.

Sequence specific polymorphism (SSP)   SSP is a rapid technique, which can be used to type a donor. A large number of PCR primer pairs are used, with each pair including a type-specific primer, which will only amplify the gene for a particular HLA type, and a degenerate primer, which will bind all alleles of the *HLA* gene to be typed. This technique can be used for low resolution typing, or using a larger number of primer pairs for high resolution typing.

Anti-HLA antibody screening and identification

Detection and identification of anti-HLA antibodies is important in solid-organ transplantation. Anti-HLA antibodies may be produced following transplantation, transfusion or pregnancy. When anti-HLA antibodies are present, transplantation of an organ bearing these antigens may result in hyperacute rejection, with graft loss. Every effort is made to identify the specificity of anti-HLA antibodies to prevent delays when an organ becomes available. Only patients with no known antibodies to the donor HLA-type are assessed by cross-matching.

Methods for detection of anti-HLA antibodies

The earliest method described for detecting anti-HLA antibodies was complement dependent cytotoxicity (CDC) and which remains important today. Patients' serum is incubated with a large panel (40+) of cells of known HLA-types. Guinea pig serum is added (as a source of complement), followed by vital dyes to facilitate distinction of living and dead cells. Each well is read to assess percentage cell kill. Presence of significant cell killing indicated the presence of antibodies to one or more of the HLA antigens expressed by cells in that well. Combining the results of several wells many anti-HLA antibodies can be defined. The overall level of sensitisation of a subject is expressed as the panel reactive antibody (PRA), which is the percentage of the cell panel killed by the patients' sera.

This technique detects only complement-fixing antibodies, and is relatively insensitive and labour-intensive. Additionally, non-HLA anti-lymphocyte antibodies interfere with the assay. Additional B cell preparations are needed to identify anti-HLA Class II antibodies.

Newer methods of anti-HLA antibody detection include ELISA and flow cytometry. Commercial reagents are available in which HLA antigens are coated on the ELISA plate. These may be purified from platelets or other cells (and therefore include mixed antigens in each well) or may be highly purified (with a single antigen per well). ELISA techniques are quicker, more sensitive and detect both complement fixing and non-complement-fixing antibodies.

Flow cytometry techniques have been adapted to detect anti-HLA antibodies, utilising either cell lines of known HLA type or beads coated with purified HLA antigens. Serum is incubated with cells or beads, and following washing FITC-conjugated anti-human antisera is added. The amount of antibody binding is assessed using flow cytometry, with fluorescence increased when antibody is present.

Lymphocyte cross-matching

Transplant threatening pre-formed anti-donor antibodies can often be identified in advance of an organ becoming available, and recipients with known antibodies against the donor HLA-type will not be considered for that donor. The final check, however, is to cross-match the donor and recipient to exclude the presence of previously unidentified anti-donor antibodies. The principle techniques used are CDC (with various enhancements to improve sensitivity) and flow cytometry.

CDC cross-matching is performed using several of the potential recipient's sera (Figure 3.15.1). Sera following potentially sensitising episodes are included, as antibody levels can wax and wane. This panel of sera is incubated with donor cells (usually B and T cells purified from lymph node or spleen), followed by guinea pig serum and vital dyes. Cell killing is assessed, and the absence of cell killing indicates absence of anti-donor antibody. Cell killing, however, indicates that anti-donor antibody or other anti-lymphocyte antibodies are present.

Flow cytometry is a more sensitive technique where donor cells are incubated with potential recipient's sera, washed and then incubated with FITC-conjugated antiserum to human

Figure 3.15.1 Use of CDC for HLA typing and cross-matching.

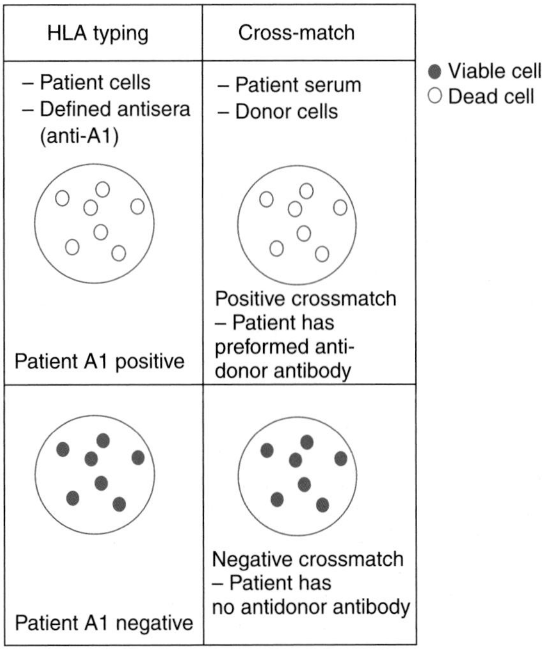

HLA typing	Cross-match	
– Patient cells – Defined antisera (anti-A1)	– Patient serum – Donor cells	● Viable cell ○ Dead cell
Patient A1 positive	Positive crossmatch – Patient has preformed anti-donor antibody	
Patient A1 negative	Negative crossmatch – Patient has no antidonor antibody	

immunoglobulin. When analysed by flow cytometry, binding similar to negative control serum indicates the absence of anti-donor antibody (i.e. the transplant can proceed) or increased fluorescence indicates the presence of anti-donor antibody, precluding transplantation.

CROSS REFERENCE
Sections 2.26–2.28   Transplantation

REFERENCE

Dyer, P. and Middleton, D. (1993) *Histocompatibility Testing. A Practical Approach.* Oxford University Press, London.

Immunophenotyping
Leukaemias and Lymphomas

Accurate diagnosis of leukaemias and lymphomas is dependent on integrated analysis of:

- Cell morphology (microscopic appearance)
- Enzyme expression (TdT – lymphoid; peroxidase/esterase – myeloid; TRAP – hairy cells etc.)
- Cytogenetic and molecular mutation profiles (chromosomal number; translocation analysis – t9:22-*Bcr*/*Abl* – chronic myeloid leukaemia (CML); t14:18 – IgH/ *Bcl-2* – follicular lymphoma etc.).

In addition to:

- Immunophenotyping – monoclonal antibodies specific for known antigens are used to 'tag' antigen-expressing cells. A variety of detection systems (fluorescence, immuno-chemical) are used to identify labelled cells. This is commonly referred to as cell marker analysis. Flow cytometry facilitates the analysis of multiple antigen expression in large numbers of cells over a short time. This technique has revolutionised leukaemia/lymphoma diagnosis and classification.

TISSUES AND TECHNIQUES USED

Immunophenotyping may be performed on any tissue or body fluid. In practice, flow cytometric analysis is frequently performed on peripheral blood and bone marrow aspirate specimens and occasionally using disaggregated lymph nodes.

Test requirements are as follows:

- Anticoagulated samples (heparinised/EDTA) – red cell lysis or mononuclear cell enrichment techniques are used to enhance white cell analysis.
- Absolute white cell differential count (same sample).
- Blood film/BM slides from fresh sample for review of the morphology of the cell of interest is essential for planning the most appropriate phenotypic analysis.

Old samples are not suitable – ideally analyse within 4 h of sampling. This is especially important if the malignancy is of probable blast or activated cell origin.

Tissues like lymph nodes can be disaggregated and single-cell suspensions analysed by flow cytometry. More often, sections of tissue are immuno-stained using MAb-based immunohistochemical methods. The range of antigens that may be detected with formalin-fixed, paraffin-embedded tissues is limited, as tissue processing alters antigenic structures. Frozen tissues are preferred for this reason. Comparison of the immuno-stained slides with routine histological analysis is always necessary.

Uses of immunophenotyping

Lineage identification Lymphoid – B/T/NK; non-lymphoid – myeloid, erythroid, megakaryocytic, etc. This is especially important in conditions where blasts are prominent and differentiation pathways are not clear from morphology – for example, distinguishing lymphoblastic leukaemia/lymphoma from undifferentiated AML – M_0 (Figure 3.16.2). More detailed marker analysis for precise classification is dictated by the initial lineage profile. Non-haematological lymphoreticular infiltrates are distinguishable from blood malignancies using appropriate immunocytochemical stains.

Stage of differentiation Malignant blood cells correlate with a distinct stage in the differentiation process. Analysis of multiple marker expression helps to clarify the approximate stage from which the malignant clone has evolved (Figure 3.16.1). The correlation is not always exact, however. Some malignant cells express inappropriate/'aberrant' antigens for the lineage or stage of morphological differentiation.

Distinct patterns of marker expression are identified for many haematological malignancies. No universal diagnostic cell marker panel is currently recommended. Specialist laboratories will advise on profiles undertaken locally. It is never justifiable to depend on marker analysis alone for diagnosis. Correlation with morphology, other diagnostic techniques and of course with the clinical features is always essential.

Clonality Morphology or CD marker expression may not be adequately discriminating to confirm lymphoid malignancy. Demonstration of monoclonality in a suspect cell population can greatly aid diagnosis. B cells will express either κ- or λ-light chain, but not both. Sole expression of one type of light chain is highly predictive of malignancy. Demonstration of T cell monoclonality is less straightforward. Monoclonal antibodies (MAbs) directed against specific families of TCR (e.g. Vβ analysis) can be used. DNA-based PCR clonality analysis of antigen receptor sequences from suspected malignant lymphoid cells is useful, sensitive and increasingly available. Monoclonal populations will have a single antigen receptor rearrangement pattern. Non-malignant populations have multiple.

Prognosis Management, responsiveness and outlook of haematological malignancies is highly variable. Immunophenotyping has enhanced the precision with which individual conditions are diagnosed. This improves planning of specific therapy and prediction of outlook. In some haematological malignancies, the pattern of expression of certain cell markers is associated with poor prognosis. CD5 positivity is usual in CLL. Loss of expression occurs in some patients undergoing transformation to a more aggressive state. CD38 and FMC-7 expression in CLL correlates with poor prognosis.

Minimal residual disease Detection of residual disease is important both for identification of patients requiring more intensive therapy or for early detection of relapse in patients in remission. Monitoring for low-level disease activity using flow cytometric immunophenotyping is highly sensitive (1 per 10^4 cells approximately). Molecular assays for malignancy-related transformations (e.g. PCR for Philadelphia chromosome, monoclonality

Figure 3.16.1 Lymphoid population and their malignant counterpart. The relationship of lymphoid malignancies to normal lymphoid counterpart is shown.

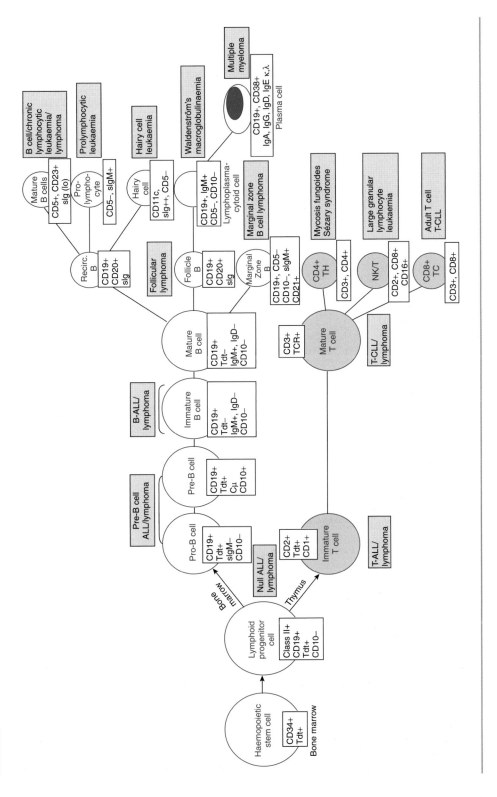

Figure 3.16.2 (a) Commonly used panels for assessment of leukaemias and lymphomas. (b) Typical patterns of important conditions

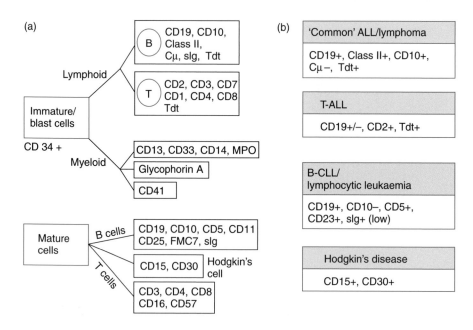

markers) can be even more sensitive. Extensive tissue gene expression analysis is now a reality. Gene expressions associated with malignancy can be assessed using DNA 'fingerprinting' technology. This can be used for both diagnosis and relapse monitoring.

CROSS REFERENCES

Section 2.29 Lymphoid Malignancies
Section 2.30 Leukaemia and Lymphoma
Section 2.31 Plasma Cell Diseases

Direct Immunofluorescence

Direct immunofluorescence (DIF) is a technique for assessing deposition of immunoreactants in tissues. This technique is part of the routine investigation of renal and selected skin biopsies. However, DIF may be applied to other tissues on an experimental basis. In general DIF is of value when diseases characterised by Type II or Type III hypersensitivity are suspected.

PRINCIPLE OF THE TEST

Normal histological fixation techniques degrade complement and some epitopes on immunoglobulins, therefore fresh tissue samples must be submitted to the laboratory. The tissue is rapidly frozen and cut into thin sections. Sections are incubated with FITC-conjugated antibodies to selected immunoreactants. Immunoreactants examined usually include C3, IgA, IgG and IgM, however the panel may be extended to include C4, fibrin, κ and λ, at least in selected cases. Following incubation, unbound antibody is washed away, the slide mounted and staining pattern assessed by fluorescence microscopy. As immunofluorescence slides fade with time, positive findings are photographed to provide a permanent record.

INTERPRETATION

Slides are interpreted by a trained pathologist and the immunofluorescence pattern must be interpreted in the context of the morphology in the biopsy (Figure 3.17.1). In general, direct binding of antibody to tissue (Type II hypersensitivity) results in linear staining with immunoglobulin, with or without complement deposits. Examples include anti-GBM disease in the kidney and pemphigus in the skin. Deposition of immune complexes (ICs) (Type III hypersensitivity) generally results in a granular pattern of positivity. Examples include membranous nephropathy in the kidney and vascular immune complex deposits in immune complex vasculitis (e.g. SLE).

Figure 3.17.1 Patterns observed on skin (a–d) and renal biopsies (e,f) by direct immunofluorescence: (a) IgA deposition in dermatitis herpetiformis, (b) immune complex vasculitis, (c) lupus band, (d) IgG binding in bullous pemphigoid, (e) mesangial IgA in IgA nephropathy and (f) IgG binding in glomerular basement membrane disease. See Plate Section for colour reproduction of these images.

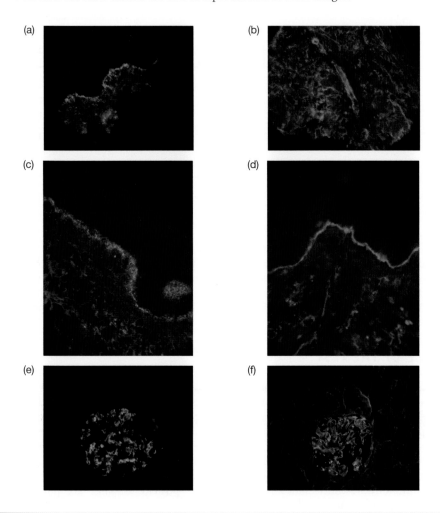

PITFALLS

Some immunoreactants are relatively rapidly degraded. Biopsies must be taken directly to the laboratory for processing. Classical findings in many skin diseases are dependent on a biopsy taken from the correct site and at the correct time. Optimum biopsy sites for some common conditions are outlined in Table 3.17.1.

False negative results may be seen in many skin conditions and it is usually advisable to request appropriate serology at the time of biopsy, as this may be sufficient to confirm a diagnosis in the presence of typical histology, even if DIF is negative.

Table 3.17.1 Typical DIF findings in skin disorders

CONDITION	TYPICAL FINDING	SITE TO BIOPSY	AGE OF LESION	ACCOMPANYING SEROLOGY
Pemphigus	Linear IgG positivity in a chicken-wire pattern in the epidermis	Perilesional skin	Close to new lesion	Antibodies to epidermal intercellular substance
Pemphigoid	Linear IgG (+/−C3) along the DEJ	Perilesional skin	Close to new lesion	Antibodies to epithelial basement membrane
Dermatitis herpetiformis	IgA(+/−C3 and fibrin) in granular or fibrillary pattern in the papillary dermis	Peri-lesional, non-erythematous skin	Close to new lesion	Coeliac serology
Vasculitis	Granular deposition of C3 (+/−C4) with at least one isotype of immunoglobulin in dermal vessels	Lesion	Fresh, preferably <24 h	C3, C4 Cryoglobulins ANA + follow-up tests ANCA RF
DLE	Granular deposition of one or more immunoreactants along the DEJ (lupus band)	Lesion	>3 months	ANA, anti-dsDNA Anti-ENA

A biopsy for DIF should always be accompanied by a sample for routine histology as DIF must be assessed by an experienced pathologist in the context of the histological appearances. False positive immunofluorescence findings may be seen, particularly in the presence of dermal inflammation.

CROSS REFERENCES

Section 2.1   Clinical Manifestations of Atopy
Section 2.20   Immune-mediated Skin Disease
Section 2.21   Immune-mediated Renal Disease

Self Assessment

Section 1

Which of the following statements are true?

3.1a. All monoclonal antibodies are monospecific.
3.1b. Antibodies are routinely conjugated to enzymes, isotopes and fluorescent tags, for use in diagnostic assays.
3.1c. Batch-to-batch variation is a significant problem when using polyclonal antibodies, but rarely a problem with monoclonal reagents.
3.1d. FITC-conjugated antibodies are only used for flow cytometry.
3.1e. Production of monoclonal antibodies relies on immortalisation of spleen cells from a vaccinated rodent.

3.2a. Agglutination techniques can be used to differentiate between different isotypes of antibody.
3.2b. Flow cytometry can only be used to measure cell surface protein expression.
3.2c. Nephelometry is a robust technique which can be automated and produce results rapidly.
3.2d. Immunoblotting can be used to investigate novel antibody systems.
3.2e. DIF is a useful method to test for autoantibodies in serum.

3.3a. Rheumatoid factors are found in approximately 90% of patients with RA and are specific for this condition.
3.3b. Anti-ribosomal P-protein antibodies are quite specific for SLE.
3.3c. Patients with polymyositis who are anti-Jo-1 positive have a high incidence of interstitial lung disease.
3.3d. Negative anti-cardiolipin antibodies exclude the anti-phospholipid syndrome.
3.3e. Most C-ANCA positivity is due to anti-PR3 antibodies, and over 60% of P-ANCA positivity is due to antibodies against myeloperoxidase.

3.4a. Anti-thyroid peroxidase antibodies play a pathogenic role in Hashimoto's thyroiditis.
3.4b. Multiple autoimmune endocrine diseases are frequently found in the same patients.
3.4c. The titre of antiepidermal basement membrane antibodies does not correlate with disease activity.
3.4d. Anti-GBM is the commonest cause of pulmonary-renal syndrome (haemopytysis with acute renal failure).
3.4e. The presence of anti-GM1 is relatively specific for GBS.

3.5a. Complement deficiency is unlikely if C3 and C4 levels are normal.
3.5b. T cell proliferation assays are useful in monitoring HIV infection.
3.5c. Normal levels of IgG, IgA and IgM indicate normal humoral immunity.
3.5d. A blood film should always be examined prior to performing neutrophil function testing.
3.5e. A paraprotein can be accurately quantified by measuring the Ig isotype involved using nephelometry.

3.6a. Absence of a serum paraprotein excludes a diagnosis of MM.
3.6b. Serum paraproteins are rarely found in patients with solitary plasmacytomas.
3.6c. BJPs are monoclonal free light chains, found in urine.
3.6d. Normal Ig levels exclude the presence of a paraprotein.
3.6e. Negative urinalysis for protein excludes the presence of BJPs.

3.7a. A negative test for nut-specific IgE excludes nut allergy, and the patient can safely resume consumption of nuts.
3.7b. Allergen-specific IgE cannot be detected if the patient is taking anti-histamines.
3.7c. A normal total IgE excludes allergy.
3.7d. Double-blinded placebo-controlled food or drug challenge is the most reliable way to exclude a food or drug allergy.
3.7e. Mast cell tryptase is usually elevated during an anaphylactic reaction, and is useful to distinguish drug allergy from other accidents during general anaesthesia.

3.8a. Cross-matching is used to identify the specificities of anti-HLA antibodies in potential recipient's sera.
3.8b. Complement-dependent cytotoxicity is a technique which can be modified for use in HLA typing, anti-HLA antibody screening, and identification and cross-matching.
3.8c. PCR-based techniques are superior to serological methods for HLA-typing at the HLA-DR locus.
3.8d. High resolution typing is routinely performed in all types of transplantation.
3.8e. Anti-HLA antibodies to a donor's HLA type predict that the cross-match with a particular donor will be positive.

3.9a. Immunophenotyping using flow cytometry can be performed on lymph nodes.
3.9b. Morphology is the most reliable diagnostic method routinely used to differentiate myeloid from T and B cell leukaemias.
3.9c. A single T cell marker and B cell marker can be used to establish the lineage of a leukaemia.
3.9d. Flow cytometry is equally useful in determining clonality of B and T cell leukaemias.
3.9e. Aberrant antigen expression is useful when detecting minimal residual disease.

3.10a. DIF is useful in the diagnosis of conditions due to Type IV hypersensitivity reactions.
3.10b. DIF can be performed on tissue which has been placed in formalin.
3.10c. Antibody binding to tissue components is associated with linear positivity, while immune complex deposition is associated with a granular pattern.
3.10d. DIF patterns must be assessed together with routine histology.
3.10e. The site and timing of the biopsy is critically important in inflammatory skin conditions.

Section 2

Match the diagnosis on the left with the typical immunophenotype on the right. Each immunophenotype may be used more than once or not at all.

1.	Chronic lymphocytic leukaemia (CLL)	a.	CD13+ CD33+
2.	Acute lymphoblastic leukaemia	b.	CD5+ CD19+
3.	Follicular lymphoma	c.	CD3+ CD4+ CD19−
4.	Acute myeloid leukaemia	d.	CD19+ CD10− Tdt+ sIg−
5.	Sézary syndrome	e.	CD19+ CD10+ bcl-2+

Match the performance characteristic of the test on the left with the correct definition from those on the right.

6.	Precision	a.	Assays ability to measure very close to the true value
7.	Accuracy	b.	Proportion of patients with positive tests who have disease
8.	Sensitivity	c.	Ability of test to indicate a positive result in the presence of disease
9.	Specificity	d.	Assays ability to obtain very tightly clustered results when repeated
10.	Positive predictive value	e.	Ability of a test to indicate negative result in the absence of disease

Match the diagnsosis on the left with the inflammatory markers on the right. Each entry on the right may be used more than once or not at all.

11.	Osteoarthritis	a.	ESR 80 mm/h; CRP 120 mg/l
12.	Multiple myeloma	b.	ESR 40 mm/h; CRP 80 mg/l
13.	Active SLE	c.	ESR 12 mm/h; CRP <5 mg/l
14.	Flare of RA	d.	ESR 120 mm/h; CRP 30 mg/l
15.	SLE with pyelonephritis	e.	ESR 60 mm/h; CRP 5 mg/l

Match the condition on the left with the typical findings on routine complement measurement on the right. Each entry on the right can be used more than once or not at all.

16.	Active SLE	a.	Normal C3; low C4
17.	Rheumatoid vasculitis	b.	Raised C3; raised C4
18.	Type II MPGN	c.	Low C3; low C4
19.	C1-Inh deficiency	d.	Low C3; normal C4
20.	RA	e.	Normal C3; normal C4

Match the condition on the left with the most useful autoantibody to establish the diagnosis from the list on the right.

21.	Sjögren's syndrome	a.	PR3-ANCA
22.	CREST syndrome	b.	Anti-Scl-70
23.	Polymyositis	c.	Anti-Ro
24.	Scleroderma	d.	Anti- Jo-1
25.	Wegener's granulomatosis	e.	Anti-centromere

Match the condition on the left with the most useful autoantibody to establish the diagnosis from the list on the right. Each entry on the right can be used more than once or not at all.

26.	Primary biliary cirrhosis	a.	Anti-LKM
27.	Type II autoimmune hepatitis	b.	Anti-Yo
28.	Stiff Man syndrome	c.	Anti-M2 mitochondrial Ab
29.	Paraneoplastic cerebellar degeneration	d.	Anti-tissue transglutaminase
30.	Coeliac disease	e.	Anti-GAD

Match the diagnostic query in the list on the left with the optimum specimen from the list on the right. Each specimen type may be used more than once or not at all.

31.	Diagnosis of multiple myeloma	a.	Clotted blood alone
32.	Monitoring paraprotein level in patient with MGUS	b.	Clotted blood and urine
33.	Assessment of oligoclonal bands	c.	Clotted blood and CSF
34.	Cryoglobulins	d.	Early morning urine
35.	Bence–Jones proteins	e.	Blood collected at 37°C

Select the most helpful test from the list on the right to further assess the clinical problems in the list on the left. Each set of tests can be used more than once or not at all.

36.	IgA deficiency and recurrent infections	a.	C3 and C4
37.	Recurrent meningococcal meningitis	b.	CD4 count
38.	Monitoring HIV therapy	c.	Test vaccination and IgG subclasses
39.	Recurrent pneumonia	d.	Lymphocyte subtyping
40.	SCID	e.	Immunoglobulins
		f.	CH100/CH50

Section 1 – Answers

3.1a.   False (all are identical. However, many cross-react with other molecules and therefore are not monospecific).

3.1b.   True.

3.1c.   True.
3.1d.   False (also used for DIF and IIF).
3.1e.   True.

3.2a.   False – detects agglutinating antibody, but cannot differentiate isotypes.
3.2b.   False – can be used to measure anything for which a fluorescent probe is available. Cell membranes can be permeabilised for intracellular staining.
3.2c.   True.
3.2d.   True.
3.2e.   False – DIF detects immunoreactants deposited in patients' tissue. IIF assesses serum autoantibodies.

3.3a.   False – Relatively non-specific test, particularly when weakly positive.
3.3b.   True – however not specific for cerebral disease as originally reported.
3.3c.   True.
3.3d.   False – lupus anti-coagulant should also be tested, as it is positive in some patients with APS who are anti-cardiolipin negative.
3.3e.   True.

3.4a.   False – in common with many autoimmune diseases, the antibodies are epiphenomena. However, they are extremely useful in establishing a diagnosis.
3.4b.   True – APGSs.
3.4c.   True.
3.4d.   False – ANCA-associated disease accounts for about 2/3 cases with only 1/3 due to anti-GBM disease.
3.4e.   False – found in several other neurological disorders also.

3.5a.   False – need to do haemolytic function assays.
3.5b.   False – HIV should be excluded before requesting proliferation assays.
3.5c.   False – only detects major hypogammaglobulinaemia.
3.5d.   True – if diagnosis can be made based on abnormal neutrophil morphology, there is little point undertaking formal neutrophil function testing.
3.5e.   False – paraproteins may not react in the same way as normal immunoglobulins with antibodies used. Also nephelometry will not differentiate residual normal Ig of the same isotype from the paraprotein. Densitometry is the method of choice.

3.6a.   False – absent in about 15% of cases.
3.6b.   False – found in 50%.
3.6c.   True.
3.6d.   False – electrophoresis should always be performed.
3.6e.   False – urinalysis sticks DO NOT detect BJPs, even when present in large quantities.

3.7a.   False – potentially fatal error.
3.7b.   False – antihistamines interfere with SPTs, not IgE measurement.
3.7c.   False – serious allergy can occur, even with normal IgE.
3.7d.   True.
3.7e.   True.

3.8a.   False – checks compatibility of donor and recipient.
3.8b.   True.
3.8c.   True.
3.8d.   False – only routine in BMT.
3.8e.   True.

3.9a.   True.
3.9b.   False.
3.9c.   False – unreliable due to aberrant expression.
3.9d.   False – less useful in T cell disease – use molecular methods.
3.9e.   True – allows differentiation of rare leukaemia cell from normal cells at similar stage of differentiation.

3.10a.   False – useful in Types II and III.
3.10b.   False – even a few seconds in formalin can denature antigens.
3.10c.   True.
3.10d.   True.
3.10e.   True.

Section 2 – Answers

1b;	2d;	3e;	4a;	5c	(see Section 3.16).
6d;	7a;	8c;	9e;	10b	(see Section 3.1).
11c;	12d;	13e;	14b;	15a	(see Section 3.9).
16c;	17c;	18d;	19a;	20b	(see Section 3.10).
21c;	22e;	23d;	24b;	25a	(see Section 3.4).
26c;	27a;	28e;	29b;	30d	(see Sections 3.6, 3.7 and 3.8).
31b;	32a;	33c;	34e;	35d	(see Section 3.12).
36c;	37f;	38b;	39e;	40d	(see Section 3.11).

PART 4

TREATMENT OF IMMUNOLOGICAL DISORDERS

INTRODUCTION

This part describes some agents commonly used to treat immunological disorders. It is not intended to replace pharmacology and therapeutics texts, but rather to provide an overview. It is also hoped that immunotherapeutics will make more sense after gaining an understanding of clinical immunology in the earlier parts of this book.

GENERAL REFERENCES FOR THIS PART INCLUDE

British National Formulary (BNF) Number 47 (March 2004). British Medical Association and Royal Pharmaceutical Society of Great Britain.

Principles of Immunosuppression

The immune system plays a vital role in protection against infection and malignancy. Therefore, the potential benefits of treating a patient with immunosuppression must be assessed in the context of the associated risks. Not all patients with immunological diseases are treated with immunosuppression. Patients with apparently similar conditions may require different treatment regimens. Decisions on appropriate therapies may be based on evidence provided by controlled trials in common disorders. However, when treating uncommon disorders evidence is often lacking. Therapy may be based on knowledge of the immunological mechanisms of the disease and the mechanisms of action of immunosuppressive agents. The following units outline different immunosuppressive drugs in common use. This parts outlines the broad principles to consider when choosing an immunosuppressive regimen for an individual patient.

WHO REQUIRES IMMUNOSUPPRESSION?

Patients with active, immune-mediated disease where suppression of the immune process is necessary to restore or improve health. The form of immunosuppression must be chosen on evidence of efficacy or likely efficacy, given the mechanism of action of the therapeutic agent and the pathogenesis of the condition to be treated. Criteria for assessing disease activity and monitoring of response to therapy are critically important. Therapeutic options other than immunosuppression may be preferable (e.g. hormone replacement in auto-immune endocrinopathies). Burnt-out disease where organ dysfunction is due to scarring will not respond to immunosuppression.

WHICH AGENTS?

High quality, randomised controlled trials of different treatment regimens may provide evidence to guide therapy. However, where evidence is lacking knowledge of the underlying mechanism of disease and natural history of the condition directs treatment decisions.

Drugs are chosen to inhibit the appropriate part(s) of the immune system. Some immunosuppressive agents take weeks to produce therapeutic effects and are not adequate where organ damage progresses rapidly.

MINIMISING DOSE AND DURATION OF IMMUNOSUPPRESSION

The risks of opportunistic infection and malignancy are related to both intensity and duration of immunosuppression. To minimise these risks the least toxic agent likely to be effective is chosen, the lowest dose likely to be effective is used, and powerful toxic agents such as cyclophosphamide are substituted with less toxic agents such as azathioprine as soon as possible. Dose reduction supervised by experienced clinicians minimises the duration of immunosuppression. However, overzealous tapering of immunosuppression may result in relapse and exposure of patients to greater cumulative doses of drugs.

PATIENT MONITORING

Patients are monitored for their response to therapy and anticipated side effects. Monitoring disease avoids over or under immunosuppression. Early detection and treatment of relapses may result in lower cumulative exposure to immunosuppression. Many immunosuppressive drugs have haematological, hepatic or renal side effects and monitoring for toxicity is required. Cyclosporin and tacrolimus levels are monitored in transplantation; however levels are less helpful in other conditions where the optimal target levels remain to be established.

APPROPRIATE PROPHYLAXIS

Many patients require long-term immunosuppression with regimens that are associated with predictable toxicity. Appropriate prophylaxis should be considered when therapy is being initiated. For example, PCP prophylaxis is indicated in patients requiring cyclophosphamide, and osteoporosis prophylaxis is routine in patients requiring chronic steroid therapy.

PATIENT EDUCATION

Compliance with treatment is higher when patients understand their treatments and the reasons for taking each drug. Additionally, patients must be aware of side effects and understand the significance of febrile illnesses or possible infection. Patients need to be aware of the importance of reporting mouth ulcers or abnormal bleeding (early symptoms of leucopaenia or thrombocytopaenia) immediately when marrow suppression is a risk. Patients should also be aware of the importance of participation in screening programmes (e.g. cervical smears) as well as UV avoidance to minimise the risk of skin cancers.

Corticosteroids

BACKGROUND

The structure and function of corticosteroids (steroids) resemble cortisol, a hormone secreted by the adrenal cortex. Cortisol (hydrocortisone) has many different actions, including mobilisation of glucose stores (glucocorticoid effects), maintenance of blood pressure control (mineralocorticoid effects) and suppression of inflammation. Cortisol protects the body during stressful events such as trauma, surgery and infection where baseline levels increase more than 10-fold.

Many different corticosteroids are used for their anti-inflammatory effects. Anti-inflammatory activity is related to glucocorticoid effects and agents with a high ratio of glucocorticoid to mineralocorticoid activity are widely used in inflammatory diseases. Prednisolone is the most commonly used oral steroid, while hydrocortisone or methyl-prednisolone are given intravenously. Steroid agents are available for local administration to the skin, respiratory tract and gastrointestinal tract. Hydrocortisone is used for replacement therapy in adrenal and pituitary failure, where endogenous steroid production is inadequate.

INDICATIONS FOR USE

Steroids are used to control inflammation in many different settings. These include:

- Post-organ transplantation – prevention and treatment of organ rejection
- Connective tissue diseases – for example, SLE; vasculitides and RA
- Autoimmune diseases – immune haematological diseases – ITP and autoimmune haemolytic anaemia; chronic active hepatitis; pemphigus; some types of glomerulonephritis
- Allergic inflammation – for example, asthma; atopic eczema; allergic rhinitis; acute allergic reactions

---

Case 4.2.1 Steroid-dependent nephrotic syndrome

A 10-year-old girl presented with progressive swelling of her ankles, and facial puffiness. Investigations showed proteinuria (++++), low serum albumin and raised cholesterol. 24-hour urine protein was 5 g/24 hours. A diagnosis of nephrotic syndrome probably due to minimal change disease was made. Steroid therapy was started and within 2 weeks proteinuria was less then 1 g/24 hours. After one month proteinuria had fully resolved and steroids were tapered. Unfortunately proteinuria quickly recurred.

Steroid therapy was restarted, remission achieved and steroids tailored again. Nephrotic syndrome recurred and a renal biopsy confirmed the clinical diagnosis of minimal change glomerulonephritis, ruling out alternative causes of nephrotic syndrome. At this stage, the child was Cushingoid, growth had fallen from the 20th to the 3rd centile and glucose tolerance was impaired.

A diagnosis of steroid dependent nephrotic syndrome, complicated by iatrogenic Cushing's syndrome was made. Steroid therapy was restarted to gain remission, with cyclosporin initially adjusting the dose based on blood levels. Steroids were successfully withdrawn. The dose of cyclosporin was slowly decreased until proteinuria recurred. The cyclosporin dose was slightly increased to achieve remission, and this dose was maintained. One year later the child remained in remission, on cyclosporin therapy.

- Inflammatory diseases – inflammatory bowel diseases; multiple sclerosis
- Malignancies – for example, treatment of leukaemias and lymphomas; intracerebral pressure reduction in brain malignancies.

MECHANISMS OF ACTION

The mechanisms by which steroids suppress inflammation include:

- Monocyte effects – impaired maturation to macrophages. Reduced antigen uptake and processing. Inflammatory cytokine production (IL-1, IL-6, TNF-α) is diminished.
- Lymphocyte effects – impaired cytokine production reducing proliferative responses and functional activity (one of the most important anti-inflammatory mechanisms of steroid therapy). Impaired recirculation causing lymphopaenia. High doses kill lymphocytes by apoptosis.
- Prostaglandin inhibition – inhibition of COX enzymes and of membrane phospholipid release.

ADMINISTERING STEROIDS

The dosage, route and duration of use of steroid medications are dependent on the clinical indication. Steroid therapy regimes are well established in many disease states and readers are referred to individual units for more information.

Figure 4.2.1 Most common side effects of steroids.

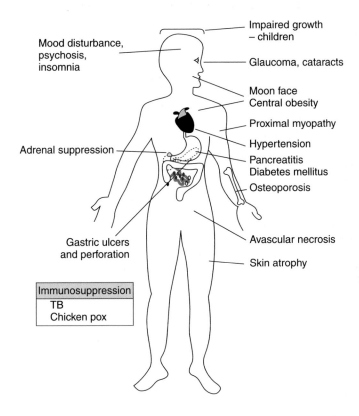

ADVERSE EFFECTS

Prolonged use of steroids or use of high doses for more than a short time (7 days) exposes patients to many potential adverse effects. Side effects can be categorised into:

◆ Exaggeration of physiological action of steroids
◆ Suppression of endogenous steroid production with relative steroid insufficiency during stress.

STEROID PRESCRIBING

Before initiating steroid therapy the following points should be noted:

◆ Consider the benefit and risks of steroid therapy and plan therapy accordingly. Use a safe, effective, non-steroid option if available.
◆ Consider objectives of therapy and plan dose and duration of treatment accordingly – the initial dose should achieve control and dose should be reduced to the lowest possible effective dose as rapidly as possible.

- Local administration (e.g. airway inhalation, application to skin or rectum) is preferred to systemic administration if possible. The side-effect profile is much less severe than with systemic steroid therapies. However, high dose inhaled steroids may cause impaired growth in children.
- Steroids are best administered in the morning, or on alternative days to limit effects on endogenous steroid production.
- Agents are not interchangeable and have different anti-inflammatory potencies (strengths). An equivalency chart is available in the British National Formulary (BNF), however equivalence values are approximate and vary in different clinical situations.
- Enteric-coated steroids may be erratically absorbed. In general, non-coated preparations are preferred if tolerated.
- Gastric and bone protection should be considered in patients at risk of peptic ulceration or osteoporosis, particularly in patients requiring long-term therapy. Bone density monitoring is indicated in patients receiving long-term therapy.
- Patients should be aware of increased steroid requirements during stress (which persists after cessation of steroid therapy), and the dangers of abrupt cessation of therapy. All healthcare providers should be aware of the history of steroid use.
- Vigilance regarding infection, especially chicken pox and tuberculosis (TB) is important for patients and doctors.
- Patients should be advised to carry a 'steroid user card' or an alert pendant to provide information in an emergency.

CROSS REFERENCES	
Section 1.7	Inflammation
Section 1.30	Atopy and Allergic Inflammation
Part 2	Many chapters describe conditions treated with steroids

Immunosuppression (I)

The drugs outlined in this section work primarily by inhibiting proliferation of lymphocytes. These agents affect T cell responses and B cell proliferation to varying degrees. Many of the side effects are due to anti-proliferative effects on other rapidly dividing cells in the body. The main differences are in potency and toxicity.

AZATHIOPRINE

First synthesised in 1961, this agent is widely used in transplantation and autoimmune disease, where it may allow substantial reduction of steroid dosage. The parent drug is inactive until metabolized in the liver to 6-mercaptopurine (6-MP). It is a moderately potent alkylating agent, whose major mechanism of action is inhibiting conversion of inosine to adenosine, leading to cellular adenosine depletion and impaired proliferation.

Azathioprine is usually administered orally. Many side effects of azathioprine are due to non-specific inhibition of proliferation, especially in the bone marrow. Patient education and monitoring of full blood count (FBC) and liver function tests allow early detection of dose-related bone marrow suppression and idiosyncratic hepatotoxicity. Other side effects include nausea, hypersensitivity reactions and hair loss. There is an increased susceptibity to infection and increased risk of malignancy, especially skin cancer. If severe nausea precludes the use of azathioprine, 6-MP may be tolerated.

METHOTREXATE

Methotrexate (MTX) interferes with DNA synthesis by blocking a critical folate pathway enzyme. It inhibits cell proliferation. It is used in large doses for the treatment of malignant conditions including some leukaemias. Bone marrow suppression, liver dysfunction and mucositis are common adverse side effects. Moderate doses given either by the oral or intramuscular routes are used with benefit in a number of immune-mediated conditions including rheumatoid disease and severe psoriasis. Gradual dose elevation from an initially small dose is undertaken once tolerance is ensured. It is important to note that MTX used in these settings is administered once weekly rather than daily. Inadvertent prescribing errors are well documented and result in critical bone marrow suppression and often death. Such unfortunate cases require admission to units where expert management of the bone marrow aplasia can be given. Folinic acid is given as a rescue treatment and works by by-passing the metabolic step inhibited by MTX.

All patients receiving MTX must be aware of the potential side effects and their likely presentations. Liver and pulmonary adverse effects are well documented in addition to the bone marrow effects. Careful and regular monitoring of the FBC and liver function tests (LFTs) is mandatory. Patients should be advised not to drink alcohol while taking this drug. MTX is associated with development of a pneumonitis which is an indication for immediate cessation. Before treatment, formal pulmonary function assessment is performed. Regular clinical and functional assessments allow early detection of pneumonitis.

MYCOPHENYLATE MOFETIL

Mycophenylate mofetil (MMF) has recently been licensed for prophylaxis of acute renal and cardiac transplant rejection. MMF is a specific, non-competitive inhibitor of inosine monophosphate dehydrogenase, a key enzyme in the *de novo* pathway of purine synthesis. Lymphocytes are highly dependent on the *de novo* pathway, and unlike most other cells cannot utilise the salvage pathway (which allows recycling of purine bases). Therefore, the anti-proliferative effect of MMF shows some lymphocyte specificity.

Dose-related gastrointestinal intolerance is common. Potential bone marrow suppression requires FBC monitoring, as well as patient education to recognise signs of possible bone marrow suppression (infections, fevers, mouth ulcers, bruising or unexplained bleeding). Infection is more commonly seen than with azathioprine, and increased incidence of malignancy is also reported. Hypersensitivity reactions and many other side effects have been reported.

The therapeutic effect of MMF appears superior to azathioprine, particularly in suppression of humoral immune responses. Although this agent is not yet licensed for use in autoimmune disease, many trials and case reports describing successful use in SLE and other antibody-mediated disorders have been published.

CYCLOPHOSPHAMIDE

Cyclophosphamide (CP) is an alkylating agent, which is widely used in cancer treatment. At lower doses it is used as a potent, but toxic immunosuppressive drug. CP cross-links DNA, inhibiting cell proliferation. This effect is not lymphocyte-specific and severe toxicity may be seen in other rapidly dividing cells. Its use is generally reserved for life-threatening or organ-threatening immunological diseases.

Administration is by a daily oral dose or pulse IV doses usually given monthly. Dose reduction may be needed in the elderly, or in severe renal or hepatic impairment.

Bone marrow suppression is commonly seen. Regular monitoring together with patient education reduce the associated risks. Haemorrhagic cystitis results from irritation of bladder epithelium by a CP metabolite, acrolein. Bladder protection by hydration or use of a drug called mesna reduces the risk of haemorrhagic cystitis. CP is generally less hepatotoxic than azathioprine, however alopaecia is seen more commonly. Prolonged treatment with CP may lead to both male and female infertility. Susceptibility to infection is marked, and prophylaxis against PCP is recommended. CP carries a significant risk of secondary cancers developing several years following therapy.

Figure 4.3.1 Immunosuppression: anti-proliferative mechanism of action of azathioprine, mycophenylate and cyclophosphamide.

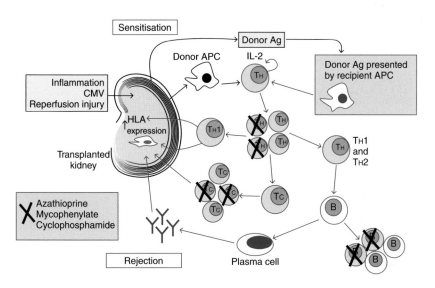

CROSS REFERENCES

Section 1.3   Cells and Organs of the Immune System
Section 1.12   Lymphocyte Maturation
Part 2   Many sections describe conditions treated with immunosuppression

Immunosuppression (II)

The agents described in this section suppress T cell responses predominantly. The oldest agent cyclosporin A, introduced in 1980, dramatically improved the results of renal transplantation and allowed the development of liver, heart and lung transplantation.

CYCLOSPORIN

Cyclosporin binds cyclophilin and inhibits activation of T lymphocytes by preventing the production of IL-2 and some other early T cell activation genes. It is a lipid-soluble drug, metabolised in the liver by CYP3A4. Cyclosporin is widely used as part of triple therapy (with steroids and azathioprine or mycophenylate) in solid organ transplantation. It is also used to prevent GvHD following bone marrow transplantation, for severe resistant atopic dermatitis and asthma, aplastic anaemia and occasionally in severe autoimmune disorders.

Two preparations are available – Sandimmune and Neoral. These are not interchangeable due to significant differences in bioavailability. In transplantation cyclosporin dosage is monitored by drug level measurement. Traditionally, this has been based on the trough level, however a 2-hour peak level may be preferable. In autoimmunity, the appropriate target level has not been defined, and so monitoring is aimed at preventing nephrotoxicity. Blood pressure and creatinine levels are maintained within predefined limits (usually creatinine should remain within 30% of pre-treatment values).

Cyclosporin interacts with many drugs, including over the counter therapies and herbal remedies. Patients must be warned about this and monitoring increased when additional therapies are required. The most serious side effect is nephropathy, which causes renal failure in over 10% of recipients of non-renal solid organ transplants. Other common side effects include hypertension, infection, impaired glucose metabolism, tremor, gastrointestinal (GI) disturbances, gingival hypertrophy, hirsutism, malignancies and neurological disorders.

TACROLIMUS

Tacrolimus (FK506) binds to FKBP-12 (FK binding protein-12) in cells, and inhibits T cell activation by a mechanism identical to cyclosporin. Absorption is bile-independent. Acute

Figure 4.4.1 Immunosuppression: mechanism of action of cyclosporin, tacrolimus and sirolimus.

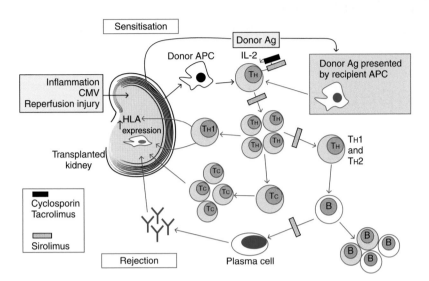

rejection rates in most solid organ transplants are lower with tacrolimus than with cyclosporin, however graft survival appears to be improved only in liver and intestinal transplants. Use of tacrolimus in autoimmune disease has not been extensively studied. Topical tacrolimus has recently become available for treatment of moderate to severe atopic dermatitis (AD). The side effect profile is similar to cyclosporin with nephropathy being a major problem. Diabetogenic potential may be greater than cyclosporin, however gingival hypertrophy and hirsutism do not occur. Dosage of tacrolimus is monitored by drug-level measurement.

RAPAMYCIN (SIROLIMUS)

Rapamycin binds to TOR (target of rapamycin) and this complex binds FKBP-12, however the mechanism of action is distinct from Tacrolimus. Rapamycin inhibits cytokine-mediated signalling in late G1 phase, and blocks the action of IL-2, IL-4 and IL-6. Rapamycin is a potent inhibitor of T cell responses, but also inhibits B cell responses and smooth muscle proliferation (potentially important in chronic rejection). Rapamycin is used in solid organ transplantation.

Rapamycin absorption is impaired by fatty food, and the drug is metabolised in the liver by CYP3A4. Because of this there is a clinically significant interaction with cyclosporin. Rapamycin dosage is guided by drug levels. Rapamycin is not nephrotoxic. Principal side effects include severe arthralgia, hyperlipidaemia and impaired wound healing.

Of interest, rapamycin does not inhibit induction of tolerance in animal studies, whereas cyclosporin and tacrolimus do. In the future, this may become an important property.

CROSS REFERENCES	
Section 1.17	Helper T Cell Activation
Section 2.28	Solid Organ Transplantation

Therapeutic Antibody Production

Antibody-based therapies are increasingly used in a growing spectrum of clinical conditions. Both polyclonal and monoclonal antibodies are used therapeutically. Antibodies raised in other species are foreign proteins, and may produce an antibody response when administered therapeutically. Immunogenicity has limited the repeated use of these agents in chronic disease. In the last decade, reshaped antibodies have been produced, in an attempt to limit immunogenicity. Principles of antibody production are described in this section; subsequent sections describe routine use of some therapeutic antibodies.

Therapeutic uses of antibodies include:

- Prevention of infectious disease
- Neutralisation of toxins
- Prevention of rhesus alloimmunisation
- Immunomodulation
- Treatment of malignancy
- T cell depletion of bone marrow for transplantation.

POLYCLONAL ANTIBODIES

Most antigens stimulate multiple lymphocytes as part of the normal immune response. Antibodies produced in such responses are polyclonal. Well-established techniques are available for isolation and purification of specific antibodies from plasma. Therapeutic antibodies may be purified from human plasma or raised in animals (usually rabbits or horses). Production of polyclonal antibodies is described in Section 3.2. There are stringent manufacturing requirements to ensure quality, purity and sterility of antibodies produced for therapeutic use.

Therapeutic polyclonal antibodies of human origin include:

- Concentrated preparations of rhesus antibodies, used to prevent rhesus alloimmunisation (Section 4.7).

- Pathogen-specific antibody concentrates (hyper-immune globulins) used as post-exposure prophylaxis (e.g. Varicella–Zoster and Hepatitis B).

Therapeutic polyclonal antibodies of animal origin include:

- Anti-thymocyte globulin (ATG) used in solid organ transplant rejection therapy
- Tetanus immune globulin for neutralisation of tetanus toxin.

MONOCLONAL ANTIBODIES (MAbs)

Production of monoclonal antibodies (MAbs) is described in Section 3.2. Besides antibody-based therapeutic agents, MAbs have also revolutionised laboratory procedures. The importance of MAbs is reflected in the award of a Nobel Prize to Kohler and Milstein, the scientists who described the technique of MAb production in 1975.

The major advantages of MAbs over polyclonal antibodies include:

- Production quantities – near-limitless amounts of antibody can be produced with stable activity over long periods of time.
- Specificity – antibody specificity remains stable. Monoclonal does not necessarily imply monospecificity. However, high-affinity antibodies without clinically relevant cross-reactivities are chosen as therapeutic agents.
- Consistency – batch-to-batch variation is rarely seen, unlike polyclonal antibody preparations.

Theoretically, MAbs could be generated using cells from any animal, however rodents are the only species in which hybridomas are produced with a high success rate. The overall structure of mouse immunoglobulin is similar, but not identical, to human immunoglobulin. This poses two problems in relation to *in vivo* use.

- Adverse reactions – antibody production against 'foreign' components can cause systemic reactions of varying severity. Fc effector components of MAbs may also trigger generalised immune activation with similar effects.
- Loss of efficacy – 'anti-antibodies' induced against species–specific components of MAbs can also impair antibody persistence and function with reducing efficacy with repeated use.

RESHAPED MAbs

Production of human MAbs is technically challenging but continues to be a goal. However, using DNA technology, chimeric and humanised MAbs have been produced and used as therapeutic agents (Figure 4.5.1).

Chimeric antibodies are produced by introducing the gene segments encoding the variable parts of both the heavy and light chains of the rodent MAb of interest into the corresponding human immunoglobulin genes. The resulting antibody is predominantly human, but still contains a significant amount of rodent protein. Approximately, 10% of human recipients of such antibodies will make human-anti-chimeric antibodies (HACAs). HACAs may inhibit antibody function. Development of antibodies is less common in patients who are receiving concomitant immunosuppression. Serum sickness reactions are rarely problematic.

Humanised antibodies were developed to further decrease the amount of rodent protein included in therapeutic antibodies. These antibodies are produced by grafting the hypervariable regions of both heavy and light chains onto the framework of a human immunoglobulin gene.

Figure 4.5.1 Comparison of MAbs, chimeric MAbs, humanised MAbs and bispecific antibodies.

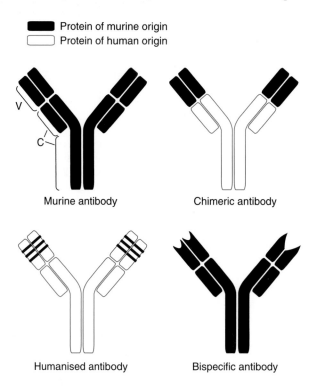

Although relatively little rodent protein remains, production of HACAs still occurs. There is a greater risk of losing antibody specificity during the protein engineering stage with this process compared with making the more straightforward chimeric protein.

Other types of engineered molecules have been produced or are in development. For example, receptors can be fused to portions of antibody molecules. This prolongs the half-life of several molecules and has been used to produce a TNF receptor-IgG protein and CTLA-4-IgG hybrid. Bispecific antibodies have also been produced where the heavy and light chains of two different molecules are joined. This produces an antibody with two different antigen-binding sites, and could be used to direct drugs, gene therapy vectors or cells to tumours or other targets.

CROSS REFERENCES

Targeted Cell Depletion

Several biological reagents have been developed in an attempt to deplete specific cells of the immune system, to facilitate more potent or more specific immunosuppression. Heterologous polyclonal antibodies, heterologous monoclonal antibodies and humanised monoclonal antibodies are in routine use. This section describes some licensed cell depleting therapies, however a large number of antibodies are currently in clinical trials.

A common side effect of all depleting antibodies is the cytokine release syndrome (CRS). This occurs as a result of cytokine release from activated lymphocytes and monocytes. Typical clinical features include fevers, chills and rigors, rash, musculoskeletal pain, bronchospasm, dyspnoea and hypotension. CRS is usually most severe after the first infusion, becoming less severe with subsequent infusions.

ANTI-THYMOCYTE GLOBULIN

Anti-thymocyte globulin (ATG) is a polyclonal heterologous antiserum, produced by immunising rabbits or horses with human T cells or a human T cell line. It is used in combination with other immunosuppressive drugs to prevent organ rejection and aplastic anaemia. In solid organ transplantation, ATG is used as prophylaxis in high-risk patients, or to treat steroid-resistant rejection.

Since ATG is a polyclonal product, there are differences between preparations, and even different batches from the same manufacturer. ATG depletes cells both by cytotoxicity and opsonisation, which results in removal of antibody-coated cells by the reticulo-endothelial system. Additionally, by binding to a number of cell surface molecules, ATG may inhibit function of the residual cells. Effectiveness may be monitored by measuring absolute T cell counts.

ATG is diluted and infused into a large vessel over several hours. Premedication with steroids and antihistamines reduces the incidence of systemic side effects. ATG is contraindicated in patients with allergy to rabbit (or horse) proteins, severe thrombocytopaenia, active infection or during pregnancy. Prior to administration, a skin test is used to rule out allergy to the heterologous antiserum. Side effects include CRS, anaphylactic reactions

Case 4.6.1 Steroid-resistant renal transplant rejection

A 39-year-old man received a second cadaveric renal transplant. He went into renal failure at the age of 25, because of anti-GBM (glomerular basement membrane) disease. He was originally treated with haemodialysis, and received three blood transfusions because of severe haemoptysis. Unfortunately he produced anti-HLA antibodies. He went on the transplant waiting list when he was 28, and anti-GBM had not been detectable for 2 years. Because of the anti-HLA antibodies he waited 3 years to receive a cross-match negative kidney. Following the first transplant he developed two episodes of rejection, which responded to steroids. Unfortunately the graft failed after 8 years. He waited a further three years on haemodialysis before receiving the current kidney. He was immunosuppressed with tacrolimus, azathioprine and steroids.

The kidney did not function for the first few days and he required two dialysis treatments. However, he then began producing urine and creatinine fell to 100 μmol/l. He was discharged after two weeks. Six weeks after his transplant, he developed severe gastroenteritis. Two days later he felt unwell with temperatures and a painful graft. He was admitted to hospital and his creatinine was 300 μmol/l. Tacrolimus was undetectable. Kidney biopsy showed severe acute cellular rejection. It was thought that this might have occurred because of inadequate immunosuppression during the episode of gastroenteritis. He was treated with a three-day course of intravenous methylprednisolone, and creatinine fell to 200 mmol/l. However, it subsequently rose to 350 μmol/l. Repeat biopsy showed worsening rejection. A course of anti-thymocyte globulin was given to reduce the number of anti-donor T cells present. During the 10-day course of treatment his T cell count dropped and creatinine gradually fell to 130 μmol/l. He was discharged on stronger maintenance therapy of tacrolimus, mycophenylate and steroids.

Cross references

Section 2.21   Immune-mediated Renal Disease
Section 2.28   Solid Organ Transplantation

(Type I hypersensitivity) and serum sickness after 8–14 days (Type III hypersensitivity). If a second course of ATG is required, antiserum from an alternative species should be chosen. If a second course is given from the same species there is a high risk of hypersensitivity and skin test results must be closely examined. The progress of T cell depletion, which can be impaired by neutralising antibodies, should be monitored.

MUROMONAB-CD3 (OKT3)

Muromonab-CD3 (commonly known as OKT3) is a murine monoclonal antibody against CD3, used to treat acute rejection (usually steroid-resistant rejection) of renal, hepatic and cardiac transplant patients.

Muromonab-CD3 results in depletion of T cells, leading to marked inhibition of cellular immune responses. Established B cell responses are not affected, however T cell help for

B cell maturation is inhibited. The effectiveness of treatment can be monitored using absolute T cell counts.

Muromonab-CD3 is administered as a daily bolus injection for 10–14 days. Methylprednisolone is given prior to the first dose to reduce the incidence and severity of the CRS, which occurs in most patients after the first dose.

Muromonab-CD3 is contraindicated in patients who are hypersensitive to mouse products, have anti-mouse titres of >1 : 1000, uncompensated heart failure or fluid overload, a history of seizures or in patients who are pregnant/breastfeeding.

Side-effects of muromonab-CD3 include anaphylaxis which may be difficult to differentiate from CRS, neuro-psychiatric events as well as complications of immunosuppression (infection, neoplasia and viral-induced lymphoproliferative disorders). Repeated treatment with muromonab-CD3 carries a risk of allergic reactions and inhibition by neutralising antibodies.

RITUXIMAB (ANTI-CD20)

Rituximab is a humanised anti-CD20 monoclonal antibody licensed for the treatment of chemotherapy-resistant follicular lymphoma. It has also been used in some antibody-mediated autoimmune diseases.

Rituximab is a cytotoxic antibody that binds to and depletes CD20-positive B cells. Plasma cells are CD20 negative, and are not depleted. Rituximab inhibits B cell maturation and may reduce autoantibody levels. Cellular immunity is not directly affected. However, B cells can present antigen to activated or memory T cells, so an indirect effect appears likely.

Rituximab is administered as an infusion, once weekly for 4 weeks. An analgesic and antihistamine, with corticosteroids are given pre-infusion. Repeated courses of treatment can be given, as humanisation of antibody reduces immunogenicity.

Side effects include infusion reactions (including CRS) and leucopaenia. Tumour pain and tumour lysis syndrome may also occur in patients with a high tumour burden.

CAMPATH-1H (ANTI-CD52)

Campath-1H is a recombinant humanised monoclonal antibody directed against CD52, a cell surface molecule, expressed on T and B cells and at low levels on NK cells. It is licensed for treatment of resistant B cell chronic lymphocytic leukaemia (B-CLL). Campath-1H has also been used for other lymphoid malignancies, autoimmune cytopaenias, RA, and induction therapy for renal transplantation.

Campath-1H depletes T and B cells *in vivo* and *in vitro*, inhibiting both cellular and humoral responses. B cell depletion lasts several months and T cell cytopaenia, persists for over a year. NK cell numbers fall temporarily, but usually recover in weeks.

Campath-1H is given as an intravenous infusion, usually after premedication with paracetamol and an antihistamine. Prophylaxis against herpes infections and *Pneumocystis carinii* is recommended.

Infusion-related side effects are commonly seen and are typical of CRS. Prolonged haematological toxicity and infections also occur.

Campath-1H is also used *in vitro* to T cell deplete bone marrow and other sources of stem cells.

Figure 4.6.1 Immunosuppression: ATG, OKT3, Campath and anti-CD20.

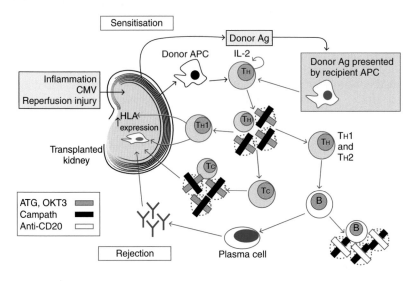

NEW AGENTS

New depleting antibodies that target specific cell populations in the immune system are under development, including antibodies to CD25, which are specific for activated lymphocytes. Additionally, non-immunological applications of targeted cell depletion include antibody-induced eradication of breast cancer cells that overexpress a growth factor receptor called herseptin.

CROSS REFERENCES	
Section 2.28	Solid Organ Transplantation
Section 2.30	Leukaemia and Lymphoma

Other Antibody Therapies

In addition to cell-depletion, therapeutic administration of antibodies is routinely used to:

◆ Prevent alloimmunisation of Rhesus-negative (Rh−) women
◆ Prevent and treat infection
◆ Immunomodulation
◆ Neutralisation of venom/digitalis overdose.

A further application of antibody therapy currently in clinical trials is treatment of allergic disease. There are many novel antibodies currently undergoing clinical trials and the range of disorders treated with antibodies is likely to expand rapidly over the next decade.

PREVENTION OF ALLOIMMUNISATION − ANTI-D(Rh$_0$) IMMUNOGLOBULIN

A major success of antibody therapy is the virtual elimination of haemolytic disease of the newborn (HDN) in the developed world. Rh− women develop antibodies to Rhesus-positive (Rh+) RBCs following transfusion or transplacental transfer of Rh+ cells. Following alloimmunisation, HDN can complicate subsequent pregnancies. HDN is a profound alloimmune haemolytic anaemia due to transplacental passage of maternal antibodies. This results in severe anaemia, congestive heart failure, generalised oedema (hydrops fetalis) and even intrauterine death. Prevention of alloimmunisation of Rh− mothers has made HDN a rare condition, usually involving rare blood group incompatibilities.

Anti-D is a human immunoglobulin solution, prepared using donors who have made high titres of anti-D antibodies following transfusion or previous pregnancies.

Anti-D is administered to non-sensitised Rh− women to remove Rh+ fetal cells before an immune response is generated. The antibody is given within 72 hours of interventions associated with possible transplacental passage of foetal cells (miscarriage, amniocentesis, other intrauterine procedures, termination and following delivery). Additionally, routine antenatal prophylaxis is recommended, with antibody given at 28 weeks and 34 weeks. Prevention of sensitisation is essential as once sensitisation occurs, it cannot be reversed.

PREVENTION OF INFECTION

The ability of antibody to neutralise toxins and organisms is exploited to prevent several infectious diseases. Antibodies used include human hyperimmune globulin, equine serum and humanised MAbs.

Indications include exposure to:

- Tetanus – the causative toxin can be neutralised by antibodies. Human hyperimmune serum is given following a high-risk injury in non-immune patients.
- Hepatitis B – the risk of infection is reduced by neutralising antibodies, which inhibit viral entry into cells. Human hyperimmune serum is administered after high-risk exposure in non-immune individuals.
- Varicella zoster (VZV) – in non-immune, immunocompromised or pregnant patients, primary infection can be fatal. Neutralising antibodies can reduce the risk of infection as well as the severity. Specific VZV immunoglobulin, or batches of intravenous immunoglobulin known to have high anti-VZV titres may be used post-exposure in high-risk groups.
- Cytomegalovirus – infection in immunosuppressed patients can cause severe disease. Immunoglobulin treatment was widely used as prophylaxis, however antiviral agents like gancyclovir are now used more commonly.
- Hepatitis A – immunoglobulin can be used in immunocompromised individuals, following exposure or prior to travel. Vaccination is preferred in immunocompetent individuals.
- Rabies and botulism – equine antibodies given post exposure may be of value in these life-threatening infections.
- Respiratory syncitial virus – RSV causes bronchiolitis in young children, and severe illness in children born prematurely, particularly if they have had bronchopulmonary dysplasia. Palivizumab, a humanised neutralizing MAb, can be administered monthly during the RSV season to reduce the risk of infection.

IMMUNOMODULATION

Cytokine activity can be inhibited by antibodies as well as soluble cytokine receptors or naturally occurring antagonists. Fusion proteins can be constructed, binding receptors to immunoglobulin Fc fragments, to increase the half-life of receptor molecules. Both TNF-α and IL-1 activity may be modified in this way.

TNF-α plays a pivotal role in many inflammatory conditions, and is intimately involved in granuloma formation. However, TNF also protects against infection.

Infliximab is a humanised MAb, which inhibits TNF, and etanercept is a TNF receptor grafted onto an IgG molecule. Anti-TNF therapy is used in rheumatoid disease, Crohn's disease and juvenile arthritis. Not surprisingly, severe infections are an important side effect, and reactivation of tuberculosis is a particular problem. Demyelinating disease of the CNS as well as occasional reports of SLE have been reported. Etanercept has also been associated with serious blood disorders.

IL-1 receptor antagonist (IL-1ra) is a naturally occurring inhibitor of IL-1. IL-1 is a cytokine produced early following infection, and in many inflammatory disorders. Anakinra (recombinant IL-1ra) is used in the treatment of severe rheumatoid disease. Severe infection, particularly in patients with asthma and neutropaenia are important side effects.

TREATMENT OF ENVENOMATION AND POISONING

These rare indications for antibody therapy demonstrate the potential versatility of antibodies as therapeutic tools. Antisera to snake venom are specific for venom produced by different

> ## Case 4.7.1 Crohn's disease
>
> A 20-year-old student presented with a 3-month history of fatigue and weightloss and a three-week history of bloody diarrhoea and abdominal pain. Colonoscopy showed discontinuous inflammation and biopsies showed granulomatous inflammation. Small bowel follow-through showed extensive inflammation in the small bowel. A diagnosis of Crohn's disease was made. Initial treatment with steroids and mesalazine produced a partial remission. However, 2 months later, despite this therapy the patient deteriorated. In an attempt to avert surgical resection of the colon, a trial of anti-TNF therapy was given.
>
> The patient received three infusions of infliximab over a 6-week period with dramatic improvement. Azathioprine was also instituted both to treat the underlying Crohn's disease, and also to reduce the risk of developing anti-chimeric antibodies. Steroids were tapered and remission was maintained using mesalazine and azathioprine.

species of snake. European venom viper antiserum is indicated for severe viper envenomation, particularly in small children and the elderly, where there is a small risk of fatality. Antiserum is used for systemic reactions and severe local reactions that extend rapidly.

Antibody fragments to digitalis are used in severe digitalis overdosage, where discontinuing digitalis and correction of electrolyte abnormalities are insufficient to stabilise the patient. The use of antibody fragments improves penetration to tissues.

ANTI-IgE – A NOVEL APPROACH TO TREATING ALLERGIC DISEASE

Type I hypersensitivity reactions result from mast cell activation through IgE bound to high-affinity IgE receptors on the cell surface. Monoclonal antibodies directed against the portion of the IgE molecule bound by the high-affinity IgE receptors prevent sensitisation of the mast cells without cross-linking cell-bound IgE. Anti-IgE therapy reduces severity of allergic rhinitis and asthma. Additionally, in patients with severe food allergies, anti-IgE increases the threshold at which reactions occur. While this would not allow return to a normal diet, the risks associated with accidental ingestion of traces of allergen may be greatly reduced.

CROSS REFERENCES

Section 2.16   Immune-mediated Haematological Conditions
Section 4.11   Vaccination and Passive Immunisation

REFERENCE

Leung, D. Y., Sampson, H. A., Yunginger, J. W. *et al.* (2003) 'Effect of anti-IgE therapy in patients with peanut allergy', *N. Engl. J. Med.*, 348(11): 986–93.

Immunoglobulin Replacement Therapy

Immunoglobulin (Ig) concentrates are prepared from pooled plasma donations from 1000–10,000 individuals. Careful donor screening, strict regulation and quality control of production, and additional anti-viral treatment of Ig concentrate, produces a very safe product. Ig contains predominantly IgG with variable levels of IgA contamination. A number of products are commercially available. Early preparations were for intramuscular administration (IMIg). Dosage was limited by pain at injection sites and side effects were common. Products suitable for intravenous use (IVIg) available since the 1980s are now widely used. Products for subcutaneous administration are also available. Ig prepared for different routes of administration, and even different IVIg products are not interchangeable. Ig is extremely expensive and supply is limited worldwide. Therefore, it is critical that its use is reserved for cases where it is clearly indicated. Clinical immunologists should be consulted prior to use outside the indications outlined in the following paragraph.

INDICATIONS FOR IVIg THERAPY

Primary antibody deficiency syndromes

IVIg is recommended therapy in CVID, XLA, CD40L deficiency, other severe genetic antibody deficiencies. Its value in IgG subclass deficiency and specific antibody deficiency is less clear. Trial use for a 12-month period may be useful. Temporary use in symptomatic transient hypogammaglobulinaemia of infancy may be useful.

Secondary antibody deficiency syndromes

IVIg is of value in patients with antibody deficiency associated with multiple myeloma and chronic lymphocytic leukaemia. Benefit of IVIg is most marked in those patients with a history of pyogenic infection or where low specific antibody levels and poor vaccine responses are demonstrated. IVIg is also used following bone marrow transplantation until immune reconstitution occurs.

Case 4.8.1 X-linked agammaglobulinaemia

A 2-year-old boy presented with recurrent chest infections and chronic diarrhoea. He had been well until the age of 6 months, following which he developed chest, and ear infections. One month prior to presentation, he developed diarrhoea, which had improved but not fully resolved. Stool examination showed *Giardia lamblia*. He was treated with metronidazole. Immunoglobulins (Igs) showed undetectable IgG and IgA with low levels of IgM. No B cells were detected in peripheral blood, suggesting a diagnosis of X-linked agammaglobulinaemia (XLA). The diagnosis was confirmed by demonstrating absence of btk, and a mutation was identified in the *btk* gene.

Intravenous immunoglobulin replacement was commenced and infections became infrequent. The family sought genetic advice and was counselled that future sons had a 50% risk of being affected. The families were keen to have the patient's older sister tested for carrier status. However, the geneticist advised against testing, as this information is of no benefit to a child. In line with guidelines on genetic testing of healthy children, predictive carrier testing for the daughter was deferred, with advice that testing could be discussed with the daughter when she would be mature enough to make her own decision.

T cell mediated immunodeficiencies

IVIg is indicated in SCID and CID syndromes where impaired antibody-mediated immunity is demonstrated.

ADMINISTRATION

Large doses of IVIg can be administered and normal levels of IgG achieved. Adverse reactions with IVIg are rare, provided care is taken with patient preparation and infusion. The average dose for replacement purposes is 0.4 g/kg every 3 weeks (half-life of IgG is 21 days). Doses and/or frequency of infusion are increased if patients do not reach normal levels of IgG after approximately 3 months of treatment. The IVIg requirement may be increased if infection is inadequately treated, with co-existent protein-losing states and rarely with hypercatabolism of Ig. Protein-losing states without associated immunodeficiency rarely require Ig replacement, despite low IgG levels. Subcutaneous administration of Ig can be useful where venous access is a problem. Intramuscular Ig is no longer used.

Initial therapy should be undertaken in a hospital setting, supervised by personnel familiar with IVIg therapy. Home therapy is an option for some patients and is organised by specialist centres that select, prepare and support patients.

Patient screening is required prior to first infusion. This includes:

* Pre-infusion IgG level
* Hepatitis virus screen (especially HCV)
* Renal and liver biochemistry
* FBC
* Infection screen

- Serum storage archive for 'look-back' studies if adverse events arise (e.g. infection transmission
- Written, informed consent covering administration, side effects and potential long-term risks of use of this blood product.

ADVERSE REACTIONS

Acute adverse reactions are most common with the first infusion of a particular IVIg product and are rare once treatment is established. Mild reactions cause headache, shivering, muscle aching and fever with severe reactions characterised by respiratory embarrassment, chest pain, hypotension, collapse and occasionally death. Symptoms occur during or within 24 hours of infusion and are usually due to immune complex formation. Causes include too rapid an infusion rate or untreated infection.

Guidelines to lessen the risk of reaction include:

- Initiate infusions at rates slower than manufacturers' recommendations
- Adequate treatment of infection prior to infusion
- Administer hydrocortisone and antihistamine before the first few infusions
- Do not change products unless absolutely essential.

Most reactions settle on slowing or stopping the infusion. Paracetamol is helpful for mild reactions. Antihistamine and adrenaline may be required for more severe reactions.

Antibody-deficient patients with complete IgA deficiency may develop anti-IgA antibodies on exposure to IVIg-containing IgA, which causes adverse effects. Products depleted of IgA are preferable for such patients.

Occasionally, patients continue to have reactions despite addressing these issues. Changing to another product may be helpful. Occasionally, continued prophylaxis with paracetamol, antihistamine or even steroid is required. Other acute reactions are usually associated with infusion of higher doses of IVIg (hdIVIg) for immunomodulation (Section 4.9).

No blood product is completely safe and transmission of blood-borne infection is a concern. Additional virucidal steps in IVIg production minimise this risk, however vigilance is always required. HIV infection has never been transmitted by IVIg. Hepatitis C virus has been transmitted by IVIg with serious consequences. Prion transmission risk (new variant Creutzfeld Jacob disease agent) is unknown but is possible in theory.

Attempts to limit the risk of blood-borne prion disease have seriously compromised the availability of plasma worldwide. Shortfalls in relation to demands are now regularly experienced posing life-threatening risks for antibody-deficient patients should supply fail.

PATIENT MONITORING

Patients receiving Ig replacement therapy should be monitored in relation to the following:

Efficacy

- Clinical status (e.g. daily diary detailing well-being, infection, antibiotic usage).
- Assessment of progress of underlying diseases – for example, pulmonary function and high resolution CT of thorax.
- Trough levels of IgG (just before infusion) should be measured regularly and dose/interval adjusted accordingly. Trough IgG should be within the normal range and

probably higher in patients with established lung disease and in CVID patients with granulomata. Clinical status rather than IgG levels are the mainstay of monitoring of patients with multiple myeloma and CLL.

Safety

- All infusions, product and batch numbers should be logged.
- Interchange of product and batch number exposure should be minimised in individual patients.
- Serial pre-infusion liver function testing and storage of samples for viral studies will allow prompt identification of infection should it occur.
- Careful records facilitate identification of the culprit product.

CROSS REFERENCES

Section 2.8   Defects in Antibody-mediated Immunity
Section 2.30   Leukaemia and Lymphoma
Section 2.31   Plasma Cell Diseases

High Dose Immunoglobulin Therapy

In several immune-mediated disorders high dose IVIg (hdIVIg) is increasingly used as an immunomodulatory therapy. The benefits of hdIVIg have been demonstrated in some conditions (e.g. immune thrombocytopaenia (ITP), Guillain–Barré syndrome (GBS), chronic inflammatory demyelinating polyneuropathy (CIDP)). High-dose IVIg is also used empirically in some situations without clear-cut evidence of effectiveness. This treatment is associated with several risks, is expensive and there is a permanent shortfall of IVIg supply.

MECHANISMS OF ACTION

There are a number of potential mechanisms by which hdIVIg may alter immune activation, including:

Fc receptor blockade

Occupation of phagocytic cell Fc receptors by infused Ig inhibits binding and destruction of antibody-bound cells.

Deactivation of pathogenic targets

Antibodies against pathogenic antibodies (anti-antibodies/anti-idiotypes) found in polyclonal IVIg may limit damaging effects of autoantibodies. Antimicrobial antibodies may similarly impair the action of pathogenic microbes.

Inhibitory effects on B cells

Polyclonal IVIg concentrate has been shown to reduce output of pathogenic antibodies by B cells.

Altered cytokine networks

Direct reduction in cytokine production, together with immune modulating effects of cytokines and cytokine receptors present in IVIg preparations may affect T cell proliferation, B cell activity and patterns of immune responses.

One mode of action may predominate as is the case in ITP where Fc receptor blockade with hdIVIg results in reduced phagocyte destruction of the platelet targets. This is a short-lived effect (5–7 days) but increases the platelet count when critically low or in advance of surgical procedures. In many instances, the precise actions of IVIg are not well-understood.

CLINICAL INDICATIONS

Indications for which at least one IVIg preparation is licensed and conditions where trials have shown effectiveness of hdIVIg (asterisked) include:

- Haematological conditions – ITP*, haemolytic anaemia, alloimmune-thrombocytopaenia
- Neurological diseases – Guillain–Barré syndrome*, CIDP*, myasthenia gravis, Eaton–Lambert syndrome
- Vasculitis – Kawasaki disease*, ANCA-related vasculitides
- Connective tissue diseases – SLE, polymyositis, dermatomyositis
- Dermatological – pemphigus, pemphigoid.

High-dose IVIg is of doubtful or no benefit in SLE, MS, intractable inflammatory bowel disease and RA, and it may be potentially harmful in some of these cases.

ADMINISTRATION

General points regarding the administration of IVIg are outlined in Section 4.8. The typical dosage for immunomodulatory indications is 2 g/kg, usually administered in five divided doses over five consecutive days, although larger doses and/or shorter periods may be used. Patients receiving hdIVIg are at risk of all the side effects outlined in Section 4.8.

Additionally, the following side effects are particularly associated with hdIVIg.

- Aseptic meningitis – headache and meningism with lymphocytic CSF inflammation.
- Renal impairment – especially in the elderly or in patients with pre-existing renal impairment. Sucrose containing products may pose increased risk.
- Hyperviscosity – increases risk of MI and CVA in predisposed patients.
- Immune complex-mediated reactions – serum sickness – in patients with immune complex disorders, for example, SLE and with high-titre rheumatoid factor (RF).
- Intravascular haemolysis.
- Severe anaphylactoid reactions.

The risk of these side effects can be lessened by avoiding hdIVIg in high-risk patients. All potential patients should be screened for renal impairment, RF activity and IgA deficiency. High-risk patients should only be treated if the indication is strong and alternative therapies are contraindicated. High-dose IVIg therapy should be administered slowly in these groups until tolerability has been assessed. Renal function should be monitored daily and therapy abandoned if a significant (>20%) rise in creatinine is seen. FBC and other indicators of immune activation in immune complex disease (e.g. serial complement levels) may also be useful during hdIVIg.

CROSS REFERENCES	
Section 2.16	Immune-mediated Haematological Conditions
Section 2.19	Immune-mediated Neurological Disease
Section 4.8	Immunoglobulin Replacement Therapy

Cytokines

Cytokines are soluble messengers, which coordinate the immune response. Physiologically, cytokines usually act in a paracrine fashion (exerting their action on nearby cells). Cytokines have many potent effects on the immune system, necessitating tight control of cytokine production during an immune response. At present, therapeutic use of cytokines cannot replicate this localisation or control of activity. Cytokines are small biologically active proteins; they cannot be administered orally due to local effects on the gut and digestion.

Despite limitations imposed by current delivery systems, cytokines are being used to treat a number of conditions:

♦   Replacement therapy in cytokine deficiency
♦   To augment or redirect the immune response
♦   As immunomodulatory therapy.

Because of their generally short half-life, these agents often require frequent administration and/or modification of the molecule to increase the half-life.

REPLACEMENT THERAPY

IL-2 deficiency is a rare cause of SCID. Regular administration of IL-2 has been associated with clinical improvement and normalisation of T cell proliferation.

Genetically transmitted IL-12 and IL-12 receptor deficiencies and defects in the IFN-γ receptor are associated with increased susceptibility to mycobacterial infections and salmonellosis. Regular treatment with subcutaneous IFN-γ can be used as an adjuvant to treatment of infection as well as prophylaxis against further infections. In patients with partial deficiency of the IFN-γ receptor high doses of IFN-γ may be effective, although not surprisingly such treatment is usually unsuccessful in complete deficiency of the IFN-γ receptor.

AUGMENTING THE IMMUNE RESPONSE

Cytokines are used in the treatment of cancers and some infections, where at least part of their therapeutic effect results from augmentation of the immune response. IL-2 is thought to have an anti-cancer effect due to immune stimulation. IFN-α has anti-tumour effects, which may be direct or related to the immunological effects of this cytokine. Interferons have also been used in a number of chronic infections. Beneficial effects are likely to be due to both immune stimulation as well as direct anti-viral effects.

Recombinant IL-2 is licensed for subcutaneous use in patients with metastatic renal cell carcinoma. It is highly toxic, and although tumour shrinkage has been documented, survival does not appear to be increased. Toxicity is universal and often severe with capillary leak syndrome, which causes pulmonary oedema and hypotension, as well as bone marrow, hepatic, renal and CNS toxicity.

IFN-α is used for treatment of haematological malignancies and solid tumours. Additionally, IFN-α is used as an adjuvant therapy for malignant melanoma as well as maintenance therapy for multiple myeloma in remission. Common side effects are dose-related and include nausea, influenza-like symptoms, lethargy and depression. Myelosuppression, cardiovascular problems, nephrotoxicity and hepatotoxicity may also occur.

IFN-α is also licensed for treatment of chronic Hepatitis B and Hepatitis C. In combination with ribavirin, IFN-α leads to clearance of virus in a significant proportion of patients with Hepatitis C. A beneficial effect of IFN-α has also been shown in lepromatous leprosy (where a predominantly T helper cell, type 2 (TH2) type response fails to control the infection), and in visceral leischmaniasis.

IMMUNOMODULATION

The original rationale for treating MS with IFN-β was based on the hypothesis that MS was due to a defective immune response to an unidentified viral pathogen. IFN-β was found to be beneficial in several types of MS. While the precise mechanism leading to clinical benefit in MS is poorly understood, the therapeutic effect of IFN-β is thought to be due to immunomodulatory effects. IFN-β rapidly restores the blood brain barrier in addition to inhibiting T cell proliferation, antigen presentation and T cell migration. Additionally, it appears to modify cytokine production towards an anti-inflammatory profile, both in the periphery and in the CNS.

IFN-β is self-administered by subcutaneous injection three times a week. The most common side effects are injection site reactions, influenza-like symptoms and depression.

The possibility of modulating or redirecting the immune response in a number of other immunological disorders using cytokines is currently under investigation, and the list of therapeutic applications of such therapies is likely to grow substantially over the next decade.

CROSS REFERENCES	
Section 2.9	Defects in T Cell-mediated Immunity
Section 2.19	Immune-mediated Neurological Disease

Vaccination and Passive Immunisation

Vaccination is the greatest success of immunology. In 1798 Jenner introduced a cowpox vaccine that protected against the antigenically related, lethal smallpox. Development of safe vaccines and mass vaccination led to the worldwide elimination of smallpox in the 1980s. The WHO aims to eliminate polio in the near future.

DEFINITIONS AND IMMUNOLOGICAL PRINCIPLES

Passive immunisation

This describes the administration of preformed antibody ('antiserum') derived from human or animal donors to the recipient. The effect is immediate but short-lived as the transferred immunoglobulin is metabolised. Immunological memory does not develop.

Vaccination (active immunisation)

During active immunisation, attenuated organisms, killed organisms or pathogen subunits are administered to the individual. The immune response develops slowly but immunological memory is evoked. Re-exposure of the subject to the pathogenic organism produces a rapid, effective secondary response, which usually prevents symptomatic infection. Effective vaccines elicit protective immune responses both in type (antibody versus cellular immunity) and in site (mucosal or systemic).

Passive immunisation – clinical uses

Passive immunisation is used in the following circumstances:

* To treat a number of serious infections.
* As a secondary prevention post-exposure in individuals at high risk of mortality.

Table 4.11.1 Some infections commonly treated with passive immunisation

INFECTION	ANTISERUM	INDICATION
Tetanus	Immune human	High-risk injury in non-immune subject
Hepatitis B	Immune human	High-risk injury in non-immune subject
Varicella Zoster	Immune human	Post-exposure in non-immune subjects who are pregnant or immunosuppressed
Botulism	Horse	Post-exposure
Rabies	Horse	Post-exposure. Vaccine also given

◆ To neutralise toxins (e.g. post-snakebite) and digitalis overdose (e.g. neutralising antibody inactivates the drug). Because the effects of passive immunisation are short-lived, vaccination is also given when available to ensure future protection.

Active immunisation (vaccination)

Vaccination produces an immune response capable of providing effective protective immunity in the absence of symptomatic infection. In any population some individuals will have contraindications to particular vaccines or will fail to respond. However, if 95% of the population are vaccinated, these non-vaccinated subjects are unlikely to come in contact with an infected subject. This protective effect is termed herd immunity.

Vaccines in routine use include live attenuated vaccines, vaccines containing killed organisms and subunit vaccines.

◆ Live attenuated organisms usually provide strong immunisation of the appropriate type and site for natural infection. In addition to developing immunity in the vaccinated subject, the attenuated organism can be passed to non-immunised subjects, eliciting protective responses and enhancing herd immunity. Live attenuated vaccines carry a risk of reversion to pathogenic strains causing disease and pose a particular risk in immunocompromised subjects.
◆ Killed vaccines do not pose a risk of infection, but generally elicit weaker responses than live attenuated vaccines. Booster doses are usually required.
◆ Subunit vaccines contain proteins, carbohydrates or inactivated toxins from organisms. They are generally less immunogenic than intact organisms, and may require adjuvants to elicit effective immune responses. Schedules usually involve multiple doses. Side effects are generally less prominent than with whole organisms. As subunit vaccines contain no viable organisms, there is no risk of vaccine-associated infections, even in immunocompromised subjects.

VACCINATION – CLINICAL USES

Some vaccines are offered to everyone, while others are reserved for people at particular risk because of an underlying medical condition, occupational risk or travel. Schedules of routine vaccination vary in different parts of the world but current UK recommendations are used as an example in this section.

Table 4.11.2 **Commonly used vaccines**

VACCINE	TYPE	INDICATIONS AND SCHEDULE
BCG	Live attenuated	Birth. Boost in teens and for occupational risk if Mantoux negative
Tetanus	Toxoid	Childhood – three doses and boost at school entry
Diphtheria	Toxoid	
Pertussis	Subunit or cellular	Tetanus boost with injury or 10 years
		Diphtheria boost for some travel
HiB	Conjugated polysaccharide	Childhood – three doses and boost at school entry
Meningococcus	Conjugated polysaccharide	
Measles	Live attenuated triple vaccine	Single dose at 15 months and boost at school entry
Mumps		
Rubella		Non-immune women offered rubella between pregnancies
Polio	Live attenuated or killed	Childhood – three doses and boost at school entry. Boost for travel
Hepatitis B	Subunit	Occupational risk. Three doses and check response serologically
Influenza	Subunit. New preparation on annual basis	Medical risk (chest disease, elderly, diabetes, immunocopromised)
		Environmental risk – nursing homes
		Occupational risk – healthcare workers
Pneumococcus	Conjugated polysaccharide/ polysaccharide	Medical risk – asplenic, chest disease, elderly
Varicella Zoster	Live attenuated	Medical risk. Non-immune children pre-transplantation
Typhoid	Polysaccharide	Travel. Single dose, Repeat at 3 years
Cholera	WHO do not recommend	Travel. Required in some countries
		Exemption certificate may be adequate
Yellow fever	Live attenuated	Travel. Single dose. Boost after 10 years

MODERN APPROACHES TO VACCINE DEVELOPMENTS

Development of more effective and safer vaccines, as well as vaccines for other diseases is a major area of research. Molecular techniques have facilitated the production of large quantities of proteins for use as subunit vaccines safely and relatively cheaply. However, development of safe effective adjuvants to enhance the effectiveness of subunit vaccines remains a challenge. Additionally, as many infections gain entry to the body via the mucosa, delivery systems that enhance mucosal immunity would offer considerable advantages. Direct injection of DNA into muscle elicits strong antibody and cellular immune responses in animal models, and is currently entering clinical trials.

Vaccination has been particularly successful in diseases where natural infection leads to sterilising immunity and long-term immunity. Many other diseases remain major public health problems. The pathogens responsible often employ several of the evasion mechanisms described in Section 1.25. While vaccination has produced several advances in public health, many challenges remain.

CROSS REFERENCES

Section 1.15   Immunoglobulin Function
Section 1.21   Maintenance of the Immune Response

REFERENCE

UK Department of Health (1996) 'Immunisation against infectious disease', *The Green Book*, The Stationary Office Books, London. Available online with new replacement chapters www.dh.gov.uk

Plasmapheresis and Plasma Exchange

Plasmapheresis (PP) and plasma exchange (PE) are physical methods for removing plasma and replacing it with donor plasma (PE) or other fluids (PP). The patient is anticoagulated, connected to an extra-corporeal circuit and plasma is removed using a membrane filter or blood cells fractionated using a cell separator. The cellular elements are then reinfused together with the chosen replacement fluid. Between 0.5 and 1.5 plasma volumes can be exchanged at each session, depending on how well the patient tolerates the procedure.

IMMUNOLOGICAL EFFECTS

PP and PE remove antibodies, intravascular immune complexes and other inflammatory mediators. PP can deplete complement and coagulation factors if this is required. The effects on antibody levels vary with the distribution of the isotype. A single plasma volume exchange will remove most IgM but only approximately 60% of IgG. The effect is short-lived as B cells become highly active in an immunoglobulin-poor environment and antibody levels may show a rebound phenomenon (antibodies rapidly climb higher than pretherapy levels) when treatment is stopped. To prevent this, immunosuppression using a powerful anti-B cell agent is usually commenced at the same time as PP.

CLINICAL INDICATIONS

PP and/or PE may be used in the following conditions:

- Antibody-mediated rejection of transplanted organs
- Anti-GBM disease
- Severe ANCA-associated vasculitis
- Cryoglobulinaemia
- Hyperviscosity syndrome
- Thrombocytopenic purpura and haemolytic uraemic syndrome

Figure 4.12.1 Plasmapheresis apparatus.

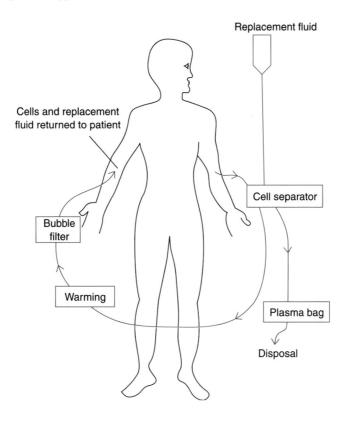

- ◆ Myasthenia gravis
- ◆ Some inflammatory neuropathies.

The use of these therapies has been reported in small numbers of patients with other conditions, with variable results.

SIDE EFFECTS

Side effects include:

- ◆ Leakage or clotting in the extra-corporeal circuit. There is a high risk of circuit occlusion in patients with cryoglobulins that precipitate at room temperature. Prior to treatment a temperature profile is performed on the cryoglobulins to establish the temperature at which precipitation can be expected, allowing equipment, fluids and the room to be pre-heated to minimise this risk.
- ◆ Bleeding due to anticoagulation and removal of coagulation factors. The risk is less with PE than PP.
- ◆ Haemolytic anaemia and thrombocytopaenia.

- Infection (due to removal of immunoglobulin). The risk can be reduced by including some intravenous immunoglobulin in the replacement fluid, particularly at the end of treatment.
- Haemodynamic instability.

Limitations in the use of these therapies include:

- Access to equipment and appropriately trained personnel.
- Patients need to be fit for the procedure. Contraindications include active bleeding, haemodynamic instability, anaemia or thrombocytopaenia or infection.
- Two sites of intravenous access capable of generating sufficient flow rates are also required.

OPTIMISING THERAPY

Most studies report results of standard courses of therapy (5 or 10 sessions). However, in many diseases the antibodies to be removed are readily measured, and the number of sessions required to remove antibody varies greatly between patients. It appears likely that close monitoring of patients during and immediately after PP to ensure that they become and remain antibody negative may improve the outcome of these therapies.

CROSS REFERENCES
Section 2.19   Immune-mediated Neurological Disease Section 2.21   Immune-mediated Renal Disease Section 2.28   Solid Organ Transplantation

Management of Acute Allergic Reactions

Clinical manifestations of allergies are described in Part 2. Acute allergic reactions cause symptoms varying from mild skin rash to life-threatening anaphylaxis. Accurate identification of the responsible allergen(s) often allows successful allergen avoidance. However, identification of unusual allergens may be impossible, particularly when reactions are infrequent and details about reactions are vague. This part describes the emergency management of an acute allergic reaction, as well as the long-term management of affected patients.

EMERGENCY MANAGEMENT OF AN ACUTE ALLERGIC REACTION

Emergency management of an acute allergic reaction is summarised in Figure 4.13.1.

The drugs used for resuscitation are primarily adrenaline, fast-acting antihistamines and corticosteroids.

Adrenaline is a physiological antagonist of many of histamine effects. Adrenaline reverses bronchospasm, reduces angioedema and increases blood pressure by reversing vasodilation and increasing cardiac output. Adrenaline is given intramuscularly in doses of 0.5–1 mg (0.01 mg/kg). This dose can be repeated every 15 minutes until a response is obtained. In patients taking non-cardioselective β-blockers, addition of IV salbutamol should be considered.

A fast-acting antihistamine such as chlorpheniramine given by slow IV injection minimises further effects of histamine. In serious reactions adrenaline should be given IM immediately, and then IV access can be secured to give other agents.

Corticosteroids, usually IV hydrocortisone, take several hours to act. Steroids prevent or reduce secondary late phase reactions. Administration of rapidly acting medications obviously takes priority.

Where there is any respiratory difficulty oxygen should be administered. Intravenous fluids and nebulised β_2-agonists are frequently required.

Patients who have a reaction requiring the use of adrenaline should be monitored for 8–24 hours in hospital as late phase reactions may cause deterioration. When discharged, patients should be given advice about further reactions and a prescription for a non-sedating,

Figure 4.13.1 Emergency management of an acute allergic reaction.

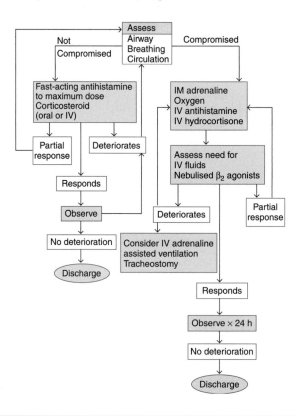

fast-acting antihistamine to take at the onset of reactions. Short-term steroid treatment is particularly useful where there is an asthmatic component to the reaction. Arrangements should also be made for a specialist allergy opinion.

NON-ACUTE ASPECTS OF MANAGEMENT

When patients have experienced an acute allergic reaction, further management aims to prevent recurrence and minimise the risks of future reactions.

Essential aspects of management of include:

- Identification of the allergen(s) responsible.
- Patient education about allergen avoidance.
- Treatment of associated asthma if present.
- Avoidance of drugs which exacerbate reactions or hinder resuscitation (especially β-blockers).
- Formulation of an individualised emergency plan, with appropriate patient education to ensure that patients can manage future reactions appropriately.
- Ensure allergies to medication are documented in a manner accessible to all healthcare providers, to prevent future avoidable reactions (e.g. MedicAlert bracelet, case note labelling).

Investigations to identify the allergen(s) responsible are described in Section 3.14. It is helpful to take a detailed history of foods and medications recently ingested as soon as possible. Full investigation may take some time, and patients should have an emergency plan while investigations are proceeding, as the risk of further reactions is highest before the allergen(s) are identified.

Underlying asthma is frequently exacerbated during an allergic reaction. Regular use of short-acting β_2 agonists is associated with reduced β_2 receptor expression in the lung, limiting the effectiveness of adrenaline and salbutamol in reversing bronchospasm, should resuscitation be required. Adequate use of inhaled steroids and other preventive medication to avoid overuse of short-acting β_2 agonists is essential.

Concomitant medications may exacerbate reactions or make resuscitation difficult. β-blockers inhibit many of the key actions of adrenaline (reversing bronchospasm and increasing cardiac output). Use of adrenaline in patients taking β-blockers and tricyclic antidepressants may be associated with severe hypertension. Angiotensin converting enzyme (ACE) inhibitors can cause angioedema, and may exacerbate allergic reactions. The risk–benefit ratio of any of the above medications should be carefully reviewed in patients who have had severe allergic reactions or where inadvertent allergen exposure is a significant risk, for example, in nut allergy. Patients should also be warned that alcohol and non-steroidal anti-inflammatory drugs (NSAIDs) may increase the severity of reactions.

Even the most conscientious patient is likely to ingest foods inadvertently, and therefore it is essential that patients understand their own emergency plan. Mild reactions may be treated with a fast-acting, non-sedating antihistamine. Patients with asthma should also use high-dose, short-acting β_2 agonist immediately. More severe reactions including laryngeal oedema, bronchospasm or symptoms of hypotension require rapid medical attention. Self-administration of adrenaline while waiting for an ambulance may be life-saving. Adrenaline in a dose suitable for self-administration (300 µg) is available in pre-filled, ready-to-use syringes.

All allergies to medications should be documented and the information transmitted to other healthcare providers. Patients with allergy to a medication commonly used in an emergency, or to latex should wear a MedicAlert bracelet.

Desensitisation is a procedure that aims to prevent allergic reactions by exposure to minute doses of allergen, which are gradually increased. Not surprisingly, this form of therapy carries a significant risk of anaphylaxis. It is contraindicated in patients with severe asthma, significant ischaemic heart disease or those who cannot discontinue β-blocker therapy. Desensitisation is used for patients who have had systemic reactions to wasp and bee venom, and occasionally for drug allergies. Desensitisation may also be used in patients with allergies to inhaled antigens, unless there is associated asthma. Unfortunately there is no safe and effective form of desensitisation available for food allergies.

CROSS REFERENCES

Section 1.30   Atopy and Allergic Inflammation
Sections 2.1–2.6   Clinical manifestations of allergy
Section 3.14   Allergy and Hypersensitivity

REFERENCE

Emergency medical treatment of anaphylactic reactions (1999) Project Team of The Resuscitation Council (UK). *Resuscitation*, 41(2): 93–9.

Self Assessment

Section 1

Provide a brief answer to the following questions indicating what you would do and why.

1. A 15-year-old boy is admitted for his fifth infusion of IVIg. IVIg was started 3 months ago, when CVID was diagnosed. Pre-treatment IgG level was 2 g/l. He has received 25 g of IVIg every 3 weeks, and weighs 70 kg. The pre-infusion IgG level before his last infusion was 5 g/l. What would you do?
2. A 55 kg woman was commenced on steroids and azathioprine 6 weeks ago for autoimmune hepatitis. She is currently on 20 mg prednisolone and 150 mg azathioprine. As her GP, you were asked to check an FBC and LFTs weekly for 6 weeks and then monthly. Her neutrophil count has remained within the normal range, however you note that it has dropped from $5 \times 10^9/l$ 3 weeks ago to $3.5 \times 10^9/l$ last week and is now $2 \times 10^9/l$. What would you do?
3. A 40-year old man recently diagnosed with Wegener's granulomatosis returns for follow-up. His original disease involved his upper airways and lungs, with no signs of renal involvement. He was treated with steroids and cyclophosphamide. Routine urinalysis shows $++++$ for blood. What would you do?
4. A 25-year-old woman had a renal transplant 5 years ago. Her renal function is normal and she is on maintenance therapy with cyclosporin, azathioprine and steroids. A routine cervical smear is abnormal and a repeat smear in 4–6 months is advised. What would you do?
5. A 48-year-old woman has had steroid therapy for the last 8 years to control mixed connective tissue disease. She is now approaching the menopause and is concerned about osteoporosis. What would you advise?
6. A 55-year-old man with RA returns for a third infusion of infliximab. He complains of a cough for the last 2 weeks and is febrile. What would you do?
7. A 22-year-old man who presents with pulmonary haemorrhage and severe renal impairment is diagnosed with anti-GBM disease and commences PP, together with cyclophosphamide and steroids. Renal function recovers and there is no evidence of further pulmonary haemorrhage. Prior to the second last plasmapheresis treatment he develops a chest infection and positive blood cultures indicating septicaemia. What would you do?

Section 2

You should be able to answer the following questions. The answers are contained in the relevant sections.

8. What are the risks associated with immunosuppression. How would you reduce these risks? (Section 4.1)
9. What are the side effects of corticosteroids? How would you minimise these risks? (Section 4.2)
10. Draw a diagram of the immune response to a transplanted organ. Indicate where each of the following agents exerts its action – azathioprine, mycophenylate, cyclosporin, rapamycin/sirolimus. (Sections 4.3 and 4.4)
11. How do humanised antibodies differ from heterologous antibodies? How does this affect the side effects seen? (Section 4.5)
12. What information would you give a patient who was commencing treatment with IVIg? (Section 4.8)

13. What are the putative actions of hdIVIg? (Section 4.9)
14. What vaccines are commonly administered? Which vaccines contain live attenuated organisms? When are live vaccines contraindicated? (Section 4.11)
15. How would you treat a patient with acute urticaria? How would you manage a patient with anaphylactic shock? (Section 4.13)

Section 1 – Answers

1. Take blood for measurement of IgG level again. Increase the dose of the infusion to 30 g/l. The aim of the treatment is to restore IgG levels to normal. The dose of IVIg is relatively low, and clearly not adequate for this patient.

2. If you are unfamiliar with the use of any immunosuppressive drug, you should seek advice from the person who prescribed the medication. Although the neutrophil count is normal (just) the progressive fall is a cause for concern and suggests that the azathioprine is causing marrow suppression. Azathioprine should be stopped or reduced to a low dose and the FBC checked in a few days. This patient will need careful monitoring and is unlikely to tolerate doses above 100 mg of azathioprine.

3. Possible causes of microscopic haematuria include haemorrhagic cystitis due to cyclophosphamide, new vasculitic renal involvement or possibly a urinary tract infection. Urine microscopy is essential. Red cell casts indicate glomerular damage (due to disease) however, absence of glomerular casts does not exclude renal involvement. Urine should also be cultured, and creatinine, acute phase markers (CRP and ESR) as well as ANCA levels should be checked urgently. If haemorrhagic cystitis appears most likely, cyclophosphamide should be stopped. If disease is in remission it may be possible to switch to azathioprine. If cyclophosphamide is essential to control disease, hyper-hydration and mesna for bladder protection will be needed.

4. Carcinoma of the cervix can progress rapidly in immunosuppressed women, and therefore a positive smear requires urgent action. A high vaginal swab to rule out infection should be taken. If infection is present it should be treated and an urgent repeat smear sent. If there is no infection or the repeat smear is abnormal the patient should be referred for colposcopy.

5. A bone density scan is helpful. Lifestyle factors contributing to osteoporosis (diet, exercise, alcohol intake and smoking) should be discussed. Supplementary calcium and vitamin D3 have some effect, however bisphosphonate therapy is more effective and is definitely indicated if there are signs of osteoporosis on bone density scan. Hormone replacement therapy slows post-menopausal bone loss, and is advised in most women requiring long-term steroids unless there are significant risk factors for breast cancer or thrombosis.

6. Do not give infliximab! Infliximab therapy is associated with the development of TB and other opportunistic infections. This gentleman requires an urgent work up to assess the cause of his symptoms, and should be isolated until it is established whether he has TB.

7. PP removes both protective and pathogenic antibodies. Many patients drop their IgG level to undetectable levels, and are unable to localise infection resulting in septicaemia. This man should not have further PP or cyclophosphamide until sepsis is controlled. A one off dose of intravenous Ig is often a very useful adjuvant when sepsis develops during PP.

Clinical Immunology – Future Prospects

Clinical immunology is a rapidly evolving specialty, which has changed dramatically over the last decade. Our rapidly advancing understanding of the immune system, together with the developments in molecular genetics, pharmacology and transplantation will continue to improve the care we can offer to patients with immunological disorders in the coming decade. This section briefly outlines some recent developments that we feel are likely to change the way we look after patients.

MOLECULAR GENETICS IN HEALTH AND DISEASE

The draft sequence of the human genome was published in 2001. A huge amount of work remains to complete our understanding of our genetic makeup, however this represents a major milestone. Available technologies allow us to research genetic changes occurring under a variety of circumstances and to determine the impact of conditions on genetic sequences even before individual genes are identified.

The genetic changes involved in many inherited and acquired diseases have been established. This knowledge will allow rational design of therapies to inhibit disease-causing molecules. A striking example is the design of STI571 in the treatment of chronic myeloid leukaemia (CML). CML is associated with the Philadelphia chromosome, a balanced reciprocal translocation that activates the *ABL* oncogene. The translocation produces expression of the *ABL* oncogene, a chronically active tyrosine kinase that produces uncontrolled myeloid cell proliferation. STI571 is a specific inhibitor of this protein, which can switch off the leukaemic process.

GENE THERAPY

Understanding the precise genetic basis of disease provides an opportunity to replace defective genes using gene therapy. This poses many challenges including delivery of genes to the appropriate cells, persistence and control of gene expression and avoiding interference with the function of other genes.

One of the first diseases to be successfully treated by gene therapy is X-linked SCID, due to defects in the common cytokine receptor γ-chain. The normal gene can be introduced into the patients own lymphoid progenitor cells, which are then infused into the patient to reconstitute the immune system. Several patients have established protective immunity following gene therapy. Unfortunately, a small number of patients have developed leukaemia, when integration of the therapeutic gene has disrupted unrelated normal genes.

VACCINATION

Vaccination harnesses immunological memory to protect against infection. Vaccination has been extremely successful in conditions where natural infections leads to lifelong protective immunity, including smallpox, poliomyelitis and measles. However, in conditions where infection does not produce sterilising, protective immunity, vaccine design has proved more challenging. Major vaccine challenges include HIV and malaria. Vaccination is immunology's greatest contribution to public health to date. Success in designing vaccines against HIV and malaria would change life for whole populations.

TARGETED IMMUNOMODULATION

Our understanding of the molecular basis of immunity has led to attempts to modulate the immune response in a highly specific way to treat autoimmune and inflammatory disorders, as well as improving outcomes in clinical transplantation. The majority of applications currently undergoing Food and Drug Administration (FDA) assessment are of biological therapeutic agents; many designed to alter the immune response. Repeated use of therapeutic antibodies has been made possible by humanising these molecules using protein-engineering techniques.

Granuloma formation is known to be critically dependent on the cytokine TNF-α. Crohn's disease, a granulomatous inflammatory bowel disease is highly responsive to biological agents which block the action of TNF-α. Additionally, the incidence of rejection following renal transplantation can be reduced by using antibodies which deplete activated T cells, by binding to CD25, a component of the IL-2 receptor.

PHARMACOGENOMICS

Racial and individual variation in the enzymes that metabolise drugs influences how well drugs work as well as the risk of drug toxicity. Knowledge of functional polymorphisms in genes encoding enzymes that metabolise drugs allows us to predict both toxicity and drug efficacy. For example, isoniazid an anti-TB agent is metabolised by acetylation. When treated with a standard dose, individuals who acetylate drugs slowly are at high risk of toxicity, while fast acetylators rarely experience toxicity, but have a poor therapeutic effect. In the future, knowledge of a patient's acetylation status may allow us individualise the dose of drug, to obtain the best balance between efficacy and toxicity. Similar assessments are beginning to be used to optimise treatment with azathioprine, an immunosuppressive drug.

XENOTRANSPLANTATION

The major limiting factor in clinical transplantation is the availability of donor organs of suitable quality. Use of organs from animals could provide an adequate supply of organs, available on a planned basis. The initial barrier to xenotransplantation was hyperacute rejection, mediated by complement, because of the species specificity of complement control proteins. Transgenic pigs have been produced which express human complement control proteins to prevent this problem. There is still a lot to learn about subsequent types of rejection xenotransplantation. However, at present the major concern delaying clinical trials is concern about transmission of infection from donor animal organs to immuno-suppressed humans. This may never happen, however the fear of an infection jumping the species barrier as HIV did in the last century is proving much more challenging than the immunological aspects of xenotransplantation.

The practice of medicine and clinical immunology will change considerably and unpredictably over the next decade. However, understanding the basics of the immune system in health and disease will remain essential for healthcare professionals looking after patients with immunological disorders.

Glossary

Adrenal insufficiency Impaired hormone production by the adrenal gland. This may be due to infection, autoimmune destruction, haemorrhage into the gland or rarely, tumours. Autoimmune destruction may occur in isolation, or in association with autoimmune destruction of other endocrine glands, in autoimmune polyglandular syndrome. Symptoms include fatigue, abnormal pigmentation and hypotension, which may be severe.

Alopaecia Abnormal hair loss. Generalised alopaecia may be associated with both non-immunological and immunological (especially autoimmune thyroid disease and SLE) causes. Patchy hair loss is seen in alopaecia areata.

Alveolitis Inflammation centred on the alveoli or airspaces in the lung. The term is usually only used when inflammation is not caused by infection. Patients present with cough and breathlessness. There may be an infiltrate on chest X-ray, however, high resolution CT picks up disease at an earlier stage. Pulmonary function tests show impaired gas transfer. Immune causes of alveolitis include extrinsic allergic alveolitis, the connective tissue diseases and cryptogenic fibrosing alveolitis. When chronic, alveolitis may progress to pulmonary fibrosis.

Anaemia Reduction in the haemoglobin content of the blood. This may be due to impaired production or increased loss or destruction of red blood cells. Size of the red blood cells may be increased (macrocytic), normal (normocytic) or reduced (microcytic) and the haemoglobin content may be normal (normocytic) or reduced (hypochromic). Patients present with fatigue and when severe, the reduced oxygen carrying capacity of the blood may cause breathlessness and angina.

Anaemia, megaloblastic Specific type of anaemia due to deficiency of folate or vitamin B_{12}. This results in impaired maturation of red blood cells and production of reduced numbers of large (macrocytic) red blood cells.

Angioedema Swelling of tissues due to increased permeability of local blood vessels. In the skin this causes visible swelling, in the gastrointestinal tract, crampy abdominal pain, and in the upper airways, airways obstruction. Causes include allergy, C1 inhibitor deficiency as well as drugs which cause histamine release and some anti-hypertensives.

Arthralgia   Joint pains in the absence of any evidence of inflammation.

Arthritis, inflammatory   Inflammation of joints. Patients present with pain and stiffness, typically worst in the morning. Joints may be swollen due to either synovial thickening or accumulation of synovial fluid, and occasionally red and hot. Causes include rheumatoid disease, connective tissue disease and seronegative spondylarthropathies.

Arthritis, reactive   Immune-mediated, sterile, inflammatory arthritis, triggered by infection, most commonly of the genitourinary or gastrointestinal tracts. Infection may be subclinical, and the arthritis may occur several weeks after the inciting infection. Sore eyes often co-exist. Reiter's syndrome refers to the triad of arthritis, conjunctivitis (red, sore eyes) and urethritis (inflammation of the urethra).

Ataxia   Inability to coordinate movements. Axial ataxia primarily involves the limbs, while truncal ataxia affects the trunk – both types cause unsteadiness when walking. Ataxia is associated with cerebellar disease, and also severe loss of sensation, particularly proprioception.

Atherosclerosis   Presence of atheroma within arteries, commonly known as 'hardening of the arteries'. Atheroma forms plaques consisting of fatty deposits in the vessel wall, induces an inflammatory reaction, as well as proliferation of smooth muscle in the medial layer of the arterial wall. Thrombus can form on the plaque surface, blocking the artery and damaging tissue or organs supplied by the vessel. Plaques can also rupture, with contents forming emboli which travel to distal vessels causing ischaemia of tissue supplied by these vessels.

Bacterial sepsis   Infection caused by bacteria, which may be localised (e.g. in the airways) or generalised (septicaemia, where bacteria enter the blood stream and continue to proliferate).

Bronchiectasis   Irreversible bronchial dilatation and inflammation, usually the result of chronic or repeated airway injury from repeated episodes of infection. Patients experience repeated frequent chest infection and often produce sputum on a daily basis, even between exacerbations. Once bronchiectasis is established infections will usually continue even if the underlying cause is identified and treated. Causes include immunodeficiency, abnormalities of the mucociliary elevator such as immotile cilia syndrome, cystic fibrosis and allergic bronchopulmonary aspergillosis.

Congestive heart failure   Results from inability of the heart to pump sufficient blood to meet metabolic demands. This results in increased venous pressure, with oedema formation. When the right side of the heart fails, oedema is in peripheral tissue, while left heart failure results in pulmonary oedema. Either side or both sides may fail. Congestive heart failure may occur in the late stages of any type of heart disease.

Encephalomyelitis   Inflammation of brain and spinal cord. Patients present with varied neurological deficits, depending on the areas within the brain and cord which are involved. Imaging generally shows extensive white matter change, and cerebrospinal fluid will have raised protein and white cells. Causes include infection and autoimmune disease.

Endocrinopathy   Abnormal function of one or more endocrine glands.

Glomerulonephritis   A group of renal disorders in which the pathological process primarily involves the glomerulus. In some, inflammation can be seen on biopsy. However, in some types of glomerulonephritis classical features of inflammation are not seen. Patients present with varying combinations of haematuria, proteinuria, impaired renal function, hypertension, nephritic or nephritic syndrome.

Gluten-sensitive enteropathy   Better-known as coeliac disease. An immune-mediated adverse reaction to gluten-containing foods results in small bowel inflammation with subsequent malabsorption. Clinical presentation is varied and can include low body weight and in children failure to thrive, anaemia, osteoporosis and in some patients it is clinically silent and is a coincidental finding. Clinical and histological abnormalities improve with exclusion of gluten-containing foods. A small proportion of patients, especially if poorly compliant with diet, develop small bowel lymphoma.

Haematuria   Presence of blood in the urine, which may be macroscopic (visible to the naked eye) or microscopic (only detected on laboratory testing). Haematuria may be due to inflammation or tumours of the kidneys or urinary tract. The presence of red blood cell casts (small tubular structures identified on microscopy) indicates bleeding from the glomerulus rather than the lower urinary tract.

Haemoptysis   The coughing-up of blood. This is an important clinical symptom. Underlying causes include lung malignancy, tuberculosis, pulmonary embolism, pneumonia, lung abscess, anti-GBM disease and vasculitic conditions such as Wegener's granulomatosus and other ANCA-positive conditions like micro-polyangiitis and Churg–Strauss syndrome. Haemoptysis always warrants further clinical evaluation.

Hyperthyroidism   Overactivity of the thyroid gland with uncontrolled and excessive production of thyroid hormone. The term thyrotoxicosis is also used to describe this clinical state. Autoimmune (Graves' disease), toxic nodular goitre and viral-induced inflammation are important underlying causes. Clinical features reflect the increase in metabolic activity induced by excess amounts of thyroid hormone and include weight loss, diarrhoea, heat intolerance, palpitations, mental nervousness and insomnia. Goitre (swelling of the thyroid gland) may be present but is not invariable.

Hypothyroidism   Underactivity of the thyroid gland with deficiency of thyroid hormone production. Autoimmune destruction is an important cause. Patients present with one or more of the following features: tiredness and excessive sleepiness, weight gain, coarsening of the facial features, hoarseness, constipation, loss of concentration and elevated cholesterol. Replacement with adequate levels of thyroid hormone brings about clinical improvement.

Impetigo   Skin infection caused by the bacteria *Staphylococcus aureus* resulting in a golden crusted pus-containing eruption, usually around the mouth or nose. Most cases respond to anti-staphylococcal antibiotics applied directly to the affected skin or by mouth.

Interstitial lung disease   An inflammatory disorder of the gas exchanging units of the lung – the alveoli – resulting from immune-mediated or toxic damage. Patients present with progressive breathlessness and in some cases progress to lung failure. Interstitial lung disease can be the sole pathology or represent one manifestation of a multi-system disease. Causes include sarcoidosis, extrinsic allergic alveolitis conditions such as farmer's lung, bird fancier's lung etc., connective tissue diseases and rheumatoid arthritis and pneumoconiosis such as occurs in coal miners.

Ischaemia   Injury to tissue or organ caused by impaired blood supply. When severe and/or sustained results in necrosis. Symptoms and signs depend on the organ or tissue involved.

Lipodystrophy   An abnormal distribution of fat tissue. Loss of fat tissue from the upper body with excess deposition in the lower body – partial lipodystrophy – is a characteristic feature in patients presenting with a particular kidney inflammatory disorder (mesangiocapillary glomerulonephritis Type II – dense deposit disease) causing nephrotic syndrome.

Livedo reticularis   A blue, mottled net-like (reticulate) discoloration of the skin seen particularly on the lower limbs. This is seen in some autoimmune conditions, most notably the anti-phospholipid syndrome, where proneness to clot formation is the predominant presenting feature, but is also seen in vasculitic disorders such as polyarteritis nodosa.

Liver disease, chronic   Liver damage resulting from an ongoing injury, usually toxic (particularly alcohol), viral, metabolic or autoimmune. Unless the cause is removed or treated, cirrhosis and portal hypertension may result. Symptoms include fatigue,

409

jaundice, abdominal discomfort and examination findings include jaundice, spider naevi, ascites, hepatic enlargement and splenomegaly due to portal hypertension.

Lymphadenopathy   Enlargement of lymph glands, which may be localised or generalised. Short-lived enlargement of regional lymph glands is appropriate during acute infection. However, persistently enlarged glands may be a sign of chronic infection, autoimmune disease, sarcoidosis, lymphoproliferative disorder or non-lymphoid malignancy. Glands in the neck, axilla and groin are palpable on clinical examination, however, imaging is required to assess nodes in the thorax and abdomen.

Lymphopaenia   Reduction in the lymphocyte count below the age-related lower limit of normal. Lymphopaenia is commonly seen in acutely ill patients. However persistent lymphopaenia may be associated with immunodeficiency, SLE as well as being induced by drugs, for example, immunosuppressants and steroids.

Mononeuritis multiplex   Abnormal function affecting two or more peripheral nerves. Involvement of motor nerves results in weakness, while disease affecting sensory nerves causes paraesthesia (pins and needles) and numbness. Usually caused by pathology of the vasa nervorum, the artery supplying blood to the nerve. Causes include vasculitis and diabetes mellitus.

Myocardial infarction   Necrosis of heart muscle (myocardium) due to impaired blood supply. This is usually a complication of atherosclerosis in the coronary arteries, but rarely occurs due to vasculitis.

Nephritic syndrome   Reduced urine output (oliguria), hypertension and haematuria. Usually caused by some types of acute glomerulonephritis, such as post-infectious glomerulonephritis.

Nephrotic syndrome   Gross proteinuria (>3 g/24 hours), reduced serum albumin level and oedema. Also usually accompanied by hypercholesterolaemia and an increased risk of thrombosis. Caused by glomerular disease including diabetic nephropathy and several types of glomerulonephritis.

Neuropathy, autonomic   Pathological process involving the nerves of the autonomic nervous system. These nerves are essential to maintain control of several essential bodily functions including blood pressure, heart rate, respiratory reflexes and gastric emptying. Autonomic functions generally do not involve conscious effort. Autonomic neuropathy can cause life-threatening abnormalities of cardiovascular or respiratory function.

Neuropathy, sensory   Abnormality of nerve fibres transmitting impulses from sensory receptors to the central nervous system. Patients present with paraesthesia (pins and needles) and numbness. This may start at the peripheries and move proximally (glove and stocking distribution) or may follow the distribution of affected nerves. Causes include toxins (including alcohol), diabetes mellitus, vitamin deficiency, autoimmune conditions and vasculitis.

Neutropaenia   Reduction in the neutrophil count, which may be due to impaired marrow production or increased destruction. When severe, neutropaenia may be associated with rapidly progressive life-threatening bacterial sepsis.

Oliguria   Reduction in urine output (<500 ml/day in an adult). This indicates acute or acute-on-chronic renal failure.

Paraesthesia   Abnormal sensation, commonly known as 'pins and needles'. This is most commonly associated with injury to peripheral sensory nerves, but may also be seen with lesions in the central nervous system. The majority of patients will have a non-immunological cause for this symptom, however, immunological causes include chronic demyelinating polyneuropathy and multiple sclerosis.

Paraneoplastic syndrome (including cerebellar degeneration)   This term refers to a number of specific syndromes where tissue-specific dysfunction arises in combination with particular tumours at other sites. The affected tissue is not invaded by tumour but rather is inflamed with resultant dysfunction or destruction. Similarities between tumour antigens and host antigens with subsequent immune mediated attack in host tissues underlie paraneoplastic disorders. Successful treatment of the tumour can result in resolution of the paraneoplastic symptoms. The nervous system is a common site where paraneoplastic syndromes occur. Specific syndromes include conditions such as the myasthenia gravis-like Lambert–Eaton syndrome with muscle fatigue and weakness, and cerebellar dysfunction.

Pericardial effusion   A collection of fluid in the pericardial space surrounding the heart muscle. A variety of causes are recognised, including tumour invasion, infections such as tuberculosis but also connective tissue diseases like SLE and rheumatoid arthritis. Patients present with varying severity of symptoms ranging from mild breathlessness through to gross heart failure when the volume of fluid surrounding the heart tissue prevents efficient heart muscle contraction. Fluid aspiration can assist in diagnosis and is used to relieve symptoms that occur in more severe cases.

Pleural effusion   A collection of fluid in the space between the two layers of pleura surrounding the lung. Patients may be asymptomatic, but usually present with breathlessness due to the reduction in lung volume with bigger effusions. Many causes are recognised. The level of protein in the pleural fluid is helpful in diagnosing the likely cause. Low levels of protein (transudative pleural effusions) occur in states where albumin levels are reduced, for example, chronic liver disease, nephrotic syndrome etc., as well as in heart and kidney failure. Exudative effusions where protein content in the pleural fluid is high, are seen in infections including tuberculosis, with lung malignancies, in pulmonary embolism and in systemic inflammatory disorders such as rheumatoid arthritis and systemic lupus erythematosus.

Polymyositis   A generalised inflammatory condition of muscles characterised by painful muscle weakness, especially notable in the upper parts of the arms and legs. Disorders of the breathing and swallowing muscles are also seen and can cause respiratory embarrassment and difficulty swallowing. Arthritis, inflammatory eye problems and very distinctive skin lesions with purplish discoloration around the eyelids and hands are also seen. Aggressive vasculitis is a feature in affected children. Some patients have co-existent malignancy and this should be considered, especially in patients presenting in later life or with suspicious clinical features. Muscle biopsy, electrical studies and autoimmune serology are useful in making the diagnosis.

Polyneuropathy   A generalised dysfunction of many nerves, most typically distal peripheral nerves, manifesting with sensory derangments such as numbness, 'pins and needles' or burning pain in a glove and stocking distribution. Weakness can also be a feature. Causes are manifold but include diabetes mellitus, kidney failure, vitamin B deficiencies, excessive alcohol intake, connective tissue diseases, paraprotein disorders, and some genetic conditions.

Pre-eclampsia   A disorder of pregnancy characterised by high blood pressure, excessive protein loss in the urine, swelling (oedema) and in severe cases seizures. Fetal growth in the womb can be impaired. The basic pathology lies in a dysfunctional placenta provoking the hypertensive and other changes outlined. This condition is a major cause of maternal and fetal morbidity and mortality and is important to recognise before it becomes severe. Bed rest, anti-hypertensive drugs and in severe cases, induced or caesarean delivery are indicated.

Protein losing enteropathy   Increased protein loss from abnormal gut mucosa resulting in low levels of albumin and oedema. Conditions such as coeliac disease, severe small bowel Crohn's disease and many unusual disorders are causative.

Pulmonary hypertension   Elevation of the normally low blood pressure within the pulmonary artery occurring as a result of chronic lung diseases such as cystic fibrosis, chronic obstructive pulmonary disease, pulmonary emboli and bronchiectasis;

congenital heart diseases and valve diseases; and rarely as a primary phenomenon. Patients present with progressive tiredness, breathlessness and features of right-sided heart failure. Outlook is poor and heart–lung transplantation may be required in some cases.

Pulmonary-renal syndrome Co-existent acute lung and kidney dysfunction occuring in the context of a systemic vasculitic disorder such as Goodpasture's syndrome, micropolyangiitis and Wegener's granulomatosis. Patients present with acute kidney failure with microscopic haematuria, and varying levels of lung failure with associated haemoptysis and pulmonary haemorrhage evident on chest X-ray. Intensive supportive management and specific therapy aimed at reversing the vasculitic inflammation is required urgently.

Raynaud's phenomenon Intermittent spasm in the small arteries of the hands, feet and other peripheries precipitated by cold and relieved by heat. Digits initially go very white due to the spasm, with a subsequent blue discoloration due to poor oxygenation followed by a red painful discoloration on heating up and vasodilatation of the blood vessels. In severe cases, digital ulcers and even necrosis requiring amputation may occur. Primary Raynaud's features without underlying pathology are usually mild and this is referred to as Raynaud's disease. However, some cases occur as part of a systemic connective tissue disease or with rheumatoid arthritis, as a result of physical injury or secondary to certain drugs such as beta-blockers. Investigation and specific management is important in such cases.

Renal failure, acute Rapid deterioration in kidney function with resultant fluid, electrolyte and acid-base upset. This can arise either because of a primary disease of the kidney itself (for example, glomerulonephritis, vasculitis, pyelonephritis, interstitial nephritis), or as a result of impaired blood supply to the kidney (such as occurs in shock states like dehydration, massive haemorrhage, or cardiac failure) or in conditions where urinary output is seriously obstructed with resultant kidney damage (for example, prostatic enlargement, ureteric damage or tumour invasion). Correction of the underlying disorder often allows kidney function to return to a baseline. Intensive management is required for optimal outcome.

Renal failure, chronic Gradual decline in kidney function over the space of months or years. Outlook depends on the nature of the underlying condition and presence and nature of other medical problems. Some disorders can be slowed down in their rate of progress more than others with specific treatments. Management of high blood pressure is an important aspect of all patients' care. Eventually most patients, if they live, will require kidney replacement therapy, for example, dialysis or kidney transplant.

Rhinitis Inflammation of the nasal passages manifesting with symptoms such as nasal congestion, discharge, itching, post-nasal drip and sore throat. Many causes are recognised including allergic, infective, vasomotor and drug-related. Correct identification of the causative agent is important for successful management.

Sarcoidosis A disorder characterised by the presence of granulomatous inflammation in various organs or tissues. Presentation is varied both in the tissues involved and in the duration and severity of the presentation. Lung involvement ranging from enlarged lymph nodes in the chest through to a progressive lung fibrosis is common. Liver, brain and renal involvement is also seen. The nature and severity of the clinical presentation dictate therapy.

Sclerodactyly Tightening of the skin of the fingers and toes giving the appearance of shiny tapered digits. This is a characteristic feature of the limited systemic sclerosis syndrome also known as CREST syndrome.

Splenomegaly Enlargement of the spleen, most commonly due to infection, autoimmune disease, lymphoproliferative disorders or liver disease. The spleen must be twice its normal size to be palpable on examination. Splenomegaly is usually asymptomatic unless the spleen is massively enlarged. When significantly enlarged the spleen is more prone to rupture, which can result in life threatening intra-abdominal haemorrhage.

Telangiectasiae   Abnormalities of the small blood vessels of the skin and mucosal surfaces manifesting as 'broken veins'. These lesions are seen in some immunological conditions, for example, systemic sclerosis, but are also seen in other disorders such as hereditary haemorrhagic telengiectasiae, where mucosal lesions in the gastrointestinal tract and less commonly the brain can be associated with fatal haemorrhage.

Thrombocytopaenia   Reduced platelet count. This may be due to impaired production by the bone marrow or excessive destruction, which is commonly immune-mediated. Thrombocytopaenia results in spontaneous bruising and abnormal bleeding.

Urticaria   Itchy, blotchy rash often associated with fluid filled lesions. Individual lesions are usually short-lived (<24 hours) and resolve without residual skin changes. Acute urticaria is a common manifestation of allergy, however, chronic (>6 weeks) urticaria is rarely associated with allergy.

Vasculitis   Inflammatory process centred on blood vessels which disrupts the internal elastic lamina of involved vessels. Vasculitis may be primary (autoimmune in origin) or secondary to other disorders. Patients present with symptoms due to generalised inflammation (fever, weight loss, fatigue) and symptoms and signs of dysfunction of involved organs (haematuria, renal failure, pulmonary haemorrhage, skin rash, etc.).

Vitiligo   Depigmentation of skin usually resulting from immune-mediated loss of melanocytes, the pigment-containing cells in the skin. Vitiligo may occur alone or in association with other autoimmune disorders.

Index

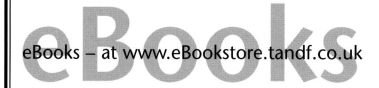